Instructor's Manual to Accompany

Maternal and Child Health Nursing

Care of the Childbearing and Childrearing Family

Second Edition

Adele Pillitteri, Ph.D, R.N.

Assistant Professor, School of Nursing
Director, Neonatal Nursing Practioner Program
State University of New York at Buffalo
Buffalo, New York

J. B. Lippincott Company
Philadelphia   Hagerstown

Sponsoring Editor: Jennifer Brogan
Coordinating Editorial Assistant: Danielle DiPalma
Ancillary Coordinator: Doris S. Wray
Compositor: Richard G. Hartley
Printer/Binder: Courier Book Company, Kendallville

ISBN: 0-397-55206-8

6   5   4   3   2   1

Any procedure or practice described in this book should be applied by the health care practitioner under
appropriate supervision in accordance with professional standards of care used with regard to the unique
circumstances that apply in each practice situation. Care has been taken to confirm the accuracy of
formation presented and to describe generally accepted practices. However, the authors, editors, and
lisher cannot accept any responsibility for errors or omissions or for any consequences from
cation of the information in this book and make no warranty, express or implied, with respect to
tents of the book.

rt has been made to ensure drug selections and dosages are in accordance with current
ations and practice. Because of ongoing research, changes in government regulations, and
ow of information on drug therapy, reactions, and interactions, the reader is cautioned to
age insert for each drug for the indications, dosages, warnings, and precautions,
drug is new or infrequently used.

Preface

*T*he following manual was designed to assist an instructor in designing classes and clinical experiences using *Maternal and Child Health Nursing: Care of the Childbearing and Childrearing Family*, Second Edition by Adele Pillitteri.

Maternal—newborn and child health nursing are expanding areas of nursing as a result of the broadening scope of practice within the nursing profession and the recognized need for better preventive and restorative care in these areas. The importance of this need is reflected in the fact that many of the year 2000 health goals for the nation focus on these areas of nursing.

At the same time that the content in these areas of nursing is increasing, less time is available in nursing programs to cover it. Students experience difficulty reading all of the material contained in two separate textbooks.

Maternal and Child Health Nursing, is written with this challenge in mind. It views maternal—newborn and child health care not as two separate disciplines but as a continuum of knowledge. It is designed to present the content of the two disciplines comprehensively, yet not redundantly. It is based on a philosophy of nursing care that respects clients as individuals and yet views them as part of families and society.

The book is designed for undergraduate student use for a combined course in maternal—newborn and child health, for concurrent use in which concepts of care are integrated throughout the program. It provides a comprehensive, in—depth discussion of the many facets of maternal—newborn and child health nursing, while it promotes a sensitive, holistic outlook on nursing practice. As such, the book will also be useful for graduate students who are interested in reviewing or expanding their knowledge in these areas.

Maternal and Child Health Nursing follows the family from the prepregnancy period, through pregnancy, labor and birth, and the postpartal period; it then follows the child in the family from birth through adolescence. Coverage includes ambulatory as well as in—patient care. It focuses on primary as well as secondary and tertiary care.

Organization of the Text

The book is organized in nine units:

Unit I discusses the area of maternal and child health nursing. National, sociocultural, and community considerations; current trends; and the importance of considering childbearing and childrearing within a family context are presented.

Unit II discusses the nursing role in preparing families for childbearing and childrearing. Reproductive and sexual health, reproductive life planning, and the concerns of the infertile family are discussed.

Unit III present the nursing role in caring for the pregnant family. Care of the woman during pregnancy and for the growing fetus is discussed. Separate chapters discuss the role of the nurse when the woman has a preexisting illness, develops a complication of pregnancy, has a special need, or will be cared for at home during pregnancy. Additional chapters detail the role of the nurse as a genetic counselor and as an advocate for fetal health.

Unit IV addresses the nursing role in caring for the family during labor and birth. Separate chapters detail the labor process, the role of the nurses in providing comfort during labor, the nursing role when a woman develops a complication of labor and birth, and during cesarean birth.

Unit V describes the nursing role in caring for the family during the postpartal period. Separate chapters discuss the care of the woman and her family, the newborn, and the changing role when a complication for either the woman or the newborn develops.

Unit VI discusses the nursing role in health promotion during childhood. Separate chapters discuss principles of growth and development and care of the child from infancy through adolescence including nutritional needs and child health assessment.

Unit VII presents the nursing role in supporting the health of ill children and their families. The effects of hospitalization on children and their families, health teaching with children, and nursing care of the child and family both in the hospital and hoe are addressed.

Unit VIII examines the nursing role in restoring and maintaining the health of children and families when illness occurs. Disorders are presented according to body systems so that students have a ready orientation for locating content.

Unit IX discusses the nursing role in restoring and maintaining the mental health of children and families. Separate chapters discuss the role of nurse with child abuse and when mental illness, long-term, or fatal illness is present.

Integrated Features of the Text

Several vital themes are emphasized throughout the text:

- The experience of wellness and illness as family—centered events
- Pregnancy and childbirth as periods of wellness
- The importance of knowing a child's developmental stage in planning nursing care
- The nursing process as the basis of nursing care
- The necessity of formatting nursing diagnoses from assessment data. Nursing diagnoses from the North American Association of Nursing Diagnosis (NANDA) are emphasized
- The importance of nursing research as a method by which nursing progresses. A box, Focus on Nursing Research, in each chapter describes an example of recent nursing research pertinent to the topic
- The importance of health teaching with families. A box in each chapter, Focus on Family Teaching, highlights teaching important to the area of care
- The importance of National Health Goals as a way to focus care. A box, Focus on National Health Goals, is shown in each chapter to highlight health goals pertinent to that area of care
- The importance of individualizing care according to sociocultural uniqueness. A box, Focus on Cultural Awareness, in each chapter describes sociocultural factors important to take into consideration when planning care in the area
- Changing areas of practice, such as the increased use of ambulatory surgery and the role of nurse—midwives and pediatric and neonatal nurse practitioners

Pedagogic Features

Each chapter in the text is organized to provide a complete learning experience for the student. Important elements include the following:

Chapter Objectives: Learning objectives are included at the beginning of each chapter to illustrate the way in which nursing process serves as the focus of nursing care and identifies the behavioral outcome expected after the material in the chapter has been mastered

Chapter Outline: This feature enables the student to gain an overview of the contents of the chapter and to focus on the location of a particular topic when reviewing material

Key Terms: Terms that would be new to a student are listed at the beginning of each chapter in a ready reference list. The terms first appear in boldface type to draw the student's attention to them and are defined as they are used. They area also defined in the glossary

Tables and Displays: These summarize important information and provide details on some topics so that the student has a ready reference

Nursing Care Planning: Nursing care plans are provided to serve as summaries and care applications of the nursing process. They are written for specific clients, not as general summaries, to stress the importance of individualized care planning

Key Points: A review of important points is highlighted at the end of each chapter in a list to help the student monitor his or her comprehension of each chapter

Critical Thinking Exercises: To involve students in the decision—making realities of the clinical setting, several questions included at the end of each chapter so students can further monitor their comprehension of the chapter's content. They could also be used as a basis for conference or class discussion

References and Suggested Readings: These provide the student with the information needed to do more in—depth reading of the sources noted in the text, as well as other relevant articles on the topics included in each chapter

Glossary: A ready reference—at—hand for the student to clarify the terminology used in the text is included at the end of the book

Appendices: Nine appendices provide quick reference to nursing diagnoses, laboratory values, growth charts, vital sign parameters, infant formulas, and drugs safe for use during pregnancy and lactation

Nursing Process

Nursing Process Overview: Each chapter begins with a review of nursing process in which specific suggestions, such as examples of nursing diagnoses and outcome criteria helpful to modifying care in the area under discussion, are given. These reviews improve students' preparation in clinical areas to focus their care planning and apply principles to practice

Nursing Process Format: A consistent nursing process format highlights the nursing diagnoses and related interventions throughout the text. A special design draws the student's attention to these sections where individual nursing diagnoses, goals, and outcome criteria are detailed for the major conditions and disorders discussed

Nursing Care Plans: Revised and redesigned in a two—column format for this section, the care plans are written with an emphasis on aiding students in applying theory to practice and making use of their critical thinking skills

Nursing Procedures: Techniques of procedures specific to maternal and child health care are boxed and presented in a two—column format that reinforces the nursing process framework

Focus on Nursing Research: These displays summarize research carried out by nurses on topics related to maternal and child health nursing and appear throughout the text to accentuate the use of research as the basis for nursing care

Focus on Family Teaching: Questions that families frequently ask during the childbearing and childrearing years are presented, followed by a list of detailed and practical information for the family, emphasizing that health teaching should be included as an intrinsic part of nursing care

Focus on Cultural Awareness: Sociocultural aspects that can influence nursing care are boxed to stress their importance and the ways that nursing care can be modified to meet individualized needs

Focus on National Health Goals: National Health Goals pertinent to each area of care that nurses can be instrumental in helping the nation achieve are boxep

d to help students appreciate the importance of national health planning and the influence that nurses can have in creating a more healthy nation

New to the Second Edition

- **Recurring Displays:** New to this edition are three displays—Focus on Cultural Awareness, Focus on Family Teaching, and Focus on National Health Goals— that place greater emphasis on the uniqueness of the nurse's role in meeting the needs of the childbearing and childrearing family and emphasize the need for individual assessment of the families

- **Two New Chapters:** The trends occurring in terms of greater diversity of ethnic groups in our nation, as well as the trends in changing health care settings, gave the impetus to provide separate chapters on the following topics:

- A new chapter, **Sociocultural Aspects of Maternal and Health Nursing**, emphasizes the need for nursing assessment and interventions to consider the unique needs of the individual, including cultural beliefs and traditions that can affect his or her response to nursing care

- **Home Care of the Pregnant Client** addresses the increase in the kinds of settings for clinical practice, including the number of pregnant women who are cared for in the home, and provides the nursing student with the knowledge necessary to provide nursing care in this setting

- **Pocket Guide.** For the second edition of *Maternal and Child Health Nursing*, a smaller volume has been prepared that focuses on the most essential information in the text and makes it easily accessible in a pocket—size format. Students will find this format very useful for day—to—day reference

- **Ancillary Package**

An accompanying **Instructor's Manual, Computerized Test Bank, Student Workbook, Transparencies,** and **Student Computerized Test Questions Disc** are provided. The **Instructor's Manual** summarizes major concepts and provides suggestions and strategies for teaching the chapter content. A case presentation that could be useful for independent nursing care planning is also included. The **Test Bank** is nursing process based and could be helpful to students to use for information review if not used by the instructor as test material. The **Student Workbook** provides additional self—learning material for students as well as suggestions for formal assignments. The **Transparencies** provided are those most apt to be helpful to illustrate concepts in a classroom setting. The **Student Computerized**

Test Questions Disc contains NCLEX-format, multiple—choice questions study or assigned to assess student knowledge.

Sections included in the Instructor's Manual are described below.

- Introduction and Objectives

  A brief summary of the chapter contents and the objectives for each chapter are presented for easy instructor reference. This should be helpful in locating specific material for class planning.

- Key Points

  Key points, as summarized at the end of each chapter, are listed for easy instructor reference.

- Definitions of Key Terms

  Key terms (words likely to be new to the student) are listed at the beginning of each chapter. These words are defined within the chapter as they are used and again in the textbook glossary. Definitions of key terms are given here to supply a ready resource for instructors.

- Nursing Process Overview

  The Nursing Process Overview for each chapter is shown. Such overviews are designed to help students focus their concept of what is important learning in the content area and specific ways that nursing care in that area can be individualized.

- Study Aids

  A list of the tabled and boxed material for each chapter is listed. The Focus displays and Critical Thinking Exercises for each chapter are shown, making this material easy to locate in order to make transparencies for class use or for quick reference. The nursing care plans from the text are also included; these are individually designed for a particular client described in a scenario preceding the care plan. This helps students appreciate that nursing care is individualized, not rote, and encouraging them to adapt nursing care plans in the text to their own clients. This allows for easier evaluation of students, since they are not simply copying a "generic" plan, and provides them with the experience of actually planning, not copying, nursing care. Nursing care plans do not necessarily include all the nursing diagnoses a designated client might have, but focus on those that illustrate the content of the particular chapter where they are placed. Nursing care plans are indexed in the text following the Table of Contents for easy student reference. They are repeated here for ready reference.

- Media Resources

  Suggestions for media to use in class or for individual learning are presented with each chapter. These lists of media sources is included in Appendix A.

- Discussion Questions

  Questions that could be used to encourage class discussion or use as examination questions are included with all chapter discussions here. A separate test bank includes 1000 multiple=choice questions to use for examination or for students to use for self—evaluation.

- Written Assignments

  Because student writing is a requirement of many university and college curricula, suggestions for written assignments that could accompany chapters are presented.

- Laboratory Experiences

  Suggestions for clinical experiences in both campus laboratories and client care settings are included.

- Care Study

  A care study pertinent to the content of the chapter is presented with major content chapters. These might be used in class to initiate discussion or assigned to students to use as data in formulate a nursing care plan. Such a care plan would be helpful in evaluating whether students have grasped content well enough to be able to apply it to actual situations. A care plan to be completed from a care study might be used as a substitute assignment for a missed clinical day or as an assignment for extra student credit. Care study questions are included to stimulate critical thinking and planning.

Table of Contents

Unit Nine The Nursing Role in Restoring and Maintaining the
Health of Children and Families with Mental Health Disorders

A Framework for Maternal and Child Health Nursing

Chapter 1 describes the concept of maternal and child health nursing as a continuum of care rather than as two separate divisions of nursing. A framework for determining care during pregnancy, delivery, and the postpartum period and continuing during childrearing years from newborn through adolescence is presented. The American Nurses' Association (ANA) standards of maternal and child health nursing practice, the year 2000 health goals for the nation, and ways that nursing research, nursing process, and nursing theory are interwoven are stressed. Roles of nurses, trends in maternal and child health care, and the importance of health-related statistics are discussed.

Chapter 1 lays a foundation for the study of maternal child health nursing and serves as a source of reference material to justify priorities of care.

Chapter Objectives

After mastering the contents of this chapter, students should be able to:

1. Describe the evolution, scope, and professional roles of maternal and child health nursing.
2. Identify the goals and philosophy of maternal and child health nursing.
3. Define common statistical terms used in the field such as infant maternal mortality.'
4. Discuss common standards of maternal and child health nursing and the health goals for the nation in terms of their implications for maternal and child health nursing.
5. Discuss the interplay of nursing process, nursing research, and nursing theory as they relate to shape the future of maternal and child health nursing practice.
6. Use critical thinking to identify areas of care that could benefit from additional nursing research.

7. Synthesize knowledge of trends in maternal and child health care with nursing process to achieve an understanding of quality maternal and child health nursing care.

Key Points

- Standards of maternal and child health nursing practice have been formulated by the ANA and the Association of Women's Health, Obstetric and Neonatal Nurses (AWHONN) to serve as guidelines for practice.
- Nursing theory and nursing research are methods by which maternal and child health nursing expands and improves.
- The most significant measure of maternal and child health is the infant mortality rate. It is the number of deaths in infants from birth to 1 year per 1000 live births. This rate is declining steadily but in the United States is still higher than 20 other nations.
- Trends in maternal and child health nursing include changes in the settings of care, increased concern about health care costs, increased preventive care, and family-centered care.
- Advanced practice roles in maternal and child health nursing include women's health, neonatal, and pediatric nurse practitioners, clinical nurse specialists, and nurse-midwives. All of these expanded roles contribute to maternal and child health care.
- Maternal and child health care involves legal and ethical considerations over and above those in other areas of practice.

Definitions of Key Terms

child health nursing: nursing care of children

clinical nurse specialist: a nurse prepared at the master's level who has a special area of clinical expertise

family-centered nursing: a nursing philosophy in which the family is considered the unit of care

fertility rate: number of births per 1000 women aged 15 to 44 years

family nurse practitioner: a nurse prepared at the master's level who has expertise in the nursing care of families

maternal-newborn nursing: nursing that concentrates on the care of a family during pregnancy, labor and birth, postpartum, and the infant immediately following birth

maternal and child health nursing: a conceptual approach to nursing care that views maternity and child health nursing as a continuum, not separate entities

mortality (infant): the number of deaths per 1000 live births occurring at birth or in the first 12 months of life

mortality (maternal): the number of maternal deaths per 100,000 live births that occur as a direct result of the reproductive process

neonatal nurse practitioner: a nurse prepared at the master's level who has expertise with nursing care of the newborn infant

neonate: an infant during the first 28 days of life

nurse-midwife: a registered nurse with extended knowledge in care of the family during the prenatal, natal, and postnatal periods. Abbreviated as C.N.M. for Certified Nurse Midwife.

nursing research: scientific investigation of topics related to nursing

pediatric nurse practitioner: a nurse prepared at the master's level with extensive skills in physical assessment, interviewing, and well-child counseling and care

puerperium: the 6 weeks following childbirth

Study Aids

Boxes

Box 1-1:   Philosophy of Maternal and Child Health Nursing

Box 1-2:   Common Measures to Ensure Family-Centered Maternal and Child Health Care

Box 1-3:   Standards of Maternal and Child Health Nursing Practice

Box 1-4:   Association of Women's Health, Obstetric and Neonatal Nurses Nursing Practice Standards

Box 1-5:   Statistical Terms Used to Report Maternal and Child Health

Tables

Table 1-1:   Definitions and Examples of Phases of Health Care

Table 1-2:   Summary of Nursing Theories

Table 1-3:   Trends in Maternal and Child Health Care and Implications for Nurses

Table 1-4:   Infant Mortality by States (per 1000 live births), United States, 1950-1990

Table 1-5:   Infant Mortality Rates per 1000 Live Births for Selected Countries, 1990

Table 1-6:   Major Causes of Death in Childhood

Displays

Focus on Nursing Research

Focus on Cultural Awareness

Critical Thinking Exercises

1. Canada has a health care delivery system based not on profit but on provision of care for all citizens through a tax-supported program. The infant mortality rate in Canada is lower than in the United States.

    a. What are some reasons that might contribute to this?

    b. How do sociocultural aspects affect the infant mortality rate?

2. The age of women having their first baby is advancing. For many women this is 30 years and above.

    a. How do you anticipate this will change care in the future?

    b. Are there special services you can anticipate that should be provided for such women?

    c. How will this trend influence childrearing in the future?

Media Resources

Hello Baby! (48 minute film, video)

Three complete films. Part I depicts three birth stories. Part II describes medical options and practices. Part III shows a cesarean birth. The role of the nurse is stressed throughout.

Source: Video Health Communications

Midwife: With Woman (16 minute film, video)

The manner in which midwifery had gained a small but important foothold in maternity care in the United States is discussed.

Source: Fanlight Productions

The Story of Eric (34 minute film)

A birth story that shows parents-to-be learning the Lamaze method for prepared childbirth and then experiencing an exhilarating birth with little medical intervention. A good introduction to the concept of family-centered birth.

Source: Centre Films

A Quiet Revolution ... The First Twenty Years (23 minute video)

The major changes and areas of progress in psychosocial care of children that have occurred during the past twenty years are discussed. The nurse's role in the health care system with emphasis on the importance of child-centered facilities is stressed. An agenda for future action to improve the quality of child health care is included.

Source: Association for the Care of Children's Health

The Pediatric Nurse as Teacher (20 minute video)

Basic childhood growth and development are reviewed with appropriate teaching strategies for children at each age. Individual developmental assessments and educational strategies to foster a child's understanding of unfamiliar hospital surroundings and procedures are presented.

Source: Medical Electronic Educational Services, Inc.

Discussion Questions

1. Including families in care is important in maternal and child health nursing. How does this change nursing care? How does it change family life when a child is ill?

2. Discuss the social, political, economic, and health care system factors which may be contributing to the high U.S. infant mortality rate as compared with other industrialized countries.

3. The United States has established health goals for the nation to guide the future of health care. If you were devising such goals what would the chief ones be? What are direct ways that nursing is affected by such goals?

Written Assignments

1. Using recent census, morbidity, and mortality statistics from your local community and/or metropolitan area, compare birth and mortality rates among various population subgroups and propose possible reasons for higher than average trends.

2. Using Table 1-4, determine the infant mortality in your state and compare this with others. What are some possible reasons that your state's rate is at that level (high or low)?

3. Bring in a recent newspaper and magazine article about an ethical issue in maternal and child health nursing such as in vitro fertilization, abortion, or death with dignity. Write a paragraph describing how you would answer a client who asked you for your opinion on one of these controversial issues.

Laboratory Experiences

1. Have students survey community resources to see what resources are available locally such as birthing rooms, intensive care nurseries, and child care centers and how many community health care agencies employ nurses in expanded roles such as nurse-midwife or pediatric nurse practitioner. Have students share this information with classmates by oral reports or by compiling a file of reports which is available to all students.

2. To help students appreciate the influence of poverty on childbearing and childrearing, play the simulation board game ''Ghetto'' (Academic Games Associates, Inc., copyright 1969; Bobbs-Merrill Company, Inc., Educational Division). The game can be played by teams. A coordinator's manual provides instructions for play and suggestions for related learning activities. Postgame discussion should focus on analyzing the availability of health care resources that could influence the health of childbearing and childrearing families.

3. Ask a nurse-midwife or nurse practitioner to describe his or her role and ways such a person can make an impact on health care at a clinical conference.

The Childbearing and Childrearing Family

Chapter 2 discusses the role of the family in both childbearing and childrearing. The chapter begins with an overview of nursing process specific to care of the family. Different family types, roles, and tasks and stages of families are discussed. Common tools for both family and community assessment are illustrated. Examples of a family genogram and a community ecogram are shown. The changing pattern of family life and the nurse's role in a changing society are stressed.

Some students may need encouragement to grasp the concept of family-centered nursing and to begin to think of the entire family as their client rather than only one individual member. Both class discussion and clinical assignments are helpful in establishing a new orientation to care.

Chapter Objectives

After mastering the contents of this chapter, students should be able to:

1. Describe family structure, function, and roles.
2. Assess a family for structure and health.
3. Formulate nursing diagnoses related to family health.
4. Plan nursing care such as helping a family modify its lifestyle to accommodate an ill child.
5. Implement nursing care such as teaching a family more effective wellness behaviors.
6. Evaluate outcom criteria established for care to be certain that goals have been achieved.
7. Identify national health goals related to the family and specific ways that nurses can help the nation achieve these goals.
8. Identify areas of care related to family nursing that could benefit from additional nursing research.
9. Use critical thinking to analyze additional ways that nursing care can be family centered or that client care can better include family members.
10. Synthesize knowledge of family nursing with nursing process to achieve quality maternal and child health nursing care.

Key Points

- A family is a group of people who share a common emotional bond and perform certain interrelated social tasks.
- Common types of families encountered are nuclear, extended, single-parent, blended, cohabitation, single alliance, gay, lesbian, and foster families.
- Common family tasks are physical maintenance, socialization of family members, allocation of resources, maintenance of order, division of labor, reproduction, recruitment and release of members, placement of members into the larger society, and maintenance of motivation and morale.
- Common life stages of families are marriage; early childbearing; families with preschool, school-age, and adolescent children; launching center and middle-years families; and the family in retirement.
- Changes in patterns of family life that are occurring are increased mobility; one-parent families; dual-parent employment; divorce; social problems such as abuse and decreased socioeconomic level; and family size.
- Considering a family as a unit (a single client) helps the nurse to plan nursing care that meets the family's total needs.
- Families exist within communities: assessment of the community and the family's place within the community yields further information on family functioning.
- Families are not always functioning at their highest level during periods of crisis; reassessing them during a period of stability may reveal a stronger family than inferred on first assessment.
- Because families work as a unit, unmet needs of any member can spread to become unmet needs of all family members.

Definitions of Key Terms

community: a limited geographic area in which the residents relate to and interact among themselves

community ecomap: a diagram of the family's interactions with the community family: two or more people who live in the same household (usually), share a common emotional bond, and perform certain interrelated social tasks

family nursing: the concept that clients do not exist outside a family; the family rather an individual is considered the client

family theory: a way of analyzing problems or concerns from a family's point of view

family of orientation: one's birth family: oneself, mother, father, and siblings

family of procreation: one's marriage family: oneself, spouse, and children

family sculpture: a technique of family assessment that creates a live portrait of family members

genogram: a diagram of family structure depicting essential family relationships: the interactive roles that exist in a family

Nursing Process Overview

Some students have difficulty centering on the family as their client and therefore may have difficulty constructing family-centered nursing diagnoses. The Nursing Process Overview in this chapter concentrates on ways to define a well family and well community and includes suggestions for family-centered diagnoses such as "family coping: potential for growth," "altered parenting," and "health seeking behaviors." The necessity to include family members in developing goals and evaluation of progress is stressed. As students begin to plan care for clients, this overview could be increasingly helpful in keeping them focused on the total family and not an individual client.

Study Aids

Boxes

Box 2-1:   Twelve Behaviors Indicating a Well Family
Box 2-2:   Methods to Help Families Deal With Stress

Tables

Table 2-1:   Family Assessment
Table 2-2:   Community Assessment

Displays

Focus on National Health Goals

Focus on Family Teaching

Focus on Nursing Research

Focus on Cultural Awareness

Critical Thinking Exercises

Marlo Hanavan is a 32-year-old bookkeeper who is pregnant with her second child. Her first child, 2-year-old Amy, has just been diagnosed by their family practitioner as having cerebral palsy. She needs long-term physical therapy and attends a special school. Mr. Hanavan is unemployed because of an accident at work. He has some income from selling woodworking products at craft shows. Mrs. Hanavan states that on many weeks she doesn't have enough money to pay bills; she is forced to choose between medical care and groceries.

1. What family stage according to Duvall have the Hanavans reached? What would a genogram of their family look like? An ecogram?

2. Why is this a particularly unfortunate time for the Hanavans to have to choose between medical care and groceries?

3. How would the Hanavan's needs change if they were an extended family? a single-parent family? a cohabitation family?

Media Resources

Adapting to Parenthood (20 minute film/video)

Parent education film about what it is really like to be a parent: "The frayed nerves and the tension, as well as the exhilaration."

Source: Polymorph Films

The Family in a Changing Society (16 minute filmstrip)

A three-part series on (1) marriage, (2) parenthood, and (3) working parents. Describes family life and methods of coping with role strain.

Source: Encyclopedia Britannica Educational

Single-Parent Families: Coping With Change (28 minute filmstrip)

The reasons for the increase in single-parent families in the United States during the past decade are explored. The controversies surrounding abortion rights, sex education, and religious rights are discussed. Techniques of successful problem solving and coping with changes in the family structure are reviewed.

Source: Random House

Stepparenting: New Families, Old Ties (25 minute film, video)

Stepparents discuss their feelings of insecurity and the conflict and confusion that accompany childrearing in blended families. Scenes realistically portray stepfamily life including problems such as weekend visitation.

Source: Polymorph Films

Fathers (23 minute film, video)

Fathering roles in three different families are portrayed. Roles include the busy working father, a father with an authoritarian approach to childrearing, and one who shares child care responsibilities in the home. Family coping styles and role prescriptions are stressed.

Source: Churchill Films

Discussion Questions

1. Use role playing and have students enact different roles of family members such as nurturer, provider, decision maker, and problem solver. Ask students to identify the roles portrayed and how the characteristic portrayed would influence family functioning.

2. Use the care study of a family presented on the following page and discuss what would be the family stage, pertinent nursing diagnoses, and interventions for the Burrows family.

3. Women are often referred to as the "keepers of the culture." How have women's health or women's liberation movements affected childbearing customs?

Written Assignments

1. Draw a family genogram of your own or a client's family and list the health risks of particular importance to that family.

2. Construct a community ecogram for your own or a client's family and write a short essay on whether you believe the family is using community resources effectively.

3. Analyze a family you care for as to their life stage according to Duvall. Justify your answer.

Laboratory Experiences

1. Have students include the type of family their clients are from as part of their client assessment data so they become used to looking at families, not individuals.

2. Ask students to include a description of the community a client is from (not just the client's address) as part of their client assessment data. This helps them to focus on problems the client will have on discharge from a hospital and possibly reasons the client has a health problem.

3. Divide students into groups and ask them to drive through different communities close to their practice setting and assess these communities as to socioeconomic status, transportation, health services available, and so forth. Ask groups to compare how a client all groups know would manage in these communities.

Care Study: The Burrows Family

The Burrows family consists of Ted Burrows, 54 years; Christina, 50 years; a maternal grandmother, Ida, 79 years; Debra, 22 years; Hank, Debra's husband, 23 years; Tina, who is Debra and Hank's child, 4 months; James, 17 years; Cheryl, 15 years; and Sandy, 6 years. They own two dogs and a cat.

The family lives in an older, four-bedroom, two-story home. The second floor is cold at night because of inadequate furnace duct work. Adequate hot water and furnishings are present; there is indoor plumbing and a city water supply is used. The telephone is in working order and neighbors they could call on for help are nearby.

Health problems in the family are experienced by the grandmother, who has considerable arthritis and so has dif-ficulty walking; Tina and Sandy, who have both had multiple allergies and ear infections over the last few months; and Hank, who recently injured his back in a motorcycle accident. Cheryl, the 15-year-old, has recently begun to suspect she is pregnant, perhaps as much as 5 months. The family has a general practitioner they see for routine health care and uses a local emergency room for accidents. Cheryl has made an appointment but has not been seen yet at a local prenatal clinic.

Ted, Christina, Hank, Debra, James, and Cheryl all smoke cigarettes. All drink beer at night with the evening meal. The family does not eat a sit-down breakfast as Christina has to leave for work too early to prepare it. Most members pack a brown bag lunch. Evening is a sit-down meal. Christina admits to "stretching" meat more than she used to as this is an expensive item in the budget. Debra is breastfeeding her daughter.

Ted works as an assistant janitor at the nearby grade school; Christina works part-time driving a school bus. Hank is currently unemployed following his back injury; Debra works part-time in a fast food restaurant. James, Cheryl, and Sandy all attend school. In addition, James works part-time as a clerk in a drug store and Cheryl part-time at a filling station.

The family describes itself as "not rich" but "not poor either." The house is rented, not owned, and Ted admits to being 2 months behind in payments. Hank owns a motorcycle and a pickup truck and Ted an older model car. An issue in the family is that James wants a car but the family can't afford this. James is planning on attending a junior college in the fall and has applied for student loans. Christina uses food stamps for grocery shopping. She is reluctant to ask for any other help as she views the family as only "temporarily in a slump."

The family attends church sporadically. They used to attend regularly until the grandmother began to have difficulty walking up the church steps. Ted and Christina belong to a weekly bowling league. They visit occasionally with neighbors for cookouts or to support school functions.

Care Study Questions

1. What type of family do the Burrows represent? What is the stage of the family according to Duvall? Can the roles of family members (nurturer, decision-maker, etc.) be determined?

2. Nutrition seems to be a concern for this family. What dietary suggestions would you make for them?

3. Lack of communication may also be a problem. How could the Burrows family develop a better relationship?

4. Complete a nursing care plan that will identify and meet the needs of the Burrows family.

Sociocultural Aspects of Maternal and Child Health Nursing

Chapter 3 discusses sociocultural aspects as they relate to childbearing and childrearing. The chapter begins with an overview of nursing process specific to care of the family. The assessment of communication patterns; use of conversational space, time, work, and family orientation; male-female roles; religion; and health and nutrition beliefs are discussed. The importance of considering families in light of their cultural background is stressed.

Some students may need encouragement to consider sociocultural aspects of care. Class discussion of how cultural aspects affect care is necessary to make them fully aware of their influence on care.

Chapter Objectives

After mastering the contents of this chapter, students should be able to:

1. Describe ways that sociocultural influences affect maternal and child nursing care.
2. Assess a family for sociocultural influences that might influence the way it responds to childbearing and childrearing.
3. Formulate nursing diagnoses that relate to culturally appropriate aspects of nursing care.
4. Plan and implement nursing care that respects sociocultural needs and wishes of families.
5. Evaluate outcome criteria to be certain that goals of care related to sociocultural aspects have been achieved.
6. Identify national health goals related to sociocultural considerations that nurses could be instrumental in helping the nation to achieve.

7. Identify areas of care related to sociocultural considerations that could benefit from additional nursing research.
8. Use critical thinking to analyze how the sociocultural aspects of care affect family functioning and develop ways to make nursing care more family centered.
9. Synthesize sociocultural aspects of care with nursing process to achieve quality maternal and child health nursing care.

Key Points

- Culture is an organized structure that guides behavior into acceptable ways for that group. Usual customs are termed mores or norms. Actions that are not acceptable to a culture are called taboos.
- Each culture differs to some degree from every other; most people are proud of these differences or cultural traits.
- Culture is transmitted by both formal and informal ways from generation to generation.
- Although cultural ideas adapt from time to time, they tend to remain constant.
- Cultural practices arise from environmental conditions.
- There is wide variation within a culture concerning values and actions because individuals make up the group and individually express their cultural heritage.
- People bring cultural values and beliefs to nursing interactions and these affect nursing care.
- Cultural aspects that are important to assess are communication patterns; use of conversational space; time, work, and family orientation; and social organization, including nutrition, family roles, and health beliefs.

Definitions of Key Terms

acculturation: the process of losing cultural beliefs and values to those of another society

assimilation: the ability to change how a set is perceived to coincide with beliefs

cultural values: beliefs generally held by the majority of people in a community or society

culture: the learned way of life of a community or society

ethnicity: a person's nationality

ethnocentrism: the belief that one's own values or beliefs are superior to others mores: customs generally accepted as right to follow by a community or society

norms: customs generally accepted as right to follow by a community or society

stereotyping: a fixed conception

taboos: actions that are prohibited in a specific culture

transcultural nursing: a philosophy of nursing that focuses on the unique cultural beliefs of people

Nursing Process Overview

The Nursing Process Overview stresses the importance of assessing for sociocultural aspects and modifying care based on these findings. Examples of nursing diagnoses and outcome criteria based on sociocultural aspects are given.

Study Aids

Boxes

Box 3-1:   Methods to Improve Health Care When Clients Do Not Speak English as Their Primary Language

Displays

Focus on National Health Goals

Focus on Family Teaching

Focus on Nursing Research

Critical Thinking Exercises

1. Anna Rodriques is a 12-year-old who is hospitalized for surgical repair of a broken tibia. She has a cast on her right leg and will be on bedrest for three days, then gradually be allowed to learn crutch walking.

   In planning care for her, you assume that because her culture is Hispanic, her family orientation will be male-dominated, her time focus will be on the present rather than the future, and nutrition preference will be Mexican American. Based on this, you concentrate on talking mainly about her current problem (bedrest) rather than future care at home. You speak to the dietitian about avoiding milk as lactase deficiency is present in many Mexican Americans. You consult with Anna's father regarding the major aspects of her care.

   You are surprised to hear Anna complain on the second day of her hospitalization that she feels like a second-class person because her father has been asked for more input about her care than she has. She says she is particularly concerned that bone healing will not take place because she has had little milk to drink.

   a. What went wrong with Anna's care? If you had actually planned care in this way, what would you have been guilty of?

   b. What would have been a better approach for determining Anna's family's cultural preferences? Supposing it is true that Anna is present-oriented, how would you approach discussions of a long-term rehabilitation program for her?

2. Miss Crawford is a woman who is 30 weeks pregnant and has not been coming regularly for prenatal care. When you visit her in her home to see why, she states that before coming to the clinic for another appointment she wants to visit a voodoo doctor who will both predict her child's sex and guarantee a safe birth.

   a. What would be a plan of care that best respects this cultural value?

   b. Would recommending that Miss Crawford have a sonogram evaluation (which also could predict the fetal sex) be likely to be as satisfying for her?

Media Resources

Streetlife: The Invisible Family (58 minute video)

A number of displaced families and their needs are discussed. The complexity of the issue is stressed.

   Source: Fanlight Productions

The Latino Family (28 minute video)

The changes in and the endurance of traditional Latino families are shown. Three generations of a Mexican American family are featured.

   Source: Films for the Humanities, Inc.

Discussion Questions

1. Adolescents may discard cultural values or beliefs as part of establishing a sense of adolescent identity. What are suggestions for strengthening cultural beliefs that would still maintain a sense of identity?

2. Mary is a Native American whose tribe has opened a gambling casino for the public. Although some people in the nearby community enjoy gambling, most people are opposed to the casino being open because they believe gambling is morally wrong. When Mary is admitted to your hospital to have a baby, her roommate, who is very opposed to gambling and anyone associated in any way with it, asks you to change her room. How would you respond to her request? What are the issues to consider?

3. Harry is a nurse who strongly believes that gays and lesbians should not be parents. You notice when you work with him that he is very cool to these parents when they bring children to the ambulatory clinic for well child maintenance. What steps could you take to help these parents receive better care? Why would a health care provider hold this type of belief?

Written Assignments

1. Give students a grocery shopping list of foods commonly found in their community and ask them to visit a market in a neighborhood that is culturally different from their own and write a description of how difficult it would be to purchase those foods if they lived in that community. What would be the implications of their discovery for nutrition counseling?

2. Billy is a 15-year-old who is severely hearing impaired. He communicates by using sign language. Billy tells you that he has been very depressed lately because a pretty girl who recently moved to his neighborhood has treated him as if he is mentally retarded since she learned of his hearing difficulty. He asks you how he could convince her that hearing, not mental retardation, is his health problem. He asks you if the problem occurred because he did not point out his problem immediately or because she is intolerant?

3. Homeless people experience a culture different from that of the average student in nursing. Ask students to describe their activities from their previous day and then how these would have been different if they had been homeless.

Laboratory Experiences

1. Ask a nurse from a culture different from the majority of students to come to a postconference and discuss with students particular beliefs or ways that interactions with health care providers can be difficult because of differing cultural beliefs.

2. Arrange for clinical experiences in culturally diverse settings such as a prenatal clinic or a child care conference that is attended by a large number of women who do not use English as their primary language. Ask students to note how they must modify their care in order to meet these clients' needs.

3. Ask an interpreter and a parent who speaks a language other than English to come to a postconference. Ask a student to volunteer to secure a prenatal or ill child history using the interpreter. Ask students afterward to evaluate the difficulties encountered in this type of setting.

Care Study: A Family With Cultural Concerns

Sue Ellen and Edward Smith were a middle-aged couple who adopted a child from Korea: 2-year-old Lon Soo, 6 months ago. Unfortunately, immediately following the adoption, Sue Ellen was killed in an automobile accident. The father brings the child to your ambulatory health center for care.

Health History

- Chief Concern: "I don't know if I can raise a child so different from myself alone, especially because she's a girl."

- History of Present Concern: Father admits that adoption of child was his wife's idea. He would have been happy to remain childfree. There are no other Korean children that he knows of in his community. Asking if changing child's name to something more "American" would help her be accepted in his community.

- Past Medical History: Child apparently well before adoption although the history is actually unknown.

Given medicine for "worms" by adoption agency on arrival in this country. Has had "colds, colds, colds" since adoption. Immunization status unknown.

- Family Medical History: Medical history of parents of child is unknown.

- Personal/Social: Father works as an airline pilot so is absent from home 3 days every week. His mother (67 years old) cares for child during this time. Child seems to have adjusted well to new home although she is very shy with strangers and is a "picky eater."

- Pregnancy History: Unknown although mother apparently had no complications. Child was placed for adoption because mother has seven others and could not give care to so many.

- Review of Symptoms: Frequent colds as mentioned above. Presently has a bad cough.

Physical Examination

- General Appearance: Thin appearing 2-year-old, coughing in paroxysms. Weight: 23 lbs. Height: 32 inches.

- HEENT: Hair: good quality and distribution. Eyes: follows well through all fields of vision; red reflex present. Ears: TMs normal color; good mobility. Nose: clear, copious rhinitis present. Skin slightly excoriated under nose. Three palpable posterior cervical chain lymph nodes present.

- Chest: Rhonchi present on auscultation. Coughed three times during examination with pattern of 5 or 6 successive coughs; no noticeable "whoop" present.

- Heart: Heart rate 100 bpm; no murmurs.

- Abdomen: Soft, nontender. Neither liver nor spleen palpable.

- Genitalia: Normal female.

- Rectum: Patent. No excoriations present.

- Extremities: Good range of motion; walks with wide-based "toddler" gait.

Care Study Questions

1. Adopting a child from another culture carries responsibilities for parents to help the child appreciate and respect her original culture. Based on this, how would you answer the father's question about changing Lon Soo's name?

2. Lon Soo is reported as being a "picky" eater. What questions would you want to ask to reveal the extent of this problem? Is the child below average in height or weight?

3. Lon Soo is diagnosed as having pertussis (whooping cough). There is always a high index of suspicion for this in children with a paroxysmal cough whose immunization status is unknown.

Complete a nursing care plan that will identify and meet the needs of the Smith family.

Reproductive and Sexual Health

*C*hapter 4 describes the anatomy and physiology of the male and female reproduction systems. The chapter begins with an overview of nursing process specific to promotion of reproductive and sexual health. The processes of ovulation and menstruation are discussed. The chapter concludes with a discussion of sexuality, the human sexual response, common methods of sexual expression, and areas of possible sexual dysfunction.

Content of the chapter is intended to help the student develop a foundation for understanding fetal development and pregnancy changes as well as counseling for sexual concerns.

Chapter Objectives

After mastering the contents of this chapter, students should be able to:

1. Describe anatomy and physiology relevant to reproductive and sexual health.

2. Assess a couple for anatomic and physiologic readiness for childbearing, biologic gender, gender role, and gender identity.

3. Formulate nursing diagnoses related to reproductive or sexual health.

4. Plan nursing care related to anatomic and physiologic readiness for childbearing or sexual health such as helping adults discuss concerns in these areas.

5. Implement nursing care related to reproductive health such as educating for menstruation.

6. Evaluate goals and outcome criteria established for care to be certain they have been achieved.

7. Identify national health goals related to reproductive health and sexuality and specific ways that nurses can help the nation achieve these goals.

8. Identify areas of care in relation to reproductive and sexual health that could benefit from additional nursing research.

9. Use critical thinking to analyze ways that clients' reproductive and sexual health can be improved.

10. Synthesize knowledge of reproductive health and sexuality with nursing process to achieve quality maternal and child health nursing care.

Key Points

- The reproductive and sexual organs form early in intrauterine life; full functioning becomes possible at puberty.

- The female internal organs of reproduction include the ovaries, fallopian tubes, uterus, and vagina.

- The female external organs of reproduction include the mons veneris, labia minora and majora, vestibule, clitoris, fourchette, perineal body, hymen, and skene's and bartholin's glands.

- The male external reproductive structures are the penis, scrotum, and testes. Internal organs are the epididymis, vas deferens, seminal vesicles, ejaculatory ducts, prostate gland, urethra, and bulbourethral glands.

- A menstrual cycle is periodic uterine bleeding in response to cyclic hormones. Menarche is the first menstrual period.

- Menstrual cycles are possible because of the interplay between the hypothalamus, pituitary, ovaries, and uterus.

- Biologic gender is determined by chromosomal content (XX or XY), which is set at conception. Gender is a person's concept of being male or female. This develops over a lifetime.

- Masters and Johnson have identified a sexual response cycle consisting of excitement, plateau, orgasm, and resolution stages. Disorders of sexual dysfunction include premature ejaculation, failure to achieve orgasm, vaginismus, dyspareunia, and inhibited sexual desire.

- Educating people about reproductive function is an important primary prevention measure because it teaches them to monitor their own health better through breast and vulvar or testicular self-examination.

- Adolescents should be taught that with sexual maturity comes sexual responsibility. The best protection against either an STD or an unintentional pregnancy is the practice of safer sex or abstinence.

Definitions of Key Terms

adrenarche: the physiologic changes that occur with puberty

andrology: the branch of medicine that treats the man and diseases specific to the male sex

anteflexion: a uterus that is bent forward just above the cervix

anteversion: a uterus that is tipped abnormally forward

aspermia: absence of sperm

bicornuate uterus: a uterus that has two fundal horns; it may have an accompanying septum

culdoscopy: the introduction of an endoscope through the posterior vaginal wall to view the pelvic organs

cystocele: pouching of the bladder into the anterior vaginal wall

dyspareunia: pain on sexual intercourse

endocervix: the inner surface of the cervix

endometrium: the inner layer of the uterus that is shed as menstruation

erectile dysfunction: the inability to achieve erection in order to complete a sex act

gonad: a sex gland; an ovary in the female; a testis in the male

gonadostat: the unknown control mechanism that stimulates the hypothalamus to begin stimulation for puberty changes

gynecology: the study of the female reproductive organs

gynecomastia: excess development of male breast tissue; a transient occurrence in normal adolescence

homologue: a structure similar in origin to another

homosexual: an individual whose sexual relations are with those of his or her own sex

laparoscopy: examination of abdominal cavity and organs by insertion of a surgical instrument through the anterior abdominal wall

lesbian: a female homosexual

menarche: the first menstrual period

mesonephric (wolffian) duct: the embryologic tissue that develops into the male reproductive organs

myometrium: the muscle layer of the uterus

oligospermia: a sperm count less than normal

oocytes: an immature ovum

paramesonephric (muellerian) ducts: the embryologic tissue that develops into the female reproductive organs

perimetrium: the outer coat of the uterus

premature ejaculation: deposition of sperm before vaginal penetration or the full enjoyment of the sexual partner

rectocele: herniation of the rectum into the posterior vaginal wall

retroflexion: a uterus that is bent backward just above the cervix

retroversion: a uterus that is tipped abnormally backwards

sadomasochism: a form of sexual expression marked by the infliction of pain

thelarche: breast development changes at puberty

transsexual: a person of one sex whose perceived identity is of the opposite sex

transvestite: a person who dresses in the clothes of the opposite sex

vaginismus: painful, involuntary spasms of the vagina

voyeurism: the practice of obtaining sexual pleasure by looking at the nude body of another

Nursing Process Overview

The Nursing Process Overview in this chapter concentrates on helping the student define sexual and reproductive health and suggests possible nursing diagnoses pertinent to this area. Stress is placed on empowering individuals to have control over this aspect of their life as they do in other areas, and the importance of the nurse in becoming comfortable discussing concerns in this life health area.

The primary role of the nurse concerning reproductive anatomy and physiology is education. Both female and male clients may feel more comfortable asking questions of the nurse than of the doctor, so it is important for a nurse to have this information readily available.

Study Aids

Boxes

Box 4-1:   Specific Questions to Include in a Sexual History

Box 4-2:   Guidelines for Safer Sex Practices

Tables

Table 4-1:   Female and Male Reproductive System Homologues

Table 4-2:   Characteristics of Normal Menstrual Cycles

Table 4-3:   Teaching About Menstrual Health

Displays

Focus on National Health Goals

Focus on Family Teaching

Focus on Nursing Research

Focus on Cultural Awareness

Critical Thinking Exercises

1. Joel is a 15-year-old you see as a school nurse. He is concerned because a number of his friends have STDs. What would you advise him regarding safer sex practices?

2. Mrs. Desmond is concerned because her daughter, age 7, seems to be a "tom boy." She asks you how she can convince her daughter to be more of a "lady." What advice would you give her? Suppose her daughter was 17? Would your advice be different? Suppose Mrs. Desmond was concerned because a son was not "boy" enough? Would your answer be any different?

Media Resources

When the Topic Is Sex (29 minute filmstrip, slides, videotransfer)

A filmstrip discussing the nurse's role in talking with clients about sexuality, emphasizing the sensitive and often anxiety-producing nature of discussing this life area. Includes an attitude and knowledge assessment questionnaire.

Source: Concept Media

Adolescent Sexuality (30 minute video)

Describes both internal factors (physiologic and psychological changes) and external factors (social, cultural demands) that influence adolescent sexual behavior.

Source: Health Sciences Consortium

Childbearing, the Classic Series (57 illustrations on charts or slides)

Illustrations of female and male anatomy, conception and fetal development, and pregnancy changes.

Source: Childbirth Graphics

Median Section of the Female Pelvis (simulated model)

Lifesize cross-section of female pelvis, uterus, bladder, and rectum; removable parts.

Source: Armstrong Medical Industries, Inc.

Discussion Questions

1. What are the advantages of the unique curve and narrow diameters of the birth canal to the fetus? To the woman?

2. A woman's sexual gender may differ from her sexual role. How might differing sexual roles affect a woman's feelings about being pregnant?

3. Should slang terms be used in discussing reproductive anatomy and physiology with clients? Why or why not?

Written Assignments

1. Ask students to write a short paragraph on how they would explain menstruation to a 12-year-old girl. Would they do it any differently for a 12-year-old boy?

2. Taking a sexual history may be awkward as a client may not feel comfortable discussing this aspect of life. Ask students to write a brief paragraph on how they would help a client to feel more comfortable responding in this area.

3. Male and female reproductive organs are analogues of each other. List the male analogues of the female organs.

Laboratory Experiences

1. Furnish anatomic models so students have the opportunity to visually see and handle simulated organs in order to better appreciate the relationship of abdominal and pelvic organs.

2. Provide for clinical experiences where students can observe surgical procedures involving the male and female reproductive systems such as laparoscopy, hysterectomy, or vasectomy so they can actually view reproductive organs.

3. Using the care study presented below, ask students to assess Cheryl Burrows and formulate nursing diagnoses appropriate to her level of understanding of sexual functioning.

Care Study: An Adolescent in Need of Safer Sex Counseling

Cheryl Burrows is a 15-year-old you see at a prenatal clinic. She is a sophomore in high school and works part-time at a filling station after school and evenings.

The Burrows family consists of Ted Burrows, 54 years; Christina, 50 years; a maternal grandmother, Ida, 79 years; Debra, 22 years; Hank, Debra's husband, 23 years; Tina, who is Debra and Hank's child, 4 months; James, 17 years; Cheryl, 15 years; and Sandy, 6 years. They own two dogs and a cat.

Cheryl's father works as an assistant janitor at the nearby grade school; her mother works part-time driving a school bus. The family lives in an older, four-bedroom, two-story home. The second floor is cold at night because of inadequate furnace duct work. Adequate hot water and furnishings are present; there is indoor plumbing and a city water supply is used. The telephone is in working order and neighbors they could call on for help are nearby.

Cheryl's menarche began at 13 years; her menstrual cycle is 30 to 32 days and her menstrual flow about 5 days in duration. She is very athletic (playing on both the soccer and softball leagues at school). She occasionally "skips" menstrual periods and she attributes this to her active participation in sports. She was pleased to notice her breasts enlarging over the last few months as she thinks they are far too small to be attractive but was also becoming worried as they are so tender.

At present it is March 16. Her last menstrual period was in October "around Halloween." Although she has been gaining weight, she states that the thought she might be pregnant "never crossed her mind."

She had sexual relations with two boys from her high school the fall before; neither of them used any contraceptive protection. The reason she states she didn't think she might be pregnant was because one of them told her that it was impossible for a girl to get pregnant after the 15th of every month. To be extra certain that wouldn't happen she douched afterward with vinegar and water.

When asked where she learned about how girls get pregnant, she laughed and said "a film in school—a bad film with everyone wearing old-fashioned clothes."

Cheryl's mother accompanied her to the prenatal clinic. When asked if she ever discussed contraception with Cheryl, she looked away, embarrassed, and finally said, "She watches enough movies, I thought she'd know enough not to get pregnant."

Care Study Questions

1. Cheryl and her mother have obviously not communicated on the topic of menstruation and the importance of safer sex practices. With so much education in schools and exposure to this on television or in movies, how much responsibility do parents have to take for this today?

2. Cheryl has support people in addition to her parents (an older sister, teachers, coaches, a school nurse). What would be a reason that she trusted a 15-year-old boy's

advice for avoiding pregnancy rather than confirming this with a better source?

3. Complete a nursing care plan that will identify and meet Cheryl's needs.

Reproductive Life Planning

*C*hapter 5 discusses common methods of reproductive life planning. The chapter begins with an overview of nursing process specific to reproductive life planning. The side effects and contraindications, effect on sexual enjoyment and future pregnancies, and use by the adolescent are discussed for each method. Oral ovulation suppressants, IUDs, barrier methods, natural family planning methods, and vasectomy and tubal ligation methods are included. Newer methods such as the use of female condoms and subdermal implants are included. The chapter concludes by discussing elective abortion, not as a reproductive life planning measure, but as a possible option if planning fails. Future possibilities for reproductive life planning and the role of the nurse in counseling for planning are included.

The term ''reproductive life planning'' is used rather than family planning throughout the chapter to accentuate the role of the nurse in counseling adolescents.

Chapter Objectives

After mastering the contents of this chapter, students should be able to:

1. Describe common methods for reproductive life planning.

2. Assess clients for reproductive life planning needs.

3. Formulate nursing diagnoses related to reproductive life planning concerns.

4. Plan nursing care related to reproductive life planning, such as helping a client select a suitable family planning measure.

5. Implement nursing care related to reproductive life planning such as educating adolescents about the use of condoms to promote safe sex practices as well as prevent unwanted pregnancy.

6. Evaluate goals and outcome criteria established for care to be certain they have been achieved.

7. Identify national health goals related to reproductive life planning that nurses can be instrumental in helping the nation achieve.

8. Identify areas related to reproductive life planning that could benefit from additional nursing research.

9. Use critical thinking to analyze methods that could be used to promote reproductive health.

10. Synthesize aspects of reproductive life planning with nursing process to achieve quality maternal and child health nursing care.

Key Points

- Reproductive life planning involves personal decisions based on an individual's background, experiences, and sociocultural beliefs. It involves thorough planning to be certain that a method chosen is acceptable and can be maintained effectively.

- Oral contraceptives are combinations of estrogen and progesterone. They provide one of the most reliable forms of contraception outside of abstinence. Women older than age 40 years who smoke are not candidates for oral contraceptive use because of the danger of cardiovascular complications. Counsel them to find a form of contraception that is reliable and allows them to remain sexually active.

- Subcutaneous implants (renewed every 5 years) and subcutaneous injections (renewed every 3 months) are new methods of contraception. These are 100% effective.

- Intrauterine devices are mechanical methods that prevent fertilization and implantation by placement in the uterus. Women with IUDs need to be aware that they are at greater risk for pelvic inflammatory disease than others. Counsel them to limit the number of sexual partners and be aware of the signs of PID as practical measures to help avoid serious illness.

- Barrier methods include the diaphragm, cervical cap, vaginal spermicides, sponge, and condom (male and female). Such methods are low cost but are not as effective as ovulation suppressant methods.

- Natural family planning (periodic abstinence) methods are varied but involve determining the fertile period each month and then avoiding sexual relations during that time.

- Permanent methods of contraception are tubal ligation in women and vasectomy in men. Counsel individuals who wish to undergo these procedures that they are largely irreversible.

- Elective termination of pregnancy is accomplished by menstrual extraction, dilatation and curettage, saline induction, or hysterotomy. Counsel women not to think of elective termination of pregnancy as a contraceptive method. It is a recourse to be used only when preventive measures fail. Women who are Rh negative need to receive $Rh_O(D)$ immune globulin following these procedures.

- When counseling clients about reproductive life planning, nurses have a responsibility to counsel them regarding safer sex practices as well such as using a condom during sexual intercourse. Even though a couple may be using another method for contraception, they should be advised to use condoms in addition to prevent sexually transmitted disease.

Definitions of Key Terms

abstinence: refraining from sexual intercourse

barrier method: a method of reproductive life planning in which sperm are prevented from entering the cervix

basal body temperature method: a method of natural family planning based on the use of the body temperature on arising

calendar method: a method of natural family planning based on the determination of fertile and nonfertile days each month

cervical cap: a latex barrier method of contraception that fits over the uterine cervix

coitus interruptus: a method of contraception in which the penis is withdrawn from the vagina before ejaculation

condom: a latex barrier method of contraception worn on the penis; provides some protection against STDs.

contraceptive: a method or device to prevent the fertilization of the human ovum

diaphragm: a mechanical barrier contraceptive device fitted over the cervix in the woman

elective termination of pregnancy: termination of a pregnancy by medical intervention

fertility awareness: a method of contraception based on analyzing the consistency of vaginal secretions

intrauterine device: a contraceptive device inserted into the uterine cavity

laparoscopy: an endoscopic examination of the abdominal cavity

natural family planning: contraception involving no medical devices or chemicals

reproductive life planning: planning to space children or prevent children from being conceived

tubal ligation: a method of contraception in which the fallopian tubes are cauterized, tied, or clamped to prevent migration of the fertilized oocyte to the uterus.

vasectomy: a surgical ligation of the vas deferens that results in male sterility

Nursing Process Overview

The Nursing Process Overview in this chapter concentrates on suggestions for nursing diagnoses pertinent to this area of health such as "decisional conflict" or "health-seeking behaviors" other than the obvious "knowledge deficit" that students may identify first. The nurse's role in educating clients about the options available to them and planning a method with them with their full input is stressed.

Study Aids

Tables

Table 5-1:   Contraceptive Failure Rates

Table 5-2:   Danger Signs Following Elective Termination of Pregnancy

Displays

Focus on National Health Goals

Focus on Family Teaching

Focus on Nursing Research

Focus on Cultural Awareness

Critical Thinking Exercises

1. Judy is a 16-year-old you care for in a family planning clinic. Would your interview differ if Judy were 39 rather than 16? Would your recommendations for a method of birth control differ?

2. John is a young adult male who is interested in playing an active role in reproductive life planning and also avoiding contracting a sexually transmitted disease. He has no regular sexual partner at present. What recommendations would you make to John? Would this be different if he had a monogamous relationship?

3. Betty Jo is a 16-year-old who has been admitted to the hospital for a saline induction for an elective termination of pregnancy. Her doctor tells you to give her only a minimum of analgesia so Betty remembers the experience as painful and, therefore, won't get pregnant again. Do you agree with this philosophy? Are there other measures you could take to help assure that she doesn't become pregnant irresponsibly again?

Media Resources

Conception and Contraception: Family Planning (20 minute slide, filmstrip, or video presentation)

Ten methods of birth control, their advantages and disadvantages, reliability, and possible side effects are included.

Source: Career Aids

Who Should Decide (13 minute video or film)

A young woman with spina bifida discovers her unborn child also has the disorder. She must decide whether or not to terminate her pregnancy in the second trimester.

Source: Pyramid Film and Video

Seasons of Sexuality (14 minute video, film)

A group of adolescents on a picnic discuss human sexuality through the life cycle and issues such as touching, loving, privacy, friendship, body image, fantasies, values clarification.

Source: Perennial Education, Inc.

Discussion Questions

1. Teaching reproductive life planning measures can be a major role for a nurse in a health maintenance setting. What are important factors to consider to ensure you will meet a couple's needs?

2. The age of a woman often influences her choice of reproductive life planning methods. How might the choice of a 16-year-old girl differ from that of a 35-year-old woman?

3. The new subdermal implants are expected to be popular with women for contraception. Discuss the advantages and disadvantages of such a method and whether you think it will gain popularity or not.

Written Assignments

1. Write a paragraph on the contraindications of specified reproductive planning methods such as ovulation suppressants? IUDs?

2. Natural planning methods are popular with some people; others are opposed to them. What qualifications do people need to use these methods effectively? Suppose one partner wants to use natural family planning and the other does not?

3. Write a paragraph explaining your understanding of the difference between the terms "family planning" and "reproductive life planning."

Laboratory Experiences

1. Obtain samples of reproductive life planning methods so students can have "hands on" time and become more familiar, especially with barrier contraceptive devices.

2. Provide clinical experiences in clinic or physician office settings where postpartum women are returning for reproductive life planning information.

3. Have students investigate what community resources there are for reproductive life planning. Share information as to whether these services are adequate for the community.

Care Study: A Woman in Need of Reproductive Planning Information

Debra Burrows is 22 years old; her husband Hank is 23. They have a 4-month-old baby, Tina. The Burrows have been married for 9 months (since Debra realized she was pregnant with Tina). They live with Debra's parents: Hank is temporarily unemployed after injuring his back in a motorcycle accident and their only source of income is Debra's part-time job at a fast food restaurant. Debra is breastfeeding Tina at present but is planning to wean her onto a formula within another month.

The couple was not using any contraceptive at the time Tina was conceived except for a condom. Hank has been insisting since Tina was born that Debra come to the clinic for a birth control pill prescription. Debra doesn't want to take pills because she has two aunts who used pills and both developed breast cancer. Hank is certain that they shouldn't have another child immediately, at least not until he is able to work again and they can get their own apartment. Debra is interested in discussing other options as long as they are "inexpensive" and "not messy."

Care Study Questions

1. Debra and Hank don't agree on what reproductive life planning method would be right for both of them. What would be a nurse's role in counseling a couple such as Debra and Hank? Should reproductive life planning be mainly Debra's or Hank's responsibility?

2. Are there other suggestions for Debra besides birth control pills? Is her worry about developing breast cancer well founded?

3. Complete a nursing care plan that will identify and meet the needs of the Burrows family.

The Infertile Family

Chapter 6 discusses common reasons for infertility in males and females and the steps of fertility assessment that are commonly carried out. The chapter begins with an overview of nursing process specific to care of the couple with a concern of infertility. The nurse's role in supporting a couple through assessment is stressed. Alternative options for the infertile couple such as in vitro fertilization, artificial insemination, surrogate motherhood, and childless living are discussed.

As infertility is an increasing problem in the United States today, students care for more and more couples with some degree of infertility. It is important for them to learn not only what are the common causes and therapies for infertility but what a devastating effect this can have on a couple's marriage or future plans.

Chapter Objectives

After mastering the contents of this chapter, students should be able to:

1. Describe common causes of infertility in men and women.
2. Describe common assessments necessary to detect infertility.
3. Formulate nursing diagnoses related to infertility.
4. Plan nursing care specific to relieving or coping with a diagnosis of infertility.
5. Assist with implementations involved in a diagnostic fertility study or assist a couple to achieve further fertility such as health teaching about the time of ovulation.
6. Evaluate outcome criteria to be certain that nursing goals were achieved.
7. Identify national health goals related to infertility that nurses can participate in helping the nation to achieve.
8. Identify areas of nursing care related to fertility that could benefit from additional nursing research.
9. Use critical thinking to analyze nursing strategies that can be used to support a couple through a fertility assessment.
10. Synthesize concern for problems of infertility with nursing process to achieve quality maternal and child health nursing care.

Key Points

- Infertility is said to exist when a pregnancy has not occurred after 1 year of unprotected coitus. Sterility refers to the inability to conceive because of a known condition.

- About 1 in 10 couples experience infertility. The incidence increases with the age of the couple.

- Male factors that contribute to infertility are inadequate sperm count, obstruction or impaired sperm motility, and problems with ejaculation.

- Female factors that cause infertility are problems with ovulation, tubal transport, impaired implantation, or interference with sperm motility.

- Infertility assessment procedures consist of a health history, physical exam, laboratory tests to document general health, and specific tests for semen analysis, ovulation, tubal patency, and hormone assessment.

- Measures to induce fertility are aimed at improving sperm number and transport, decreasing infections, and regulating hormones.

- Artificial insemination, in vitro fertilization, adoption, surrogate motherhood, and childfree living may all be suggested as solutions for infertility.

- Infertility testing is an intense psychological stress period for couples. Support from health care personnel is necessary during this time not only to help couples through the experience on an individual basis but to help them maintain their relationship as a couple.

- Couples who are told that an infertility problem has been discovered are apt to suffer a great loss of self-esteem. Offer support to help them look at other aspects of their lives where they do achieve to help them feel that they are productive, healthy people in many ways.

Definitions of Key Terms

anovulation: the absence of ovulation

cryptorchidism: undescended testes

endometriosis: abnormal implantation sites of endometrial cells outside the uterus

failure to achieve ejaculation: the failure to accomplish deposition of sperm with a sex act infertility: the state of being unable to reproduce; sterile

mumps orchitis: inflammation of the testis from invasion of the mumps virus

primary infertility: the state of never being able to conceive

secondary infertility: the state of being unable to conceive although the ability was previously present

sperm count: the number of sperm present in a single ejaculation

sperm motility: the documented movement of sperm after ejaculation

spermatogenesis: the formation and maturation of spermatozoa

Nursing Process Overview

The Nursing Process Overview in this chapter concentrates on helping students understand the impact that infertility has on families. This allows them to formulate nursing diagnoses at a deeper level than they might otherwise choose to do. The nursing role as a member of a health care team and the need for coordinated planning and interventions is stressed. The addresses of resources available for securing more information on infertility for students or families are given.

Study Aids

Tables

Table 6-1:   Cervical Mucus Scoring

Displays

Focus on National Health Goals

Focus on Family Teaching

Focus on Nursing Research

Focus on Cultural Awareness

Critical Thinking Exercises

1. Joanne Bigwan is a 30-year-old woman who has just been married; she wants to have a child as soon as possible. What advice would you give her to help increase her chances of conceiving quickly?

2. When Joanne doesn't conceive within a year, she is scheduled for a hysterosalpingogram and an endometrial biopsy. How would you prepare her for these procedures? What should she expect following them?

3. Joanne states that she feels fertility testing is extremely stressful. What are measures you could take to make the process easier for her?

Media Resources

Fertility (20 minute video)

The biologic requirements for human pregnancy and the reasons for infertility are discussed; methods of screening are illustrated.

Source: ACOG Distribution Center

Infertility in Women (14 minute video)

Basic descriptions of infertility for client education; diagrams and animation are used to illustrate basal body temperature, post-coital testing, endometrial biopsy, a hysterosalpingogram, and diagnostic laparoscopy.

Source: Polymorph Films, Inc.

In Search of a Child (27 minute video)

The psychological effects of infertility on three couples who want to have children are explored. The workings of the normal male and female reproductive systems, causes of infertility, and treatment options are discussed.

Source: Health Sciences Consortium

Discussion Questions

1. A hysterosalpingogram is a test frequently used to establish tubal patency. How would you prepare a woman for this?

2. Artificial insemination is not an easy concept for some couples to comprehend. How would you explain this option to a couple? Is there any risk to the couple involved?

3. Surrogate motherhood can result in dilemmas if the outcome is not as expected or if one party fails to honor the agreement. What moral, ethical, and legal principles should a couple consider before choosing this option?

Written Assignments

1. Infertility assessment can stress a couple's relationship. List ways a nurse can help a couple adapt to this stress in a healthy way.

2. Childless living is not appealing to everyone. What would be advantages and disadvantages of this? How might a couple's perceptions change over time?

3. A popular term for in vitro fertilization is ''test-tube babies.'' Explain how this term is a misnomer.

Laboratory Experiences

1. Ask students to have a significant other record (or record their own) basal body temperature. Discuss in a conference if a time of ovulation can be readily observed from these records.

2. Ask students to survey local drug stores or book stores to determine the quantity of products or literature available to the average couple on fertility so they can be aware how extensive a concern this problem is to the general public.

3. Ask a couple that is undergoing or has recently completed a fertility series to explain their feelings about the experience. How could health care providers have been more helpful or supportive to them? (If no couple wants to do this in person, ask permission to tape record their voices).

Care Study: A Family With an Infertility Concern

Andrea Newman is a 37-year-old woman attending an infertility clinic. She has been married for 5 years and has a 3-year-old and a 4-year-old child at home. She and her husband had planned on having three children; because they were married when they were both 32, they planned on having them close together.

Andrea had been not using a contraceptive for a year and a half and is concerned because she is apparently unable to conceive a third child.

Health History

- Chief Concern: "I want to get pregnant again."
- History of Present Illness: Client and husband have been trying for a third child for $1\frac{1}{2}$ years. Both are very discouraged and concerned at the delay because Mrs. Newman is 37.
- Past Medical History: Rubella at 6 years; appendectomy at 16 years. "Bad" adolescent acne treated with tetracycline during adolescence.
- Family Medical History: Husband's father has hypertension; a mother's cousin has renal failure.
- Personal/Social: Is independently employed as she owns a craft shop. Admits to long hours of standing to meet needs of customers; Drinks 6 cups of coffee daily; "occasional" wine; does not smoke. 24-hour nutrition recall reveals a diet light in protein and possibly iron.

  Husband works at a desk job as a stock broker. Client visibly upset discussing her inability to have a third child. Asked, "Do you realize what a good mother I would be to a girl? Why can't I have one?"

- Gynecologic History: Menarche at 13 years; cycle 30-32 days, duration of flow, 7 days. Has "terrible" dysmenorrhea she treats with Motrin. Last menstrual period: $2\frac{1}{2}$ weeks ago. Used vaginal sponge as method of contraception up until a year and a half ago. Papanicolaou smear negative as of 1 month ago; basal body temperature shows biphasic reaction with a drop in temperature preceding a sustained rise on day 15 of three successive cycles. Endometrial biopsy performed on first day of menstruation revealed progesterone stimulated endometrium. A hysterosalpingogram on the 9th day of cycle showed normal uterine cavity and patent tubes.

- Obstetric History: Therapeutic abortion at 18 years; Male, 7' 13'', born 4 years ago, vertex presentation, alive and well. Male, 8' 3'', born 3 years ago, vertex presentation, alive and well. Membranes were ruptured longer than 24 hours and labor was induced. Andrea had a mild endometritis treated with intravenous antibiotics for 4 days following birth. Feels this is the reason for her infertility now.

- Review of Systems: Essentially negative; one urinary tract infection 5 years ago shortly after marriage.

Physical Examination

- General Appearance: Mildly overweight, distressed appearing Caucasian woman; Height: 5'6'' Weight: 140 pounds.
- HEENT: Grossly negative; one "shotty" lymph node present on posterior cervical chain.
- Chest: Normal breast development; lungs clear to auscultation
- Abdomen: Soft, no masses; uterus not palpable
- Extremities: Mild varicose vein on medial aspect of left leg; full range of motion in all joints; deep tendon reflexes 2+
- Pelvic Exam: Performed as post-coital exam. Cervical mucus thin and with spinnbarkeit properties; a few sperm with reduced motility present; uterus and tubes palpable; normal size and shape.

Care Study Questions

1. Many couples discover that infertility has resulted in them not being able to have children at all. Is Mrs. Newman's anxiety at not being able to have a third child warranted in light of this? Suppose she doesn't conceive again? Could there be psychological repercussions on the second boy, knowing a girl was wanted more?

2. What are the risk factors for infertility that the Newmans evidence?

3. Complete a nursing care plan that will identify and meet the needs of the Newman family.

Genetic Assessment and Counseling

Chapter 7 discusses the nursing role in genetic assessment and counseling. The chapter begins with an overview of nursing process specific to care of the couple with a genetic concern. The nature of inheritance including dominant, recessive, X-linked, polygenic, and nondisjunction inheritance is discussed. The role of the nurse as a member of a genetic counseling team and the legal and ethical implications of genetic counseling are stressed.

Most students have a basic understanding of genetics gained from previous science courses but their knowledge is often too abstract for them to appreciate the impact a genetic disorder can have on a specific family. Studying a number of specific syndromes and how they affect families helps students refine their knowledge in this area.

Chapter Objectives

After mastering the contents of this chapter, students should be able to:

1. Describe the nature of inheritance, patterns of recessive and dominant Mendelian inheritance, and common chromosomal aberrations such as nondisjunction syndromes.

2. Assess a family for the probability of inheriting a genetic disorder.

3. Formulate nursing diagnoses related to genetic disorders.

4. Plan nursing care related to an alteration in genetic health, such as assisting with an amniocentesis.

5. Implement nursing care related to identification of or counseling for a genetic disorder.

6. Evaluate outcome criteria to be certain that nursing goals were achieved.

7. Identify national health goals and specific measures that nurses can take to help the nation achieve these goals.

8. Identify areas related to genetic assessment that could benefit from additional nursing research.

9. Use critical thinking to analyze ways that nurses can contribute to health education and counseling as genetic counselors.

10. Synthesize knowledge of genetic inheritance with nursing process to achieve quality maternal and child health nursing care.

Key Points

- Genetic disorders are ones that result from malstructure or abnormal number of genes or chromosomes. Genetics is the study of how and why such disorders occur.

- A person's phenotype is the outward appearance. Genotype refers to actual gene composition. A person's genome is the complete set of genes present. A karyotype is a graphic representation of chromosomes present.

- A person is homozygous if he or she has two like genes for a trait, and heterozygous if he or she has two unlike genes for a trait.

- Mendelian laws can predict the likely incidence of recessive or dominant diseases in offspring. Division disorders including nondisjunction abnormalities, deletion, translocation, and mosaicism abnormalities also create genetic disorders.

- Genetic counseling can be a role for nurses if they are well versed in genetics. Assessment of genetic disorders consists of a health history, physical examination, laboratory studies such as chorionic villi sampling, amniocentesis, and buccal smears.

- Some karyotyping tests such as chorionic villi sampling and amniocentesis introduce a risk of initiating labor. Be certain that women undergoing these tests remain in the health care facility for at least 30 minutes following a procedure to be certain that complications such as vaginal bleeding or labor contractions are not initiated.

- Women with an Rh-negative blood type need Rh immune globulin administration following procedures such as chorionic villi sampling and amniocentesis.

- An important aspect of genetic counseling is respecting a couple's right to privacy. Be certain that information is not given indiscriminately to other family members.

- People who are told that a genetic abnormality does exist in their family are apt to suffer a loss of self-esteem. Offer support to help them look at other positive aspects of their lives.

- Common nondisjunction genetic disorders are Down syndrome (trisomy 21), trisomy 13, trisomy 18, Turner's syndrome, and Klinefelter's syndrome. Most of these syndromes include mental retardation (discussed in Chapter 56).

Definitions of Key Terms

acrocentric chromosome: a chromosome with the "arms" crossing at a center point

alleles: alternate forms of genes found at the same chromosome locus

centromere: the point of attachment of the "arms" of chromosomes

chromosomes: the rod-shaped structures composed of DNA and found within the nuclei of cells that carry genetic information

dermatoglyphics: the patterns of skin configurations on fingers and toes

dominant gene: a gene that will be expressed in a heterozygous union

genes: segments of DNA material that carry character traits from generation to generation

genetics: the study of gene transmission of characteristics from generation to generation

genome: the total gene complement of an individual

genotype: the genetic constitution of an individual

heterozygous trait: possessing two different genes for a character trait

homozygous trait: possessing two like genes for a character trait

imprinting: the differential expression of genetic material that makes it possible to identify whether chromosomal material was inherited from the male or female parent

karyotype: a display of the number, size, and shape of chromosomes of a representative body cell

meiosis: a process whereby a cell divides and reduces its chromosome number by half; reduction cell division

metrocentric chromosome: a chromosome with a central centromere

nondisjunction: failure of two paired chromosomes to separate during cell division; leads to trisomy disorders

phenotype: the appearance of an individual in relation to genetic makeup

recessive gene: a gene that will not be expressed unless a homozygous gene for the trait is present

submetrocentric chromosome: a chromosome with the centromere below the midpoint so "arms" of unequal length are created

Nursing Process Overview

The Nursing Process Overview in this chapter concentrates on helping the student appreciate what a unique experience pregnancy is to women so they can better understand the importance of individualizing prenatal care. Examples of nursing diagnoses involving changes of pregnancy are given. The necessity for changing diagnoses as pregnancy progresses is stressed.

Study Aids

Boxes

Box 7-1:   Legal Guidelines for Genetic Screening

Tables

Table 7-1:   Selected Examples of Single-Gene Disorders

Table 7-2:   Common Physical Characteristics of Children With Chromosomal Syndromes

Table 7-3:   Chromosomally Determined Diseases That Can Be Detected by Amniocentesis or CVS

Displays

Focus on National Health Goals

Focus on Family Teaching

Focus on Nursing Research

Focus on Cultural Awareness

Media Resources

Our Genetic Heritage (14 minute video)

An overview of human genetics including the basics of DNA to prenatal testing; a variety of genetic diseases and parents' reactions are discussed.

Source: March of Dimes Birth Defects Foundation

Healthier Babies: The Genetic Era (20 minute video)

An overview of clinical genetics; diagnosis, treatment, and prevention is stressed. Prenatal diagnosis and a number of genetic disorders are shown.

Source: March of Dimes Birth Defect Foundation

Prenatal Diagnosis: To Be or Not to Be (45 minute film)

Amniocentesis, fetoscopy, and ultrasound and their use in prenatal diagnosis are demonstrated. A couple who lost one child to Tay-Sachs disease is shown rejoicing when amniocentesis reveals that a second child is a healthy girl. The overall ethics of prenatal decision-making and the ethical dilemmas inherent in genetic testing are discussed.

Source: Filmmakers Library

Between Joy and Sorrow: Parents of Children With Serious Genetic Conditions (27 minute video)

A glimpse into the lives of five sets of parents whose children were born with serious genetic conditions. Parents discuss how they handled their individual situations and the strategies they used to meet the challenge of having such a child.

Source: Health Sciences Consortium

Discussion Questions

1. Parents who have a child with a chromosomal abnormality may develop a severe loss of self-esteem. What are ways you could reinforce a sense of high self-esteem in such parents?

2. A client asks you to tell her what proportion of her children are apt to have a disease you recognize as being autosomally recessively inherited. How would you explain this to her?

3. Deciding to have a procedure such as chorionic villi sampling (CVS) done is difficult for parents because this procedure may result in the loss of a normal fetus. What would be your role in helping parents make this decision?

Written Assignments

1. Research one of the common chromosomal syndromes such as Down syndrome and write a paragraph describing common features of the disorder.

2. Analyze a genogram of a particular family and write a paragraph describing the type of inheritance pattern you think is in the family. Justify your conclusions.

3. Write to a national organization such as the March of Dimes foundation or to facilities in the local community to survey what resources are available to parents to obtain information on a genetic disorder. How much information does the local library system have available to parents?

Laboratory Experiences

1. Schedule students for an experience at an antepartal clinic or a physician's office where they are able to view sonograms or amniocentesis for genetic analysis being completed. If these experiences are not available to all students, ask those who do see these procedures to report their observations in conference.

2. Ask students to interview clients about their reactions to being scheduled for alpha fetoprotein serum levels or amniocentesis during pregnancy. If a client's reaction was fright or worry, how could a health care provider have made the experience easier for them?

3. Schedule students for an observational experience at a local genetic screening center. Ask them to note particularly how genetic screening and counseling is a team effort of various health professionals.

Care Study: A Woman Concerned About a Genetic Abnormality

Cheryl Burrows is a 15-year-old pregnant woman you care for at a prenatal clinic. She asks to be referred to a genetic screening clinic to have an amniocentesis done because she is concerned that her baby will inherit one of the diseases that runs in the two families. Cheryl has two paternal aunts who have breast cancer and a paternal uncle with prostate cancer. Her sister's baby was born with an extra finger which was ligated at birth. The boy she thinks is the baby's father—Tony Vallo—had a brother die of thalassemia as an infant. Although she doesn't want any further association with him, Cheryl also is interested in having it proven that Tony is the father of the baby.

Care Study Questions

1. Are Cheryl's concerns about there being inherited genetic diseases warranted? Would an amniocentesis be helpful to her?

2. Is proof of paternity a sufficient reason to have an amniocentesis? Would you want to know more about Cheryl's reasons for wanting proof Tony is the father?

3. Complete a nursing care plan that will identify and meet Cheryl's needs.

Psychological and Physiologic Changes of Pregnancy

Chapter 8 discusses the psychological reactions and physiologic changes of pregnancy and how they affect the woman and her family. The chapter begins with an overview of nursing process specific to care of the family during pregnancy. Initial psychological reactions as well as psychological tasks of pregnancy are included. Physiologic changes in body systems and the signs and symptoms that lead to the diagnosis of pregnancy are discussed. The effect of psychological and physiologic changes on the entire family and ways that nurses can intervene with health education are stressed.

Most students are interested in learning about psychological and physiologic changes of pregnancy from a personal as well as a professional viewpoint. Some students need help in understanding how the theoretical changes produce common symptoms or moving from a general knowledge level to counseling individual women during pregnancy.

Chapter Objectives

After mastering the contents of this chapter, students should be able to:

1. Describe the psychological and physiologic changes that occur with pregnancy, the underlying principles for these changes, and the relationship of the changes to the pregnancy diagnosis.
2. Assess a woman for the psychological and physiologic changes that occur with pregnancy through health history and physical examination.
3. Formulate nursing diagnoses related to psychological and physiologic changes of pregnancy.
4. Plan nursing care related to the changes and diagnosis of pregnancy such as helping women plan to get adequate rest.
5. Implement nursing care such as health teaching related to the expected changes of pregnancy.
6. Evaluate outcome criteria to be certain that nursing goals established for care were achieved.
7. Identify national health goals that nurses could be instrumental in helping the nation achieve.
8. Identify areas of nursing care related to the psychological and physiologic changes of pregnancy that could benefit from additional nursing research.
9. Use critical thinking to analyze how the physical and psychological changes of pregnancy affect family functioning and develop ways to make nursing care more family centered.
10. Synthesize knowledge of psychological and physiologic changes in pregnancy with nursing process to achieve quality maternal and child health nursing care.

Key Points

- The ability of a woman to accept a pregnancy depends on social, cultural, family, and individual influences.
- The psychological tasks of pregnancy are centered on ensuring safe passage for the fetus. These consist of accepting the pregnancy (first trimester), accepting the baby (second trimester), and preparing for parenthood (third trimester). Fathers undergo the same steps.
- Common emotional responses that occur with pregnancy can be grief, narcissism, introversion or extroversion, decreased decision making ability, body image and boundary confusion, emotional lability, and changes in sexual desire.
- Physiologic changes that occur with pregnancy are both local (uterine, ovarian, and vaginal) and systemic (respiratory, cardiovascular, urinary, and skin).
- The diagnosis of pregnancy is rated according to three types of findings: presumptive, probable, and positive.
- The positive signs of pregnancy are demonstration of a fetal heart separate from the mother's, fetal movement felt by an examiner, and visualization of the fetus by ultrasound.
- Women may have read about the expected psychological and physiologic changes of pregnancy, but once these changes are actually being experienced, the effects may be more intense than anticipated.
- Although a woman may be in a physician's office or prenatal clinic for only an hour, if her pregnancy was confirmed at that visit, she invariably feels ''more

pregnant'' when she leaves. From that day, most women try to eat a proper diet and give up cigarette smoking, alcohol ingestion, and over-the-counter medication. Because a woman may not take these measures before confirmation of her pregnancy, early diagnosis is important. If the woman does not wish to continue the pregnancy, early diagnosis is imperative; elective termination of pregnancy always should be carried out at the earliest stage possible for the safest outcome.

Definitions of Key Terms

ballottement: the sensation of an object rebounding after being pushed by an examining hand. Used for pregnancy diagnosis

Braxton Hicks contractions: painless, erratic uterine contractions that occur toward the end of pregnancy. They ready the cervix for labor but cervical dilation does not occur with them

couvade syndrome: somatic symptoms experienced by the father during pregnancy simulating those of the pregnant mother

diastasis: a separation of the rectus abdominis muscle

Goodell's sign: softening of the cervix; a probable sign of pregnancy

Hegar's sign: softening of the lower uterine segment; a probable sign of pregnancy

hyperptyalism: Excessive secretion of saliva

lightening: descent of the fetus into the pelvis about 2 weeks prior to delivery; also engagement

melasma: excessive body pigment that occurs during pregnancy

multipara: a woman who has delivered more than one child past the age of viability

operculum: the mucus plug formed in the cervical canal during pregnancy

polyuria: excessive amount of urine output

positive signs of pregnancy: findings that definitely indicate a pregnancy is present

presumptive signs of pregnancy: findings, largely subjective in nature, that suggest but do not confirm that a pregnancy is present

probable signs of pregnancy: findings, largely objective in nature, that suggest but do not confirm that a pregnancy is present

pseudoanemia: the apparent anemia that occurs early in pregnancy due to rapid expansion of blood volume

Nursing Process Overview

The Nursing Process Overview in this chapter concentrates on helping the student appreciate what a unique experience pregnancy is to women so they can better understand the importance of individualizing prenatal care. Examples of nursing diagnoses involving changes of pregnancy are given. The necessity for changing diagnoses as pregnancy progresses is stressed.

Study Aids

Boxes

Box 8-1:   Possible Life Events That Could Contribute to Difficulty Accepting a Pregnancy

Tables

Table 8-1:   Timetable for Physiologic Changes of Pregnancy

Table 8-2:   Respiratory Changes During Pregnancy

Table 8-3:   Changes in the Cardiovascular System During Pregnancy

Table 8-4:   Urinary Tract Changes During Pregnancy

Table 8-5:   Presumptive and Probable Signs of Pregnancy

Displays

Focus on National Health Goals

Focus on Family Teaching

Focus on Nursing Research

Focus on Cultural Awareness

Critical Thinking Exercises

1. Molly is a young adult woman you care for in a prenatal setting. She tells you that she ''hates'' her parents and ''would die'' if she thought she might be the same type of parent they were. Has Molly completed the psychological development tasks of pregnancy? Are there suggestions you could make to her to help her be a better parent?

2. Teresa is a 15-year-old adolescent you know who is 4 months pregnant. She tells you she has had almost constant heartburn or nausea since she became pregnant. How would you explain why these symptoms happen with pregnancy?

3. Teresa used a home test kit to determine that she is pregnant and has not been to a health care setting because she says the most important reason for going would be to learn whether she is pregnant or not and she already knows that. What argument could you use to convince her that prenatal care is important for more than pregnancy diagnosis?

Media Resources

Growing Into Parenthood (28 minute video)

The adjustment to pregnancy, birth, and new parenthood of four couples of various backgrounds expecting their first child is explored.

Source: Educational Graphic Aids

Family Bonding: Pregnancy, Birth and the First Hours (20 minute video, slides, filmstrip)

The vital nature of family attachment and interaction is demonstrated. The beginning of maternal and family bonding with the baby through pregnancy, birth, and the first hours is explored. The development of family support and the significance of active participation are stressed.

Source: Educational Graphic Aids

<u>Maternal Changes and Prenatal Care</u> (30 minute video)

Physical changes of pregnancy in each trimester are reviewed. A case study following a pregnant woman through prenatal assessment, care, and teaching is shown.

Source: Medcom

<u>Pregnancy Model</u> (simulated model)

Life-size model of pregnant abdomen including 14 parts and 8 fetal models. Each month of pregnancy can be illustrated.

Source: Armstrong Medical Industries, Inc.

Discussion Questions

1. Almost all body systems accommodate to meet the requirements of pregnancy. How do respiratory adjustments aid fetal growth?

2. The emotional changes that a woman experiences during pregnancy can interfere with a marriage relationship. What changes would you want to be certain to include in anticipatory guidance at a prenatal visit?

3. Some women are reluctant to discuss emotional responses to pregnancy in a health care setting. What environment would be most conducive to helping a woman discuss her feelings about pregnancy?

Written Assignments

1. Fatigue in early pregnancy is a symptom that many women find distressing. Write a paragraph describing the physiologic adjustments that account for such extreme fatigue.

2. Some women with cardiac disease are unable to complete a pregnancy successfully because of the necessary cardiovascular adjustments. List these adjustments.

3. "Nest building" is an outward sign that a woman is actively planning on having a child. What activities would you assess at a prenatal visit to determine if a woman is engaged in this?

Laboratory Experiences

1. Assign students to prenatal settings so they have opportunities to interview pregnant women as to psychological and physiologic changes of pregnancy.

2. Invite a pregnant woman who is experiencing a major role change with pregnancy or who has common symptoms of pregnancy such as nausea and vomiting to come to postconference and discuss how she is resolving these concerns.

3. Ask students to survey pregnant women they care for as to how many used home-test kits to see if they were pregnant rather than waiting for a physician visit for pregnancy confirmation. Discuss the pros and cons of such home testing.

The Growing Fetus

*C*hapter 9 describes growth and development from fertilization until birth. The chapter begins with an overview of nursing process specific to fetal growth. The development of major organ systems and the structure and function of accessory organs of fetal growth are discussed. Methods of estimating fetal well being and age are described. Milestones of fetal growth and development are presented for each lunar month of pregnancy. Gaining knowledge of fetal growth in order to be an effective health educator is stressed.

Chapter Objectives

After mastering the contents of this chapter, students should be able to:

1. Describe the growth and development of the fetus by gestation weeks.

2. Assess fetal growth and development through maternal and pregnancy landmarks.

3. Formulate nursing diagnoses related to the needs of the pregnant woman and developing baby.

4. Plan nursing care that promotes healthy fetal growth.

5. Implement nursing care to help ensure a safe pregnancy outcome and a safe fetal environment.

6. Evaluate outcome criteria established in relation to fetal growth to be certain that nursing goals have been achieved.

7. Identify national health goals related to fetal growth that nurses can help the nation to achieve.

8. Identify areas of fetal health that could benefit from additional nursing research.

9. Use critical thinking to analyze ways to promote fetal growth and development appropriate for individual families.

10. Synthesize knowledge of growth and development of the fetus with nursing process to achieve quality maternal and child health nursing care.

Key Points

- The union of a single sperm and egg (fertilization) signals the beginning of pregnancy. The fertilized ovum (a zygote) travels by way of the fallopian tubes to the uterus where implantation takes place in about 8 days. From implantation to 5 to 8 weeks, the growing structure is called an embryo. The period following this until birth is the fetal period.

- Growth of the umbilical cord, amniotic fluid, and amniotic membranes proceed in concert with fetal growth. The placenta produces a number of important hormones: estrogen, progesterone, chorionic somatomammotropin, and human chorionic gonadotropin.

- Various methods used to assess fetal growth and development are fundal height, fetal movement, fetal heart tones, ultrasound, magnetic resonance imaging, alpha fetoprotein analysis, amniocentesis, percutaneous umbilical blood sampling, amnioscopy, and fetoscopy. A biophysical profile is a combination of fetal assessments that better predict fetal well being than single parameters.

- A fetus needs protection from teratogens such as drugs in order to grow well. Remind women that nicotine and alcohol are drugs so they know to avoid these.

- Fetal growth can be demonstrated by x-ray, but it is not assessed this way in order to avoid exposing the fetus to x-ray. Remind women to tell health care providers that they are pregnant before they have an x-ray for any reason so they can be furnished with a lead apron for the procedure to protect the fetus.

Definitions of Key Terms

amniocentesis: the withdrawal of amniotic fluid from the uterus by means of introduction of a needle through the abdominal wall

amniotic cavity: space in the developing conceptus from which the ectodermal cells develop

amniotic membrane: the innermost membrane surrounding the fetus that secretes amniotic fluid

blastocyst: a hollow sphere of cells that forms in very early fetal development

cephalocaudal: relating to head and tail; progression of development in a fetus

chorionic membrane: the outer fetal membrane

chorionic villi: projections of the trophoblast that produce human chorionic gonadotropin and begin osmosis of nutrients to the embryo

coelocentesis: the transvaginal aspiration of fluid collected in the extraembryonic cavity early in pregnancy for analysis

corona radiata: the crown-like grouping of cells that surrounds the ovum immediately after ovulation

cotyledons: a subdivision of the maternal surface of the placenta; filled with maternal blood to allow for osmosis of nutrients to the fetal placental villi

decidua basalis: the endometrium portion under the implanted blastocyst

decidua capsularis: the endometrium portion that covers the blastocyst

decidua vera: the endometrium portion that covers the nonimplanted portion of the uterus

ductus arteriosus: a blood vessel joining the pulmonary artery and aorta in fetal life; closes at birth

ductus venosus: a blood vessel joining the umbilical vein and the inferior vena cava in fetal life; closes at birth

ectoderm: one of the layers of primary germ cell tissue in the embryo

embryo: the intrauterine growth period from the time following implantation until organogenesis is complete (tenth day to 5 to 8 weeks)

entoderm: one of the layers of primary germ cells in the embryo

expected date of birth: calculated date on which birth can be predicted to occur

fertilization: the union of the sperm and ovum

fetoscopy: the visualization of the fetus by inspection through a fetoscope

fetus: the developing structure from the eighth week postfertilization until birth

foramen ovale: an opening between the atria of the heart during intrauterine life

hydramnios: an excessive amount of amniotic fluid (generally over 2,000 mL)

implantation: nidation; the attachment of the zygote to the uterine endometrium

lightening: descent of the fetus into the pelvis at about 2 weeks prior to delivery; also engagement

McDonald's Rule: the fundus to symphysis distance in centimeters is equal to the week of gestation between the 20th to 31st week of pregnancy

mesoderm: one of the layers of primary germ cell tissue in the embryo

morula: the developing blastomere structure as it multiplies rapidly and forms a bumpy surface

neural plate: the embryonic structure from which the nervous system develops

nonstress test: an assessment of fetal well being determined from examination of the fetal heart rate in relation to fetal activity

oligohydramnios: a decreased amount of amniotic fluid

quickening: the first movement of the fetus perceived by the mother

surfactant: a lipoprotein secreted by the alveoli cells to reduce surface tension on expiration

trophoblast: the outer layer of the lining of the trophoblast villi

umbilical cord: the structure composed of two veins and one artery that connects the placenta to the fetus

Wharton's jelly: the gelatinous substance that gives bulk to the umbilical cord

yolk sac: the space in embryonic life from which the hemopoietic system develops

zona pellucida: a layer of fluid that surrounds the ovum at ovulation

zygote: a fertilized ovum

Nursing Process Overview

The Nursing Process Overview in this chapter concentrates on helping students appreciate the unique care they must devise when they have a "hidden" client present. Examples of nursing diagnoses pertinent to fetal health are given. The role of the nurse in educating about fetal health and necessity to involve the mother in planning care is stressed.

Study Aids

Box 9-1:	Nagele's Rule

Tables

Table 9-1:	Terms Used to Denote Fetal Growth
Table 9-2:	Mechanisms by Which Nutrients Cross the Placenta
Table 9-3:	Origin of Body Tissue
Table 9-4:	Comparison of Nonstress and Contraction Tests
Table 9-5:	Timing of Amniocentesis Procedures
Table 9-6:	Biophysical Profile Scoring

Displays

Focus on National Health Goals

Focus on Family Teaching

Focus on Nursing Research

Critical Thinking Exercises

1. Jessica Ayers is a woman who is 6 weeks pregnant. She asks you how big her fetus is at this point. What would be the best way to illustrate this for her?

2. Jessica is scheduled for an ultrasound at 20 weeks gestation to assess fetal growth. She states she does not want to know her fetus' sex if it is revealed by the test. Why do you think some women want to know the sex of a fetus and some don't? Is there an advantage to knowing or not knowing?

3. Late in pregnancy, Jessica is scheduled for a number of nonstress and contraction stress tests. She states she

hates to have these done because they are time consuming and boring. What are ways you could make such tests more appealing and so increase compliance?

Media Resources

Life in the Womb: The First Stages of Human Development (filmstrip or video)

A two-part series that chronicles the course of human development from fertilization to birth. The Course of Development focuses on the growth of the ovum and discusses the role of the placenta. Influences of Prenatal Development covers prenatal growth including genetic inheritance and disorders, blood type, age of mother, diet, medications, pollutants, and health.

Source: Career Aids

Miracle of Life (15 minute video)

Microscopic photography is used to show the reproductive process of fertilization, cell division, and development of the fetus.

Source: Pyramid Film and Video

Knowing the Unborn (29 minute video)

Ultrasound images and photography of developing fetuses are interwoven with interviews of leading authorities on fetal development to illustrate fetal growth and capabilities.

Source: Childbirth Graphics

Human Reproduction and Development Kit (simulated fetal models; filmstrip)

Fetal models plus a filmstrip on fetal growth allow students two opportunities to visualize fetal growth.

Source: Nasco Health Care

Ultrasound: A Window to the Womb (15 minute video)

The physics of ultrasound and how to perform the procedure are explained. Three case studies illustrate why ultrasound examinations are used during each of the trimesters of pregnancy.

Source: Health Sciences Consortium

Discussion Questions

1. Amniocentesis is a commonly used assessment procedure for fetal well being. What are nursing responsibilities during such a procedure?
2. The placenta is indispensable to fetal life. What are the body organs that it is replacing?
3. The ability of low-birthweight infants to survive depends on their level of development at birth. What would be the differences in a 20-week and a 26-week fetus?

Written Assignments

1. Write a brief paragraph tracing the development of one body system in utero. Compare this development with your previous expectations of fetal growth.

2. Interview a pregnant woman you care for as to her lifestyle and then write a short report on whether you feel her lifestyle is optimal to encourage fetal growth.
3. Investigate the effects of a teratogen such as drug ingestion or smoking and then write a report on the specific harmful effects of the teratogen on fetal growth.

Laboratory Experiences

1. Using a simulated teaching model, hold a contest asking students to estimate which month of pregnancy and fetal development the model is adjusted to illustrate. Give a prize for the best rationale for the estimation.
2. Assign students to experiences in prenatal settings where they can view sonograms for gestational age being recorded. Provide time in class for discussions of observations, including the mother's comments on the size or health of her fetus.
3. Have students interview pregnant clients they care for and ask them about their impression of how well developed their fetus is at that point in pregnancy. Provide class discussion time to contrast these expectations with actual fetal growth and development.

Care Study: A Pregnant Woman With Concern for the Fetus

Jessica Menendez is a 20-year-old woman who is 20 weeks pregnant. You care for her in an emergency room. She has a stab wound of the upper abdomen from an argument with her boyfriend.

Health History

- Chief Concern: "Do you think my baby's all right? What if the knife hit it?"
- History of Chief Concern: Client and boyfriend were arguing over who should have the last piece of popcorn in a bowl when he stabbed her with a kitchen paring knife. Client has felt the fetus move since the incident; movement is "same as always."
- Past Medical History: Client had nephrosis as a preschooler; no apparent sequelae. One previous incident of domestic violence when a previous boyfriend beat her and left her for dead on a roadway. Had no childhood diseases.
- Family Medical History: Mother died at age 36 of uterine cancer. Father's health history unknown. An aunt has "some kind of heart condition."
- Personal/Social: Client lives in one-bedroom apartment; finances are provided by government assistance. Has a high school education; unable to find employment, especially since she has become pregnant. Named her landlord (Mrs. Rubins) as her most accessible support person. When asked if she intended to continue relation with boyfriend she answered, "He ain't a bad dude; he just got a bad temper." Does not intend to press charges against him for stabbing.
- Pregnancy History: Pregnancy planned to "make boyfriend settle down." Has had no prenatal care; not taking

prenatal vitamins. Alcohol consumption: ''a beer to help me sleep at night''; smokes two packs of cigarettes a day; states she takes no recreational or prescription drugs.

- Gynecologic History: Menarche at age 11 years; mild dysmenorrhea each month. Gonorrhea at age 13 years; treated at Health Center. Does not use contraception; as relationship with boyfriend is monogamous, does not ask him to use condom.

- Review of Systems: Essentially negative; occasional constipation.

Physical Examination

- General Appearance: Pregnant-appearing young adult woman in obvious emotional distress from recent incident. Clothing is blood-stained over abdomen.

- HEENT: Normocephalic. Eyes: Follows to 5 positions of gaze; red reflex present. Mucous membrane appears pale. Ears: No redness; TMs mobile. Mouth: Midline uvula; two cavities present in lower teeth. Four keloid linear scars, each approximately 2 cm long, present on left cheek.

- Chest: Respiratory rate: 22/min. No rales or rhonchi present. Good aeration all lobes.

- Abdomen: One inch long linear incisional type wound present 2 inches above umbilicus at midline; wound oozing slight serosanguineous drainage. Uterus palpable at umbilicus. Fetal movement felt by examiner. FHR: 155/bpm by fetal heart rate monitor. No uterine contractions present on monitor.

- Genitalia: Normal female; no discharge, lesions, or redness.

- Extremities: Ecchymotic marks in the impression of a hand present on both upper arms. Well demarcated ecchymotic marks approximately 2 X 3 cm present over tibia on both legs.

Care Study Questions

1. Jessica's reason for having a baby was to ''help her boyfriend settle down.'' Does it sound as if her technique is working? Do you feel as if Jessica and the fetus will remain safe from violence following this incident?

2. Jessica's fetus is in danger from sources other than the recent stab sound. What are these?

3. Complete a nursing care plan that identifies and meets the needs of Jessica and her fetus.

Assessing Fetal and Maternal Health: The First Prenatal Visit

Chapter 10 discusses the importance of and the nursing role in prenatal care. The chapter begins with an overview of nursing process specific to prenatal care. Health interviewing, physical examination including a pelvic examination, laboratory analysis, and establishment of an antepartum fetal risk score are discussed. Emphasis is on individualizing prenatal care and including support people in care so it best fulfills women's needs.

Students are aware that women receive care during pregnancy before they study this content but are generally unaware of the extent of assessment which is undertaken and especially how much of antenatal assessment is completed by nurses. Learning this role can enrich the student's perception of the capabilities of nurses as well as increase knowledge of pregnancy and prenatal care.

Chapter Objectives

After mastering the contents of this chapter, students should be able to:

1. Describe health assessment measures commonly included in a first prenatal visit.
2. Assess a pregnant woman for optimal health status by obtaining a health history.
3. Formulate nursing diagnoses related to health status for pregnancy.
4. Plan nursing care such as preparing a woman for a pelvic examination or fundal measurement.
5. Implement nursing care such as establishing a risk score for pregnancy.
6. Evaluate outcome criteria related to fetal or maternal health to be certain goals of care were achieved.
7. Identify national health goals that nurses can be instrumental in helping the nation to achieve.

8. Identify areas of prenatal care that could benefit from additional nursing research.
9. Use critical thinking to analyze ways that the family can be included in prenatal care to keep care family centered.
10. Synthesize knowledge of pregnancy health assessment with nursing process to achieve quality maternal and child health care.

Key Points

- Prenatal care has the potential to reduce congenital anomalies and the infant mortality rate. The purposes of prenatal care are to establish a baseline of present health, determine gestation age of the fetus, monitor fetal development, identify the woman at risk for complications, minimize the risk of possible complications by anticipating and preventing problems before they occur, and provide time for education about pregnancy and possible dangers.

- A first visit for prenatal care not only confirms a pregnancy but provides a time to assess client needs and educate about pregnancy. Assessments consist of a health history, physical examination, and laboratory tests. The physical exam could include measurement of fundal height and assessment of fetal heart sounds, a pelvic examination (including a pap test), and perhaps estimation of pelvic size.

- Common types of pelves are gynecoid (well rounded with wide pubic arch), anthropoid (narrow), platypelloid (flattened), and android (male or with a sharp pubic arch). A gynecoid pelvis is ideal for childbearing.

- The true conjugate (conjugate vera) is the measurement between the anterior surface of the sacral prominence and the posterior surface of the inferior margin of the symphysis pubis (the anterior-posterior diameter of the pelvic inlet). The average is 10.5 to 11 cm. The ischial tuberosity diameter is the distance between the ischial tuberosities or the transverse diameter of the outlet. The average is 11 cm.

- A first prenatal visit sets the tone for visits to follow. Maintaining a supportive manner is helpful in establishing rapport and allowing the woman to feel comfortable to return for future care.

- Remember that a family, not a woman alone, is having a baby and include family members in procedures and health teaching as desired.

- Pregnant women have decreased balance. For safety, help them to positions on examining tables as needed. Pregnant women should remain in a lithotomy position as short a time as possible to help prevent thromboembolism and supine hypotension.

Definitions of Key Terms

abortion: the expulsion of the products of conception before 20 weeks gestation or before an age of viability

age of viability: the age at which a fetus is likely to be able to live if born at that point; 20 to 24 weeks gestation

conjugate vera: the pelvic measurement from the upper margin of the symphysis pubis to the sacral promontory, a distance of about 10.5 to 11.5 cm

diagonal conjugate: distance from the sacral promontory to the lower posterior border of the symphysis pubis

erosion: cell changes of the uterine cervix associated with irritation or infection

gravida: the number of pregnancies a woman has had; a pregnant woman

ischial tuberosity: the projections of the pelvic bone that mark the transverse diameter of the pelvic outlet

lithotomy position: an examining or delivery position with the client lying supine; knees are flexed and heels are elevated in stirrups

multigravida: a woman who is having or has had more than one pregnancy

multipara: a woman who has delivered more than one child past the age of viability

nulligravida: a woman who has never been pregnant

para: a live birth

primigravida: a woman who is having her first pregnancy

primipara: a woman who has given birth to one live born child

speculum: an instrument with curved blades designed for examination of the vagina and cervix

true conjugate: the distance between the interior surface of the symphysis pubis and the sacral prominence

viability: the state of being capable of living outside the uterus

Nursing Process Overview

The Nursing Process Overview in this chapter concentrates on helping students plan care comprehensively so care meets the needs of both the fetus and the parents. The importance of long-term planning (9 months) is also stressed. Without this emphasis, students may set only an immediate goal and therefore miss the concept that what they are teaching must be retained for the entire pregnancy and probably during future pregnancies as well.

Study Aids

Boxes

Box 10-1:   Suggestions for Improving Prenatal Care

Tables

Table 10-1:   Danger Signs of Pregnancy

Table 10-2:   Gynecologic Disorders

Table 10-3:   Terms Related to Pregnancy Status

Table 10-4:   Classification of Papanicolaou Smears

Table 10-5:   Assessments for a First Pregnancy Visit

Table 10-6:   Antepartum Fetal Risk Score

Procedures

Procedure 10-1:   Instructions to Help a Woman Obtain a Clean-Catch Urine Specimen

Displays

Focus on National Health Goals

Focus on Family Teaching

Focus on Nursing Research

Critical Thinking Exercises

1. It is important to ask enough questions during a health history to be able to estimate health risks. The client, Jessine Wardall, described in the Nursing Care Plan, works as a Spanish teacher for grade school students. Are there any special risks you can think of associated with this occupation? Is there a greater opportunity than normal for her to develop upper respiratory infections, for example? Is this a job that probably keeps her on her feet for long periods? Is she apt to be exposed to toxic substances at work?

2. Some women don't come early in pregnancy for prenatal care because they know a first visit includes a pelvic examination. What are techniques you can use to help women better accept this procedure?

3. What are things about Jessine Wardall's lifestyle you would like to see her change during a pregnancy that you would stress in pregnancy education for her? Are there factors to make you believe she will comply with instructions well? Are there reasons to think she might not comply?

Media Resources

Growing Into Parenthood (28 minute video)

The adjustment to pregnancy, birth, and new parenthood of four couples of various backgrounds expecting their first child are explored.

Source: Educational Graphic Aids

Family Bonding: Pregnancy, Birth and the First Hours (20 minute video, filmstrip, or slides)

The concept of family attachment and interaction is demonstrated. The beginning of maternal and family bonding with the baby through pregnancy, birth, and the early hours which follow are explored. The development of family support and the significance of active participation are emphasized.

Source: Educational Graphic Aids

Maternal Changes and Prenatal Care (30 minute video)

The physical changes of pregnancy in each trimester are reviewed. A case study follows a woman through prenatal assessment, care, and teaching.

> Source: Medcom

The Breast and Pelvic Examination: A Sensible Approach (27 minute video)

An instructional program to teach health care providers how to perform breast and pelvic examinations.

> Source: University of Arizona Biomedical Communications

The Growing Uterus (charts, slides)

Charts illustrating the relationship of the growing uterus to other body organs and the resultant objective and subjective symptoms of pregnancy.

> Source: Childbirth Graphics

Pregnancy (model)

Life-size model of a pregnant abdomen including 14 parts and 8 models with embryo and fetus. Provides ability to illustrate each month of pregnancy.

> Source: Armstrong Medical Industries, Inc.

Expectancy Vest (simulated teaching model)

A weighted garment that when worn will enable the wearer to experience temporarily more than 20 of the typical symptoms and effects of pregnancy.

> Source: Birthways Childbirth Resource Center, Inc

Maternity Game (Game)

A board game that reviews care for a client through prenatal, labor and delivery, and postnatal periods. Players devise assessment data and formulate nursing diagnoses, goals/interventions, and teaching strategies. For 3 to 6 players or teams.

> Source: Nasca Health Care

Discussion Questions

1. Mrs. Rodriquez has the following pregnancy history: an induced abortion, a boy born at term, a girl born at term, a spontaneous abortion, and an infant born at 32 weeks. What is her TPAL classification?

2. It is important to encourage support people to accompany women to prenatal visits. What are measures you would use to make these people feel welcome in a prenatal setting?

3. Women generally enjoy the feeling of control that comes with being an active participant in health care. What are some activities that you could initiate in a prenatal setting to encourage women to participate in their own care?

Written Assignments

1. Most women voice that they do not enjoy having pelvic examinations done at health assessments. List measures that can be used to make these exams better tolerated by women.

2. An important teaching point at prenatal visits is to inform women about the danger signs of pregnancy. List these and the importance of the finding.

3. The time clients spend in prenatal settings waiting for health personnel can be enriched if audio-visual materials are available. Design a poster that explains some aspect of pregnancy care that would be appropriate for your care setting. Be certain to consider the educational level of the women attending the care setting.

Laboratory Experiences

1. Provide students with simulated urine that tests positive for sugar and protein or blood and ask them to practice testing the specimens. Ask them to state whether they would report the finding as abnormal for pregnancy or not. Create simulated urine by boiling weak tea; add gelatin powder as a source of protein, karo syrup for sugar, vinegar for ketones.

2. Assign students to a prenatal setting so students have the opportunity to interview clients for an initial prenatal history.

3. Ask a pregnant woman to come to a postconference and discuss her expectations of prenatal care. How could health care personnel be most helpful to her?

Care Study: A Pregnant Woman at a First Prenatal Visit

Andrea Newman comes to an obstetrician's office because she has completed a home-test assessment and is certain she is pregnant. Mrs. Newman has been married for $6\frac{1}{2}$ years; she has a $3\frac{1}{2}$- and a $4\frac{1}{2}$-year-old child at home. She works as the owner of a craft store; her husband works as a stock broker.

Health History

- Chief Concern: "I think I'm pregnant."

- History of Present Illness: Present pregnancy was planned. Couple was attending a fertility clinic because they had not been using a contraceptive for $2\frac{1}{2}$ years and could not seem to conceive. Husband's sperm count was found to be subnormal. Couple was advised to space coitus further apart (no closer than 1 X week). Pregnancy occurred after 4th month of new regimen.

- History of Past Illnesses: Appendectomy at age 16. "Bad" adolescent acne treated with tetracycline during adolescence; no major illnesses, hospitalizations except for previous childbirths.

- Family Medical History: Husband's father has hypertension; a mother's cousin has renal failure.

- Personal/Social: Is independently employed as she owns a craft shop. Admits to long hours of standing to meet needs of customers; Drinks 6 cups of coffee daily; no alcohol since she thought she might be pregnant; does not smoke. Takes no medication except for occasional acetaminophen for headache. Walks a city block daily from bus to store. Twenty-four hour recall nutrition history reveals a diet seemingly low in protein and possibly iron.

- Gynecologic History: Menarche at 13 years; cycle 30—32 days, duration of flow, 7 days. Has "terrible" dysmenorrhea she treats with Motrin. Last menstrual period: 6 weeks ago. Papanicolaou smear negative as of 6 months ago.

- Obstetric History: G4P2. Therapeutic abortion at age 18. Male born 4 years ago, vertex presentation, alive and well. Male, born 3 years ago, vertex presentation; alive and well. Membranes were ruptured longer than 24 hours and labor was induced. Andrea had a mild endometritis treated with intravenous antibiotics for four days following birth. Feels this was the reason for her infertility.

- Review of Systems: negative except for urinary tract infection 6 years ago following marriage.

Physical Examination

- General Appearance: Mildly overweight, pleasant-appearing Caucasian woman; Height: 5'6" Weight: 138 pounds

- HEENT: Normocephalic; slight bleeding at gumlines. Conjunctiva of eyelids appear pale.

- Chest: Normal breast development; areola darkened; occasional veins present. Lungs clear to auscultation; heart sounds normal and at 76/minute; blood pressure 130/80.

- Abdomen: Soft, no masses; uterus not palpable; suggestion of linea nigra present.

- Extremities: Mild varicose vein on medial aspect of left leg; full range of motion in all joints; deep tendon reflexes 2+.

- Pelvic Exam: Vagina and cervix deep purple in color; uterus slightly enlarged; Hegar's sign present.

Laboratory Reports

- Hemoglobin: 10 mg/dL

- Hematocrit: 39%

- Urinalysis: Negative for protein, glucose, and ketones.

Care Study Questions

1. Andrea has some risk factors for herself during her pregnancy. What precautions does she need to take to reduce the possibility of varicose veins? Will it be easy for her to get adequate rest during pregnancy?

2. Andrea's nutrition is less than adequate and her hemoglobin is 10 mg/dL. What suggestions would you make to help her increase her protein intake? Her overall nutrition?

3. Complete a nursing care plan that will identify and meet the needs of the Newman family.

Promoting Fetal and Maternal Health

Chapter 11 discusses ways to promote fetal and maternal health during pregnancy. The chapter begins with an overview of nursing process specific to the maintenance of fetal and maternal health. Self care needs, precautions necessary to take in work settings, common discomforts of pregnancy, prevention of complications of pregnancy, signs of beginning labor, and prevention of fetal exposure to teratogens are discussed. Emphasis is placed on making the woman a knowledgeable participant in her care through health teaching and guidance.

Chapter Objectives

After mastering the contents of this chapter, students should be able to:

1. Describe health practices important for a positive pregnancy outcome.
2. Assess a woman during pregnancy for health practices and concerns.
3. Formulate nursing diagnoses related to health promotion during pregnancy.
4. Plan pregnancy health promotion measures such as ways to limit exposure to teratogens or reduce the minor symptoms of pregnancy.
5. Implement care to promote positive health practices during pregnancy.
6. Evaluate outcome criteria related to health promotion goals to be certain that goals of care were achieved.
7. Identify national health goals related to pregnancy care that nurses can help the nation to achieve.
8. Identify areas of prenatal care that could benefit from additional nursing research.
9. Use critical thinking to analyze ways that prenatal care can be made individualized and more family centered to achieve maximum effectiveness.

10. Synthesize knowledge of health promotion measures with the nursing process to achieve quality maternal and child health nursing care.

Key Points

- Women need discussion periods during pregnancy on such topics as bathing, sexual activity, sleep, and exercise.
- Women who work outside of their homes need to make provisions for rest periods during their day and to be aware of any potential teratogens at their work site such as radiation or heavy metals. Women who travel should plan for break periods to avoid congestion in their lower extremities and to be certain to use seatbelts.
- Discomforts of early pregnancy that women may notice are breast tenderness, constipation, palmar erythema, nausea and vomiting, fatigue, muscle cramps, pain from varicosities or hemorrhoids, heart palpitations, frequency of urination, pruritus, and leukorrhea. If women know that these symptoms occur they will not interpret them as complications of pregnancy.
- Minor discomforts of middle or late pregnancy may include backache, dyspnea, ankle edema, and uterine contractions.
- The more women know about monitoring their own health, the more likely they will enter a pregnancy in good health. This makes intrapartal or prepregnancy counseling as important as counseling during pregnancy.
- The more women know about measures they should take during pregnancy to safeguard their health, the more likely they will avoid substances or activities harmful to fetal growth. This makes prenatal education an important part of prenatal care.
- Teaching women those signs or symptoms that indicate a complication of pregnancy allows them to monitor their own health and alert health care providers at the first instance of danger.
- Danger signs that women should be aware of are vaginal bleeding, persistent vomiting, chills and fever, sudden escape of fluid from the vagina, abdominal or chest pain, and signs of pregnancy-induced hypertension such as swelling of the face or fingers, flashes of light, blurring of vision, or continuous headache.
- Beginning signs of labor that women should be made aware of are lightening, show, rupture of membranes, and uterine contractions.

- Women need to be made aware of the danger to the fetus during pregnancy of infectious diseases such as rubella, HIV, cytomegalovirus, herpes genitalis, syphilis, Lyme disease, and toxoplasmosis and how to avoid these illnesses.

- All women should also be counseled about the necessity to avoid recreational drug use, alcohol, and cigarettes during pregnancy.

- Women enter pregnancy with a wide variety of knowledge about good pregnancy care. Assess each woman individually to establish how much education is necessary.

- Urge women to find the best way for them to modify their lifestyle for pregnancy. Pregnancy is 9 months long, so modifications must be agreeable to the woman or she will not maintain them over this long a time span.

- It is almost impossible for a woman to modify a lifestyle, such as stopping smoking, if her support person does not agree to the change (and usually change also). Including the family in care is an important way of helping support persons understand the necessity for the modification and increase cooperation.

Definitions of Key Terms

Braxton Hicks contractions: painless, erratic uterine contractions that occur toward the end of pregnancy to ready the cervix for labor

cytomegalovirus: an organism representing a large, herpestype virus that causes serious neurological illnesses in newborns

fetal alcohol syndrome: a syndrome marked by growth retardation, mental deficiencies, and facial, cardiac, and joint anomalies caused by the mother's consumption of alcohol during pregnancy

leukorrhea: a whitish vaginal discharge

organogenesis period: the period of fetal life during which the major organs are forming; the 5th to 8th weeks

Sims' position: a resting position with the mother lying on her side, tipped slightly forward so the weight of the fetus rests on the bed surface

teratogen: an agent capable of causing harm to a fetus

teratogenicity: the state of causing fetal harm

toxoplasmosis: an infection caused by a protozoan parasite and characterized by severe liver and brain involvement in the newborn; spread commonly by cat feces

Nursing Process Overview

The Nursing Process Overview in this chapter concentrates on encouraging the student to make parents active participants in their prenatal care, not only so they can learn optimally about the pregnancy, but to help strengthen the family unit. The importance of helping women to avoid teratogens is stressed. The importance of modeling a healthy lifestyle such as not smoking is included.

Study Aids

Boxes

Box 11-1:   Guidelines for Exercise in Pregnancy

Box 11-2:   Employment Rights of Pregnant Women

Box 11-3:   Kegel Exercises

Tables

Table 11-1:   Common Discomforts of Pregnancy

Table 11-2:   Embryologic Abnormalities by Time in Ovulation Weeks

Table 11-2:   Pregnancy Risk Categories of Drugs

Table 11-3:   Some Potentially or Positively Teratogenic Drugs

Table 11-4:   Selected Real or Suspected Chemical Hazards to Reproductive Health and Where They May Be Found in the Workplace

Displays

Focus on National Health Goals

Focus on Family Teaching

Focus on Nursing Research

Focus on Cultural Awareness

Critical Thinking Exercises

1. Jackie is a 19-year-old college student you care for in a prenatal clinic. She is unmarried and lives in a college dormitory. She admits she has not been taking her prenatal vitamins and describes a day to you that involves long periods of sitting with almost no exercise.

   a.   What would be some recommendations you could make to help Jackie increase her exercise level?

   b.   What suggestions could you make to improve her medication compliance?

   c.   Jackie mentioned no support person that she relies on for advice during pregnancy. Would you make any recommendations for who she might consult on a college campus?

2. Mel and Harriet are a young couple you see in an obstetrician's office. They report that Harriet's pregnancy has been "terrible—one ache or pain or problem after another." Harriet's record shows that the only symptoms she reported to the doctor were mild nausea, some constipation, and occasional backache that he considered all within normal parameters. Why do you think this discrepancy in the perceived seriousness of Harriet's concerns has occurred? Are there measures that could have been employed to make Harriet's pregnancy a better experience for her?

Media Resources

Mrs. Kathy Shaw: Antenatal Care for a Primigravida Client (45—60 minute CAI)

Clinical simulation designed to develop decision-making abilities for the antenatal client through realistic nurse-client interactions.

Source: J.B. Lippincott Company

Pregnancy: Antepartum (30 minute CAI)

Maternity simulation designed to build decision-making and problem-solving skills while interacting with a prepartal client.

Source: MediSim

Prenatal Care (12 minute video)

A video for client education in early pregnancy describing the events of prenatal visits and discussing concerns and body changes of pregnancy.

Source: Polymorph Films

Discussion Questions

1. Pregnant women usually have many questions on self care. What advice would you give them in relation to bathing? Clothing? Exercise?

2. Couples may have to modify sexual relations during pregnancy. What suggestions you would make in this area?

3. A woman at a first pregnancy visit tells you that she must catch a bus and can spend only 15 minutes. What counseling information would be most important to offer her as priority information? How would this differ from a 34th week visit?

Written Assignments

1. As many as 90 percent of women work at least part-time today. List the actions in terms of rest or nutrition that a working woman should take to help ensure a safe pregnancy.

2. Most women are able to discuss some areas of their health more easily than others. What areas of pregnancy health care would you be certain to ask about because they are often difficult for a woman to broach spontaneously?

3. Design a "pregnancy game" or flash cards similar to those described under Media Resources, including those items most pertinent to women in your practice setting or local community. Play it in the waiting room of a prenatal setting both to assess women's needs and educate regarding prenatal care.

Laboratory Experiences

1. Using a learning aid such as the Expectancy Vest ask students to describe what symptoms they experience. Have them elaborate on what would be their first thought to relieve such a symptom and compare this with established pregnancy care recommendations.

2. Using charts or slides that show physiologic changes during pregnancy, ask students to determine which month of pregnancy is being illustrated. Give a prize for the most correct answers.

3. Assign students to prenatal settings so they can participate in care of women during pregnancy. Stress that maintaining a welcoming tone in a prenatal setting is critically important to encouraging women to come for care.

Care Study: A Woman With Midpregnancy Concerns

Juanita Harper is a 26-year-old woman who comes to a prenatal clinic for care. She works as an executive secretary for a major corporation in the inner city. Her husband, Jose, 30 years old, works as a carpenter. This is Juanita's first pregnancy. She is 28 weeks pregnant.

Health History

- Chief Concern: "Tired and my back aches."

- History of Present Illness: Tiredness has been present from early pregnancy. Back ache has been noticeable over the last week. Pain is sharp and mostly on right side, noticed most at end of day.

- Past Medical History: Had mumps at 8 years; rheumatic fever at 12 years; no residual heart disease; appendectomy at 16 years.

- Gynecologic History: Menarche at 11 years; cycle of 28 days; duration of flow 5 days, moderately heavy. Slight dysmenorrhea. No sexually transmitted diseases. Was using a diaphragm and foam as contraceptive measure before pregnancy.

- Obstetric History: No previous pregnancies. This pregnancy was planned.

- Family Medical History: Father died at age 43 of arteriosclerotic heart disease; paternal grandmother has mature onset diabetes mellitus.

- Personal/Social: Works a 40 hour week; job consists of sitting at desk for long stretches or else filing for long stretches. Fair degree of stress as she is secretary to two people who compete for her time. Does not smoke; has taken no alcohol since pregnancy began; no teratogenic exposure at work she is aware of. Exercise is limited to occasional walks on Saturday or Sunday.

  Client lives with husband in a one-bedroom apartment. Describes finances as "adequate." Has begun to prepare a section of the bedroom for the baby. Unwilling to move because of the price of a bigger apartment and because present one is close to mother's house. Plans to return to work following birth; a sister will care for baby during the day.

- Nutrition: 24-hour recall:

  Breakfast: 1 cup coffee (decaffeinated) with cream; 2 slices toast; 1 glass orange juice; prenatal vitamin

  Lunch: 1 cup fat-free yogurt; small green salad

  Snack: 1 dish ice cream; 1 glass cola (caffeine free)

  Dinner: 1 bowl onion soup; a serving vegetable lasagna, 1 serving green peas; 1 slice bread.

  Snack: 1 piece apple pie; 1 glass skim milk

- Review of Systems: Head: occasional headache if she works too long at a computer; Eyes: no blurring of vision; GI: has noticed "heartburn" off and on during pregnancy; some tendency toward constipation during pregnancy. Genitourinary: slight discomfort on voiding for last three days; no vaginal discharge. Blood type: A positive. Has never had a transfusion.

Physical Examination

- General Appearance: Well-dressed, alert young adult woman.

- Height: 5' 2''; Weight: 125 (15 lb gain in pregnancy); Blood pressure: 114/74.

- HEENT: Normocephalic; red reflex; reads fine print without difficulty; hearing adequate for normal conversation. Nose: mucous membrane slightly swollen but not reddened; No palpable lymph nodes present.

- Chest: Areolae of breasts enlarged; colostrum present on nipples. Numerous veins distinguishable. Lung sounds clear to auscultation. Occasional systolic heart murmur present; heart rate: 78/minute.

- Abdomen: Linea nigra and numerous striae present. Fundal height: 22 cm; fetal movements palpated; FHR = 178/minute.

- Back: Area tender over right kidney; no tenderness at spinal column.

- Extremities: Slight varicosity formation on medial surface of right leg; occasional spider angiomas.

- Rectum: Slight internal hemorrhoids present.

Laboratory Reports

- Hemoglobin: 10.5 g/dL

- Hematocrit: 36%

- Urinalysis by reagent strip: pH: 9; protein, trace; glucose: trace; ketones: negative; blood: +2.

Care Study Questions

1. Juanita is reporting symptoms suggestive of a pyelonephritis. What findings on physical examination support this?

2. Is Juanita's lifestyle ideal for pregnancy? Could she benefit from more exercise? Better prevention measures to prevent varicosities? Is her nutrition adequate?

3. Complete a nursing care plan that will identify and meet the needs of the Harper family.

Promoting Nutritional Health During Pregnancy

Chapter 12 discusses ways to promote nutritional health during pregnancy. The relationship of maternal diet to infant health, the constituents of a healthful pregnancy diet, and assessment techniques to obtain an accurate nutrition history are discussed. The necessity of avoiding foods such as excess caffeine and alcohol are stressed. Interventions for common problems with nutrition such as nausea and vomiting, constipation, and pyrosis are included. Care of women who are categorized as high risk because of faulty nutrition patterns such as the woman who is under or over weight are included.

Most students have knowledge of what is a good nutritional intake from previous course work. Their most important task, therefore, is to adapt that knowledge to pregnancy counseling. Some students need to obtain a client's poor nutrition history before they can appreciate that not everyone knows as much as they do about good nutrition and that counseling in this area is needed.

Chapter Objectives

After mastering the contents of this chapter, students should be able to

1. Describe the requirements of healthy pregnancy nutrition.
2. Assess a woman's nutritional intake during pregnancy.
3. Formulate nursing diagnoses related to nutritional concerns during pregnancy.
4. Plan health teaching for nutritional intake during pregnancy, including ways a woman can increase her iron and calcium intake.
5. Implement nursing care that encourages healthy nutritional practices during pregnancy such as eating a high protein diet.
6. Evaluate outcome criteria related to nutritional care goals to be certain that goals were achieved.

7. Identify national health goals related to nutrition and pregnancy that nurses can be instrumental in helping the nation achieve.
8. Identify areas related to nutrition and pregnancy that could benefit from additional nursing research.
9. Use critical thinking to analyze the effects of different life situations on nutrition patterns and ways nutritional health can be improved.
10. Synthesize nutrition knowledge with nursing process to achieve quality maternal and child health nursing care.

Key Points

- The old saying that a pregnant woman must eat for two is not a myth; women must add additional calories, protein, and certain vitamins during pregnancy to help ensure fetal growth.
- Nutrition during pregnancy should be high in calories to provide for protein sparing and high in protein for fetal growth.
- Important minerals necessary for pregnancy are iron, iodine, calcium, fluoride, and sodium. Most women need to take an iron supplement to supply enough of this mineral to prevent iron deficiency anemia.
- Women should work to reduce caffeine and artificial sweeteners during pregnancy.
- Assessment of nutritional health consists of a health history (24-hour recall) as well as physical examination.
- Women who are at high risk for nutritional problems are those who are adolescent or over age 35; have decreased nutritional stores, multiple pregnancy, or lactose intolerance; are underweight, overweight, or on a special diet; use drugs including alcohol or cigarettes; or have hyperemesis gravidarum.
- Hyperemesis gravidarum is nausea and vomiting of pregnancy that extends past 16 weeks of pregnancy or is too extreme to allow for adequate nutrition. Women with this may need nutrition supplemented by total parenteral nutrition or enteral feedings.
- Common nutritional concerns associated with pregnancy are nausea and vomiting, constipation, cravings (pica), pyrosis, and cholelithiasis.
- Advise women during pregnancy not to go longer than 12 hours between meals to avoid hypoglycemia.
- Pregnancy vitamins contain additional folic acid supplements so should be used instead of regular vitamins during pregnancy. Adequate folic acid in the diet pre-

vents megaloblastic anemia and possibly birth defects. Be certain women regard vitamins as medication and follow the medication rule concerning them: take none besides that recommended by their primary care provider.

Definitions of Key Terms

body mass index: weight (in kg) divided by height (in meters^2)

complete protein: protein that contains all essential amino acids necessary for cell growth

Hawthorne effect: the phenomenon that people behave differently when they know they are being observed

hypercholesterolemia: elevated cholesterol levels in serum

hyperplasia: an increase in the number of cells

hypertrophy:: an increase in the size of body cells

incomplete protein: protein that does not contain all the essential amino acids

lactase: the enzyme that breaks down lactose

obesity: a body weight over 200 lbs or 50% above ideal body weight

overweight: a weight greater than 20% above ideal weight or a body mass index over 26.1

pica: the indiscriminate eating of nonfood substances

pyrosis: heartburn

underweight: the state of being 10 to 20% less than ideal weight

Nursing Process Overview

The Nursing Process Overview in this chapter concentrates on helping students identify other nursing diagnoses than the obvious one of "altered nutrition." Suggestions for securing dietary recall histories are given. The importance of ongoing evaluation to be certain an improved diet is maintained for 9 months is stressed.

Study Aids

Tables

Table 12-1: Recommended Daily Dietary Allowances for Pregnant and Nonpregnant Women

Table 12-2: Quantities of Food Necessary During Pregnancy

Table 12-3: Nutritional Risk Factors During Pregnancy

Table 12-4: Areas to be Assessed for a Total Nutrition History

Table 12-5: Physical Signs and Symptoms of Adequate Pregnancy Nutrition

Displays

Focus on National Health Goals

Focus on Family Teaching

Focus on Nursing Research

Focus on Cultural Awareness

Critical Thinking Exercises

1. Mary is a 30-year-old woman who is 2 months pregnant. She works as a cashier at a supermarket from 6 AM to 2 PM daily. She states she is too nauseated in the morning to eat before she leaves for work; she is too tired of seeing food go by her to prepare a good meal after work. What suggestions could you make to Mary to help her increase her food intake?

2. Anita is a 21-year-old who rarely eats vegetables. When she does she fries them in butter. How would you use a food pyramid to explain better pregnancy nutrition to Anita?

3. Chris is a 19-year-old college student. The food plan she subscribes to provides for only lunch and dinner and these must be obtained from the college cafeteria. What suggestions could you make to Chris to be certain she obtains adequate nutrition during a pregnancy?

Media Resources

Nutrition During Pregnancy for Mother and Child (20 minute filmstrip, slide/tape, video)

The basics of good nutrition are outlined. Food groups and methods of selecting, storing, and preparing foods are discussed. Various common cultural/ethnic diet patterns are included.

Source: Career Aids, Inc.

Pregnancy and Nutrition (12 minute film, video)

A presentation intended for client education. Basic proper nutrition before and during pregnancy; common discomforts associated with pregnancy; negative effects of sugar, nicotine, alcohol, and caffeine; and positive effects of exercise are explained. Available in Spanish.

Source: Polymorph Films, Inc.

Nutritional Assessment of the Pregnant Woman (CAI)

A case study that provides practice in the application of knowledge necessary to counsel a woman regarding nutrition during a normal pregnancy.

Source: Nasco Health Care Education Materials

Discussion Questions

1. Many women know little about nutrition planning even though they prepare all their family's meals. What nutrition planning would you want to discuss with a woman at the beginning of pregnancy? At the 28th week of pregnancy?

2. Using a list of recommended food allowances for pregnancy, form teams and have each team design a day's menus for pregnant women with varying circumstances such as one who packs a lunch, a homeless one with no stove, a vegetarian, or an adolescent. Elect a judge to decide which team's menus seem best.

3. Debate the basis for cravings during pregnancy. Would a hunger for oranges be considered a craving or only foods such as pickles and chocolate?

Written Assignments

1. Many women never drink milk. List ways you can encourage an adequate calcium intake under these circumstances.

2. Ingesting enough iron during pregnancy may be a major problem for women. List suggestions you would make to help a woman solve this problem.

3. Nausea and vomiting are universal symptoms of pregnancy. What are practical suggestions you would make to help a woman maintain adequate nutrition while this is present.

Laboratory Experiences

1. Assign students to a prenatal setting and have them show a film on nutrition during pregnancy to clients. Allow discussion following the presentation so misperceptions of nutrition can be corrected.

2. Assign students to a prenatal setting. Ask them to interview a client for a 24-hour nutrition recall history. Have the student compare the foods ingested to common food values from a nutrition text and calculate the adequacy of the diet. Asking the student to provide suggestions on how she or he would improve the client's nutrition helps to enlarge knowledge of nutrition counseling.

3. Ask students to interview clients in a prenatal setting about their cultural or ethnic beliefs about nutrition during pregnancy. Ask them to give possible rationales for the development of these practices and to evaluate whether there would be any advantage in changing the practice during pregnancy.

Care Study: A Pregnant Woman in Need of Nutritional Counseling

Maria Vallo is a 34-year-old woman having her fourth pregnancy. Her prepregnancy weight was 144; today at 12 weeks since her last menstrual period it is 156. Her hemoglobin is 11.5 g. Maria is an excellent cook and has won prizes at the county fair for her cakes and pies. She is a housewife; she cooks for a husband and three other children. Culture: Italian. Finances are adequate.

24 hour nutrition recall:

> Breakfast: 1 serv. oatmeal with milk and honey, 1 glass orange juice, 2 slices cinnamon toast with butter; pregnancy vitamin
>
> Snack: 4 peanut butter cookies and 1 glass milk.
>
> Lunch: 1 serv. tomato soup, 1 bacon and cheese sandwich; 2 pieces cherry pie, 1 glass lemonade.
>
> Dinner: 1 serv. spaghetti and meatballs, 1 serv. green salad, 2 slices bread and butter, 2 pieces carrot cake, 1 glass milk, 1 cup tea.
>
> Snack: 2 slices cinnamon toast, 2 oranges.

Care Study Questions

1. Maria has already gained 12 pounds in the period of pregnancy when most women gain 3 pounds. Assess her 24-hour recall history. Does her intake seem excessive? What suggestions would you want to make to her to modify her intake?

2. Many women who cook for others as well as themselves have difficulty modifying their intake during pregnancy because they have to change their family member's intake as well. What questions would you want to ask Maria to see if her family is overweight as well? Suppose other family members don't want to change? How could you help Maria change?

3. Complete a nursing care plan that would identify and meet the needs of the Vallo family.

Preparation for Childbirth and Parenting

*C*hapter 13 discusses various methods that couples can use to prepare for childbirth. The content of preparation classes, including exercises, methods to reduce pain, choice of birth settings, and advantages and disadvantages of different birth settings, is discussed. Preparation by the Lamaze psychoprophylactic method is stressed.

Most students are interested in learning more about preparation for childbirth as they anticipate using or supporting a person using these techniques in their future personal life as well as their professional one. As they care for women in labor and see these techniques being effectively used, the content becomes even more pertinent to them.

Chapter Objectives

After mastering the contents of this chapter, students should be able to:

1. Describe common alternative settings for birth and preparation necessary for childbirth and parenting.
2. Assess a couple for readiness for childbirth in regard to choice of birth attendant or setting.
3. Formulate nursing diagnoses related to preparation for childbirth.
4. Plan nursing care such as teaching exercises that are effective for strengthening muscles for childbirth.
5. Implement nursing care such as supporting a woman during labor by the Lamaze (psychoprophylactic) method of prepared childbirth or helping a couple select and prepare for an alternative birth setting such as the home.
6. Evaluate outcome criteria to be certain that goals of nursing care were achieved.
7. Identify national health goals related to preparation for parenthood that nurses could be instrumental in helping the nation to achieve.
8. Identify areas related to preparation for childbirth that could benefit from additional nursing research.

9. Use critical thinking to analyze ways that birth can be made more family centered through the use of expectant parent's prepared childbirth classes and alternative birth settings.
10. Synthesize the principles of prepared childbirth with nursing process to achieve quality maternal and child health nursing care.

Key Points

*   Couples should be encouraged to make a childbirth plan early in pregnancy including birth attendant and place for birth.
*   Common exercises taught in pregnancy to strengthen perineal muscles are tailor sitting, squatting, and Kegel exercises. Abdominal muscle contraction and pelvic rocking exercises strengthen abdominal muscles and relieve backache.
*   Types of childbirth preparation include the Bradley (husband coached), psychosexual (Kitzinger), and Dick-Read and Lamaze (psychoprophylactic) methods.
*   Commonly used techniques for pain relief in labor are conscious relaxation, consciously controlled breathing, effleurage, focusing, and imaging.
*   Expectant parents' classes provide information on pregnancy, birth, and child care.
*   Common sites for childbirth range from the hospital to alternative birthing centers and home.
*   The Leboyer method is a method of birth that stresses a quiet, calm atmosphere in order to avoid sudden shock to the newborn.

Definitions of Key Terms

alternative birthing center (ABC): a free-standing facility for birth which encourages active maternal and family participation in labor and birth

birthing bed: a bed designed for labor and birth

birthing chair: a chair designed for labor and birth in an upright position

birthing room: a room specially designed for labor and birth

cleansing breath: a deep breath taken at the beginning and end of breathing exercises to prevent hyperventilation

conditioned response: a response that occurs when a secondary stimulant is substituted for an original stimulant

consciously controlled breathing: deliberately paced breathing

conscious relaxation: the deliberate release of tension in muscle groups

cutaneous stimulation: massage of the skin to interfere with the transmission of painful sensations

distraction: focus on an alternate point or thought to block out an incoming sensation

effleurage: light massage

gating theory of pain perception: the theory that pain sensation can be interrupted from being interpreted as pain

labor-delivery-recovery-postpartum room: a room designed to accommodate a family during an entire birth experience hospital stay

Leboyer method: a method of birth that encourages subdued light and a welcoming bath for the baby at birth

psychoprophylaxis: the Lamaze technique of prepared childbirth

vaginal birth after cesarean birth (VBAC): a planned vaginal birth following a previous cesarean birth

Nursing Process Overview

The Nursing Process Overview in this chapter concentrates on helping students to view their role in childbirth preparation as one of informing parents about the options available to then and then allowing clients to make informed personal choices based on this knowledge. Addresses of resources to secure additional information for students or parents are given.

Study Aids

Boxes

Box 13-1: Safety Precautions for Exercises During Pregnancy

Box 13-2: Sample Content for Expectant Parents Class

Box 13-3: Advantages and Disadvantages of Hospital Birth

Box 13-4: Advantages and Disadvantages of ABCs

Box 13-5: Advantages and Disadvantages of Home Birth

Box 13-6: Supplies Necessary for a Home Delivery

Tables

Table 13-1: Supplies to Prepare for Labor

Displays

Focus on National Health Goals

Focus on Family Teaching

Focus on Nursing Research

Focus on Cultural Awareness

Critical Thinking Exercises

1. Avery is a 19-year-old expecting her first baby who states she does not intend to attend a preparation for labor class because she wants to have epidural anesthesia as soon as she is admitted to the hospital in labor. Would you advise her to attend a class or not?

2. You are working at a hospital where traditional labor and delivery rooms are available. You would like to see the hospital convert to a labor-delivery-recovery room pattern. How would you go about this? What are reasons that might make a hospital reluctant to let go of such a traditional pattern?

3. Bob and Rae are a couple having their third child. They ask you if they should allow their oldest child to view the birth. How would you advise them? What further information would you need to give informed advice?

Media Resources

Childbirth Preparation Program (52 minute video)

A two-segment program that includes training in techniques for muscle relaxation, massage, breathing, and visual imagery in part one. The second segment includes scenes from 14 actual labors and births.

Source: Feeling Fine ASPO/Lamaze

Gentle Birth (15 minute film, video)

"Nonviolent" (Leboyer) birth is depicted included scenes of the warm bath and breastfeeding at delivery.

Source: Polymorph Films, Inc.

Family Choices: Hospital Options (35 minute slide/script presentation)

Five births illustrate the opportunities for choices in selecting a birthing setting. VBAC and C-birth with sibling and grandmother sharing in the experience are included.

Source: Childbirth Graphics

Traditional Birthing: Maude Bryant (19 minute video)

Maude Bryant, retired midwife, reflects on her experiences at over 100 births in rural North Carolina. She discusses her procedure for preparing for a birth, the basic diet she suggests for expectant mothers, and herbal teas and salves she prepares.

Source: Health Sciences Consortium

The Joy of Natural Childbirth (60 minute video)

A program hosted by Lorenzo and Michele Lamas that examines personal experiences of childbirth with such people as Kenny Rogers, John Ritter, and Jane Seymour. Emphasis is placed on the Lamaze method. A Lamaze birth is shown.

Source: Cambridge Educational

Tender Loving Care: The Coach's Role in Labor and Delivery (26 minute video)

First-time parents are followed from their arrival at the hospital through the birth of their 8 lb, 9 oz girl. Important coaching variations are demonstrated. A live birthing experience and coaching model is offered.

Source: AJN Educational Services

Discussion Questions

1. Prepared childbirth was not well accepted by nurses in the United States at first. What are some reasons for this?

2. A coach in labor can easily feel unwelcome on a busy maternity service. What are definite ways you could make such a person feel welcome?

3. Preparation for parenthood classes vary depending on the individual people in attendance. What modifications would you make if a class was mostly teenage girls? Career women?

Written Assignments

1. Not all women are interested in taking preparation for childbirth classes. List the advantages of being prepared. Are there any disadvantages?

2. You are caring for a woman in labor who has had no preparation for labor. List some specific measures you could take to help her control the discomfort of labor in the light of no prior preparation.

3. Women today make informed choices about the setting for birth. List the advantages and disadvantages of the various settings. Include Leboyer birth and water births.

Laboratory Experiences

1. Assign students to attend a series of classes on preparation for parenthood. Insist they participate in doing exercises with class members to learn the techniques.

2. Assign students to women in labor who are well prepared and also those who are not so they can contrast the difference preparation makes.

3. Ask a woman who used a preparation method to come to a postconference and share her experiences with students. What surprised her during labor that she wasn't prepared for? How could health care personnel have been more helpful to her?

Care Study: Preparation of a Woman for Labor

Cheryl Burrows is a 15-year-old, having her first baby, who is taking a series of preparation for labor classes. Cheryl is not married and because the father of her child is not supportive, her sister, Debra, will support her in labor. Cheryl states she ''wants to learn everything there is to know about labor so I'll not have to take any medicine.''

Teresa Mollison is 28-year-old also having her first baby. Teresa is married and her husband would like to serve as a labor coach. Teresa states ''I don't mind practicing for natural childbirth but I can't stand pain. I know I'll need something besides breathing exercises during labor.''

Care Study Questions

1. Women differ a great deal in their response to preparation for labor. Which of the two women above do you anticipate will practice breathing exercises most?

2. Teresa sounds as if she believes accepting some medication during labor will completely rule out also using breathing exercises. Is this true? What if she has epidural anesthesia?

3. Complete nursing care plans that would identify and meet the differing needs of Cheryl and Teresa.

High-Risk Pregnancy: The Woman With a Preexisting or Newly Acquired Illness

Chapter 14 discusses the effect of a preexisting or newly acquired illness on pregnancy. Heart disease; the anemias; urinary and renal tract disorders; respiratory, rheumatic, gastrointestinal, neurologic, endocrine, and musculoskeletal disorders; cancer; sexually transmitted diseases including HIV infection; psychiatric illness; and trauma including battering are discussed. Cardiopulmonary resuscitation and chest thrust techniques to relieve choking for the pregnant woman are reviewed. The role of the nurse in assisting a family cope with the psychological stress of having a secondary illness superimposed on a pregnancy as well as the nurse's role in providing direct care is stressed. Students may not be able to care for pregnant women with these complications of pregnancy because clients with these disorders are cared for on high-risk care units, sometimes at distant sites from their primary care provider. It is important for students to be familiar with the disorders, however, because they add to a student's knowledge of general nursing care and help students understand the importance of assessing all woman during pregnancy for common findings such as blood pressure or proteinuria.

Chapter Objectives

After mastering the contents of this chapter, students should be able to:

1. Define high-risk pregnancy and identify factors that can make a pregnancy high risk.

2. Describe common illnesses such as heart disease, diabetes mellitus, or renal and blood disorders that can cause complications when they exist with pregnancy.

3. Assess the woman with an illness during pregnancy for changes occurring because of the pregnancy.

4. State nursing diagnoses related to the effect of a preexisting or newly acquired illness on pregnancy.

5. Plan interventions that will contribute to a safe pregnancy outcome when illness occurs with pregnancy (eg, planning ways a woman can secure more rest).

6. Implement a plan of care for the woman with an illness during pregnancy (eg, teaching insulin administration to a woman newly diagnosed with diabetes).

7. Evaluate outcome criteria to be certain nursing goals related to care for the high-risk pregnant woman have been achieved.

8. Identify national health goals related to complications of pregnancy and ways that nurses can be instrumental in helping the nation achieve these goals.

9. Identify areas related to illness and pregnancy that could benefit from additional nursing research.

10. Use critical thinking to analyze ways that nursing care can remain family centered when a preexisting or newly acquired illness develops.

11. Synthesize knowledge of high-risk pregnancy and nursing process to achieve quality maternal and child health nursing care.

Key Points

- A High-risk pregnancy is one in which some maternal or fetal factor, either psychological or physiologic, may result in the birth of a high-risk infant or in some way cause harm to the woman herself.

- Pregnancy is a stress to any family because it involves financial expenses plus changes in family roles. If a complication of pregnancy develops, this stress is almost automatically intensified. Families need support during this time to be able to cope with the increased burden.

- When women with a preexisting disease become pregnant, it is important that a thorough history and physical examination is done at their first prenatal visit to establish a baseline of information on their condition and vital signs such as blood pressure. Documentation of any medication being taken for a secondary condition is also necessary to protect against adverse drug interactions and the possibility of terogenic action on the fetus.

- Teaching is an important nursing concern because the woman with a preexisting illness must make modifications in her usual therapy to adjust to pregnancy. Pregnancy often stimulates women to learn more about their primary disease as well.

- Women who have a complication early in pregnancy may continue to worry about the health of their fetus all during pregnancy. They need to be assured (appropriately) that the episode was temporary and that with continued monitoring, the fetus should not suffer harm. After giving birth, they may need additional time to spend with their newborn to convince themselves that the infant is healthy so bonding can begin.

- Because blood volume increases by as much as 50% during pregnancy, cardiac function may become inadequate if cardivascular disease is present. Illnesses that cause difficulty can be either acquired disorders such as Kawasaki disease and rheumatic fever or congenital disorders such a mitral valve prolapse and coarctation of the aorta.

- Various forms of anemia can cause complications of pregnancy; iron deficiency, sickle cell, and folic acid deficiency are examples. All these anemias can result in fetal distress because of inadequate oxygen transport.

- Urinary tract disorders can lead to pregnancy complications because pregnancy increases the workload of the kidneys. Urinary tract infection and chronic renal disease are two disorders that may lead to early pregnancy loss.

- Acute nasopharyngitis, asthma, pneumonia, influenza, and tuberculosis are respiratory disorders seen in pregnancy. Because tuberculosis is on the increase, it needs special assessment and care.

- Juvenile rheumatoid arthritis and systemic lupus erythematosus are examples of rheumatic disorders seen in pregnancy. These disorders generally require large doses of salicylate and nonsteroidal antiinflammatory agents for therapy; women are usually advised to discontinue NSAID agents during pregnancy. They are advised to decrease use of salicylates 2 weeks before birth to avoid bleeding disorders in the newborn.

- Some gastrointestinal illnesses that occur with pregnancy are hiatal hernia, cholecystitis, viral hepatitis, inflammatory bowel disease, and appendicitis. If surgery is necessary for conditions such as cholecystitis or appendicitis, this can be scheduled during pregnancy but may result in preterm labor.

- Recurrent seizure is the most frequently seen neurologic condition during pregnancy. Many drugs used to control seizures are teratogenic; women need to have their medical reginmen evaluated prior to pregnancy to be certain that they are regulated on the lowest number of medications possible.

- The major endocrine disorder seen during pregnancy is diabetes mellitus. Gestational diabetes is diabetes that occurs during pregnancy and fades following it.

- Sexually transmitted diseases such as candidiasis, trichomoniasis, chlamydia, syphilis, herpes type 2, gonorrhea, papilloma, and HIV may occur during pregnancy. These illnesses   need prompt treatment when they occur. Women need to follow   safer sex practices to help prevent these diseases.

- Trauma in pregnancy includes automobile accidents and falls. Women with traumatic injuries need to be carefully assessed to determine if spouse abuse was the cause of the trauma.

Definitions of Key Terms

deep vein thrombosis: a clot in an underlying vein such as the ovarian

glucose tolerance test: a test of the body's ability to metabolize carbohydrate in reaction to a standardized dose of glucose

glycosuria: the presence of glucose in the urine

glycosylated hemoglobin: hemoglobin or hemoglobin with attached glucose

high-risk pregnancy: any pregnancy in which some maternal or fetal factor is apt to result in the birth of a high-risk infant or in some way harm the mother

hyperglycemia: a greater than normal amount of glucose in the blood

hypoglycemia: a lesser than normal amount of glucose in the blood

insulin pump therapy: the administration of insulin using a continuous subcutaneous infusion pump

iron deficiency anemia: a microcytic, hypochromic anemia caused by an inadequate supply of iron

megaloblastic anemia: a hematologic disorder characterized by the production of immature, nonfunctional, but large erythrocytes

orthopnea: the condition in which a person must sit upright in order to breathe comfortably

paroxysmal nocturnal dyspnea: sudden attacks of shortness of breath and tachycardia that awaken a person from sleep

peripartal cardiomyopathy: a unique form of heart disease that occurs only with pregnancy

proteinuria: protein in the urine

sexually transmitted disease: an illness spread by sexual relations

trauma: physical injury caused by a violent action

Nursing Process Overview

The Nursing Process Overview in this chapter concentrates on helping students to appreciate that a complication of pregnancy leads to a stressed state for an entire family, not just one woman. Realizing this, a student is better able to formulate nursing diagnoses that speak to the entire family or conceptualize the wide area of care necessary. Planning realistic goals in light of the woman's health needs and the restrictions placed on her by her health concern are stressed.

The importance of changing goals and outcome criteria as an illness improves or increases in severity is included. A reminder that all pregnancy outcomes will not be optimal should help students to keep their perspective on the importance of support should this occur.

Study Aids

Boxes

Box 14-1: Factors That Categorize a Pregnancy as High Risk

Box 14-2: Signs and Symptoms of Urinary Tract Infection

Tables

Table 14-1: Classification of Heart Disease

Table 14-2: Risks for Maternal Mortality by Various Heart Diseases

Table 14-3: Classification of Diabetes Mellitus

Table 14-4: Oral Glucose Tolerance Test Values

Table 14-5: Initial Assessments Following Trauma During Pregnancy

Table 14-6: CPR During Pregnancy

Displays

Focus on National Health Goals

Focus on Family Teaching

Focus on Nursing Research

Focus on Cultural Awareness

Critical Thinking Exercises

1. Mary G. is a 23-year-old you care for who has gestational diabetes. Mary is resistant to teaching about her condition because she knows that the condition is only temporary and will fade at the end of pregnancy. What type of teaching plan would you devise to help Mary learn in the face of this attitude?

2. In the past many women with heart disease were advised not to attempt pregnancy. What has changed to make this advice different in most instances today? What are the modifications an average woman with heart disease would have to make in her lifestyle if she were required to rest at least 4 hours every day? How difficult do you anticipate this is for the average woman?

3. One of the most devastating medical diagnoses today is that of acquired immune deficiency syndrome (HIV). How is this illness a threat to the newborn as well as the mother? What are the measures nurses can use to help prevent the spread of this disorder? Are there changes a prenatal clinic would have to make to care for an HIV positive woman?

Media Resources

Diabetes Mellitus in Pregnancy (slides/audiocassette)

A multispecialty approach to the prevention of perinatal mortality and morbidity associated with diabetes in pregnancy.

Source: ACOG Distribution Center

Diabetes in Pregnancy: Caring for the Childbearing Woman (30 minute video)

Current information on the nursing management of diabetes in pregnancy covering the antepartal period in detail. Included are an overview of the disease, adaptation during pregnancy, and proper antepartum management and nursing care.

Source: Polymorph Films

Gestational Diabetes: You Are in Charge! (20 minute video)

A pregnant woman talks about her experiences with gestational diabetes. Her visits with her obstetrician and dietitian serve as a reinforcement for other diabetic mothers that gestational diabetes is a controllable problem that will probably not affect their babies. Diet changes and blood testing procedures are discussed.

Source: Health Sciences Consortium

Management of Herpes Simplex in Pregnant Women and Neonates (58 minute video)

The increasing problems associated with herpes simplex virus (HSV) are discussed as they relate to the pregnant woman and the neonate. Appropriate diagnostic methodology and a detailed decision-making approach to case management is presented.

Source: Health Sciences Consortium

Perinatal AIDS: Infection Control for Hospital Personnel (17 minute video)

Which body fluids are most infectious, ways of identifying patients at high risk, and the appropriate infection control measures specific to prenatal, labor and delivery, postpartum, and nursery settings are shown. Nurses' fears are reviewed. An accompanying handout provides a summary of the content.

Source: Polymorph Films

The ABC's of STD's (20 minute video)

Basic information on STDs is offered in a nonthreatening manner and in simple language. The diseases, how they are transmitted, what are the symptoms, and what to do if someone thinks he or she has one are shown.

Source: Polymorph Films

Toxoplasmosis: A Hidden Epidemic (10 minute video)

A presentation of interviews with mothers who have children affected by toxoplasmosis. Characteristics of the disease and ways to avoid it are discussed.

Source: Health Sciences Consortium

Discussion Questions

1. Following trauma, pregnant women are afraid for both their own safety and fetal safety. What are ways to assure a woman that the fetus' health is not compromised?

2. A quiet, darkened setting should be provided for the woman with severe preeclampsia. What factors would you need to consider in order to arrange for this at your care setting?

3. Discovery of a hydatidiform mole is always perplexing for a woman. How would you explain the development of this and the care the woman must take during the following year?

Written Assignments

1. A woman with heart disease tells you that she is having trouble getting enough rest daily because of two small children she must care for. List suggestions you might make to her.

2. Because of the physiologic changes of pregnancy, pregnant women need special precautions following trauma. Write a paragraph detailing these precautions.

3. Both placenta previa and premature separation of the placenta occur as third trimester bleeding. What is the difference in presentations in terms of pain, vaginal bleeding, and timing?

Laboratory Experiences

1. If opportunities are available, assign students to care of clients with high-risk status. If such opportunities are not available, encouraging students to participate in physician rounds helps them appreciate the care of high-risk clients. Reviewing the chart of a high-risk client is another possibility. Use of a care study such as that shown below can help with nursing care planning.

2. Assign students to prenatal clinic settings where fetal assessment procedures such as nonstress testing can be observed. Ask students to report to the clinical group not only the procedure observed but the health problem of the mother that necessitated the test.

3. Collect fetal monitoring strips that are not being saved as part of the permanent record. Ask students to analyze them as to fetal well being. Discuss conditions in the mother such as diabetes mellitus that could lead to poor variability on a rhythm strip.

Care Study: A Woman With Early-Pregnancy Concerns

Connie Taylor is a 38-year old gravida 1, para 0 seen during the 12th week of pregnancy.

Health History

- Chief Concern: "I can't sleep at night I am so short of breath."

- History of Present Illness: Client entered pregnancy without any feeling of shortness of breath. Since 2 weeks ago, she has been extremely fatigued and has mild constant swelling in her ankles, a persistent cough, inability to walk upstairs without becoming breathless, and orthopnea so severe at night she cannot sleep without four pillows.

- Past Medical Illnesses: Had rheumatic fever at 8 years; was aware she had a mild mitral stenosis as a result of this. Took prophylactic penicillin until she was 18 years old. No other major illnesses; has never been hospitalized.

- Family Medical History: One aunt with breast cancer; an uncle with arteriosclerotic heart disease.

- Personal/Social: Client works in a department store as a clerk. States she has to continue working as her husband does not earn enough to continue to pay the mortgage on their house without her help. Husband works as a real estate salesman. Does not smoke; no alcohol ingestion since pregnant.

- Nutrition: 24-hour recall evidences adequate pregnancy diet. Is taking a prenatal vitamin daily.

- Gynecologic History: Menarche at 13 years; cycle duration, 30 days; flow duration, 6 days. Moderately heavy; mild dysmenorrhea.

  Became sexually active at 16; had therapy for gonorrhea shortly afterward. Has been using a vaginal sponge for 2 years of marriage.

- Obstetric History: No previous pregnancies. Present pregnancy was not planned but is wanted. Couple was planning on waiting 3 more months and then starting a family.

- Review of Symptoms: Negative except for symptoms of chief concern.

Physical Examination

- General Appearance: Extremely worried and tired appearing pregnant Caucasian woman. Height: 5'4''; Weight 180 lbs.; BP: 135/88.

- HEENT: Negative

- Chest: Prominent grade II diastolic murmur heard at left sternal margin; apical first heart sound is accentuated; second sound is split. Cardiac enlargement suggested by percussion. Rhonchi heard on lung auscultation; respiratory rate: 22/minute. Abdomen: Fundal height: 28 cm; linea nigra and striae present on abdomen; FHR at 158/min.

- Pelvic: Deferred

- Rectum: Two 1 cm hemorrhoids present; no bleeding

- Extremities: Edema 2+ present on both legs extending from feet to midcalf.

- Neurologic: Deep tendon reflexes 2+.

Laboratory Results

- Hemoglobin: 12 g/dL

- Hematocrit: 41%

- Urinalysis: Protein and glucose, negative.

Care Study Questions

1. Women with heart disease need to consult their internist before becoming pregnant to be certain that their heart

is as healthy as possible. Assuming Mrs. Taylor didn't do this, what measures should she have taken early in pregnancy to improve her heart function? Is her weight appropriate for her height? Was this an area she could have improved before pregnancy?

2. Mrs. Taylor states she has to work although this may be difficult for her to continue during pregnancy. Would it have been wiser for her to postpone this pregnancy until she was more financially stable? Would her age have influenced this decision?

3. Design a nursing care plan that will identify and meet the needs of the Taylor family.

High-Risk Pregnancy: The Woman Who Develops a Complication of Pregnancy

*C*hapter 15 discusses care of the woman who develops a complication of pregnancy. Bleeding during pregnancy, pregnancy-induced hypertension, multiple gestation, postmature pregnancy, hyperemesis gravidarum, pseudocyesis, Rh incompatibility, and fetal death are discussed. The nurse's role in supporting the woman and her family through a complication of pregnancy as well as immediate interventions for these situations are stressed.

Students are not apt to see a pregnant woman with a bleeding disorder of pregnancy except after the fact as these are emergency situations and managed immediately by experienced hospital personnel. It is important for students to appreciate the impact that bleeding can have on a pregnancy, however, so they can give accurate advice to women regarding bleeding in pregnancy. Appreciating the effect of Rh sensitization helps them to understand the importance of administering RHIG injections in the postpartum period; being aware of the effect of hyperemesis gravidarum helps them to understand the importance of assessing nutritional intake in pregnant women.

Chapter Objectives

After mastering the contents of this chapter, students should be able to:

1. Identify complications of pregnancy such as bleeding, premature rupture of membranes, postmature labor, and hypertension of pregnancy.
2. Assess the woman with a complication of pregnancy.

3. Formulate nursing diagnoses that address the needs of the woman with a complication of pregnancy as well as the needs of her family.
4. Plan nursing interventions that address both short-term and long-term goals and that allow the woman to feel a measure of control in her daily life.
5. Implement nursing actions specific to complications of pregnancy (eg, begin intravenous fluid, prepare for an emergency cesarean birth).
6. Evaluate outcome criteria to be certain that nursing goals established for care were achieved.
7. Identify national health goals related to complications of pregnancy and specific measures nurses can take to help the nation achieve these goals.
8. Identify areas of nursing care related to high-risk pregnancy that could benefit from additional nursing research.
9. Use critical thinking to analyze ways that nurses can help prevent complications of pregnancy through health teaching and risk assessment as well as keep nursing care family centered in the midst of a pregnancy complication.
10. Synthesize knowledge of complications of pregnancy with nursing process to achieve quality maternal and child health nursing care.

Key Points

- As the uterus is such a vascular organ during pregnancy, a major complication that can occur all during pregnancy is bleeding. First trimester causes of this are abortion (the spontaneous loss of a pregnancy) and ectopic pregnancy (pregnancy outside the uterus).
- The bleeding evident with bleeding disorders of pregnancy is not indicative of the actual amount of blood loss because a great deal of internal bleeding also occurs. As a rule, women with bleeding of pregnancy should be positioned flat on their left side to help improve placenta circulation.
- Vaginal bleeding during pregnancy is always serious until ruled otherwise as it has the potential to diminish the blood supply of both the mother and fetus.
- Spontaneous abortion is the loss of a pregnancy before viability of the fetus (20 to 24 weeks). The majority of these early pregnancy losses are attributed to chromosomal abnormality. Abortions are classified as threatened, inevitable, complete, incomplete, missed, or recurrent.

Women who have a spontaneous abortion at home should bring any tissue passed with them to the hospital for an analysis for gestational trophoblastic tissue.

- Ectopic pregnancy is pregnancy implantation outside the uterus, usually in a fallopian tube. If discovered before the tube ruptures, this can be treated with methotrexate. If not discovered early, it produces sharp lower quadrant pain at about 6 to 12 weeks as the tube ruptures. Surgery is removal or repair of the tube to halt bleeding.

- Common causes of bleeding in the second trimester are gestational trophoblastic disease (abnormal growth of trophoblastic tissue) and incompetent cervix (cervical dilatation before fetal maturity).

- An incompetent cervix is a cervix that dilates early in pregnancy before viability of the fetus. Sutures (cervical cerclage) can be placed to prevent the cervix from dilating prematurely in a second pregnancy.

- Common causes of third trimester bleeding are placenta previa (low implantation of the placenta) and premature separation of the placenta.

- Placenta previa is low implantation of the placenta so it crosses the cervical os. If not discovered before labor, cervical dilatation may cause the placenta to tear and result in extreme blood loss. Women who have symptoms of placenta previa (painless vaginal bleeding in the third trimester) should not have routine vaginal examinations to avoid tearing the low placenta.

- Premature separation of the placenta (abruptio placenta) usually occurs late in pregnancy and means the placenta has separated from the uterus before the fetus is born. This separation immediately cuts off blood supply to the fetus. Women over age 35, those with previous uterine surgery, and those who use cocaine are at highest risk for this. It is manifested by sudden sharp fundal pain, then a continuing dull pain and vaginal bleeding.

- Gestational trophoblastic disease is abnormal growth of the trophoblast tissue. If not discovered earlier by sonogram, bleeding will occur at about the 16th week of pregnancy. Women need close follow-up as this can lead to choriocarcinoma, a malignancy.

- Pregnancy-induced hypertension is a unique disorder that occurs with pregnancy. The three classical symptoms are hypertension, edema, and proteinuria. A sudden increase in weight (more than 1 lb per week) or facial or finger edema are the first symptoms a woman usually reports. It is categorized as preeclampsia or eclampsia. If mild (blood pressure not over 140/90), treatment is bedrest. If severe (BP over 160/110), bedrest plus administration of magnesium sulfate is necessary. If a convulsion occurs the condition is eclampsia. The mortality of the fetus is high following eclampsia. Helping prevent disease progress to this stage is an important nursing responsibility.

- The HELLP syndrome is a unique form of preeclampsia marked by hemolysis of red blood cells, elevated liver enzymes, and low platelet count.

- Multiple gestation puts an additional strain on a woman's physical resources and may lead to birth complications or immaturity of the infants. Helping a woman obtain adequate nutrition and rest during pregnancy are nursing responsibilities.

- Postterm pregnancy is pregnancy that extends beyond 42 weeks. As the placenta is a timed organ, the fetus may receive decreased nutrients postterm.

- Hydramnios is overproduction of amniotic fluid (above 2000 mL). This can lead to premature labor from ruptured membranes because of increased intrauterine pressure. Newborns must be assessed carefully to be certain a swallowing defect wasn't present to cause the hydramnios.

- Disseminated intravascular coagulation is a blood disorder that can occur with any degree of trauma. It can accompany premature separation of the placenta and pregnancy-induced hypertension. Blood coagulation is so extreme at one point in the circulatory system that clotting factors are used up and absent in the remainder of the system. Beginning symptoms of this are easy bruising, petechiae, and oozing from intravenous sites. A woman with DIC can bleed profusely. Therapy is treatment with heparin to stop the coagulation and free up clotting factors for systemic use.

- Rh incompatibility is a possibility when the woman is Rh negative and the fetus is Rh positive. When this happens, maternal antibodies form that can actually destroy fetal red blood cells leading to anemia, edema, and jaundice in the newborn. Being certain that women are screened for blood type early in pregnancy is a nursing responsibility.

Definitions of Key Terms

abortion: the expulsion of the products of conception before 20 weeks gestation or before an age of viability

abruptio placentae: a normally implanted placenta that separates prematurely (between the 20th week of gestation and birth of the infant)

cervical cerclage: a procedure in which a suture is placed in the uterine cervix to prevent it from dilating prematurely

cervical ripening: softening of the cervix prior to the onset of labor

complete abortion: the expulsion of all the products of conception before 20 weeks gestation or before an age of viability

Couvelaire uterus: board-like rigidity and discoloration of the uterus due to accumulation of blood in the myometrium from hemorrhage into the muscle wall; can occur with premature separation of the placenta

eclampsia: severe pregnancy-induced hypertension after the point a woman has convulsed

ectopic pregnancy: a pregnancy implanted outside the uterine cavity; generally located in a fallopian tube

erythroblastosis fetalis: hemolytic disease of the newborn caused by isoimmunization resulting from Rh or ABO incompatibility.

gestational trophoblastic disease: abnormal growth or proliferation of the trophoblast cells; no fetus forms and clear, fluid-filled, grape-like vesicles form in place of the placenta

HELLP syndrome: a condition characterized by hemolysis, elevated liver enzymes, and a low platelet count

hemolytic disease of the newborn: erythroblastosis fetalis; anemia caused by an incompatibility between mother and fetus

hydatidiform mole: gestational trophoblastic disease

hydramnios: an excessive amount of amniotic fluid (generally over 2000 mL)

hyperemesis gravidarum: extreme vomiting during pregnancy or vomiting beyond the first trimester of pregnancy

imminent abortion: a situation where irreversible uterine evacuation has begun; the internal cervical os is dilated. At this point the pregnancy will inevitably be lost.

incompetent cervix: a defect of the cervix that makes it unable to remain closed through pregnancy; premature delivery occurs at about 20 weeks

incomplete abortion: an abortion in which not all of the products of conception are expelled. Further therapy is necessary to halt potential hemorrhage

isoimmunization: the development of antibodies against antigens from the same species such as the development of anti-Rh antibodies

missed abortion: a fetal death in which the products of conception have not yet been expelled

placenta previa: a placenta that is implanted in the lower uterine segment so that it touches or covers the internal os of the cervix

postterm pregnancy: a pregnancy that extends beyond 42 weeks

preeclampsia: a former name for pregnancy-induced hypertension

premature separation of the placenta: abruptio placentae.

pseudocyesis: a psychological condition in which a woman believes she is pregnant when she is not

Rh incompatibility: sensitization to the Rh antigen by an Rh-negative woman; antibodies produced by the woman destroy the red blood cells of an Rh-positive fetus

spontaneous abortion: the expulsion of the products of conception before 20 weeks gestation or an age of viability; a "miscarriage"

threatened abortion: unexplained vaginal bleeding but without cramping or cervical os dilatation

Nursing Process Overview

The Nursing Process Overview for this chapter concentrates on helping the student identify when a woman is developing a complication of pregnancy and the immediate measures to take at this time. The necessity for establishing nursing diagnoses that meet immediate needs and the necessity to modify them later as the woman's condition changes

are both included. Suggestions for including nursing diagnoses that represent the mother's psychological state, ie, "fear" or "anxiety," should help the student consider the effect of the complication in pregnancy on the entire family.

Study Aids

Boxes

Box 15-1: Drugs Used in Pregnancy-Induced Hypertension

Box 15-2: Eliciting a Patellar Reflex and Ankle Clonus

Tables

Table 15-1: Summary of Causes of Bleeding During Pregnancy

Table 15-2: Signs and Symptoms of Hypovolemic Shock

Table 15-3: Emergency Implementations for Bleeding in Pregnancy

Table 15-4: Immediate Assessment of Vaginal Bleeding During Pregnancy

Table 15-5: Premature Separation of the Placenta: Degrees of Separation

Table 15-6: Symptoms of Pregnancy-Induced Hypertension

Table 15-7: Effects of Increasing Magnesium Sulfate Serum Levels

Displays

Focus on National Health Goals

Focus on Family Teaching

Focus on Nursing Research

Focus on Cultural Awareness

Critical Thinking Exercises

1. Mrs. Graver is a 30-year-old G_1P_0 admitted to the labor service with a probable diagnosis of placenta previa. Everyone else on the unit is at lunch so you are alone. You know you shouldn't do a pelvic exam with a placenta previa. How would you estimate her amount of blood loss? How would you determine that the blood loss wasn't affecting the fetus?

2. Alu Wu is a college student who has just been diagnosed as having gestational trophoblastic disease. She tells you she thinks the sonogram she had in early pregnancy caused this. How would you explain gestational trophoblastic disease to her? Was the sonogram responsible for this?

3. Berta is a 30-year-old woman with signs of pregnancy-induced hypertension. Her doctor asks you to explain the necessity for bedrest to her as she insists that she has to continue her job as a lawyer or she will be passed over for promotion to a full partner in her firm. How would you explain this to her? If Berta is prescribed bedrest, what suggestions would you give her so she could achieve this? Does Berta have an ethical obligation to rest? What about a legal obligation?

4. Jessica is a 25-year-old who is pregnant for the second time. A first pregnancy ended in an early spontaneous

abortion 2 years ago. Because she felt well following the abortion, she didn't see a health care provider at the time. You realize looking at Jessica's prenatal record that she is Rh negative. Is she high risk for Rh incompatibility with this pregnancy?

Media Resources

Nursing Interventions for the Client With Pregnancy Induced Hypertension (30-45 minute CAI)

A simulated case study of Ann, a 20-year-old primigravida with hypertension of pregnancy. The student is asked to apply problem-solving techniques as well as knowledge of the manifestations of PIH and related therapies.

Source: J.B. Lippincott Company

Nursing Interventions for the Client With Abruptio Placentae (30 minute CAI)

By means of a simulated case study of Joy, a 37-year-old multipara client, the student is asked to apply problem-solving techniques as well as knowledge of the manifestations of the condition and related therapies.

Source : J.B. Lippincott Company

What Is Preterm Labor?

A presentation of the characteristics of women who are at greater risk of preterm labor than usual, physical signs that indicate preterm labor, steps that can be taken to prevent preterm labor, and common myths about preterm labor are included.

Source: Health Sciences Consortium

Understanding Preterm Labor (17 minute video)

The major risk factors are identified and early warning signs and symptoms of preterm labor are explained. Uterine contractions and cervical changes are illustrated. Tocolytics and bedrest treatments are discussed. Early detection and open communication with health care professionals are stressed.

Source: Polymorph Films

Nursing Management of Hypertension of Pregnancy (28 minute video)

The possible causes of hypertension, how to screen patients at risk, and how to recognize the condition at the onset are explained. Included are the importance of family education, emotional support, rest, and therapy. Steps to prevent and treat seizures, indications for immediate delivery, and possible complications in the newborn are stressed.

Source: AJN Educational Services

Dating the Pregnancy: Some Consequences of Post Maturity (15 minute video)

The characteristics and stages of postmaturity are discussed. Causes of mortality and morbidity and theories relating to the evaluation of gestational age with emphasis on the use of ultrasound are presented.

Source: Health Sciences Consortium

Discussion Questions

1. A quiet, darkened setting should be provided for the woman with severe preeclampsia. What factors would you need to consider in order to arrange for this on a hospital unit?

2. Discovery of a hydatidiform mole is always perplexing for a woman. How would you explain the development of this and the care the woman must take during the following year?

3. Discuss the problem of Rh incompatibility. What factors are necessary to cause incompatibility? What are the preventive measures that should be taken?

Written Assignments

1. Both placenta previa and premature separation of the placenta present as third trimester bleeding. List how these two happenings can be differentiated in terms of pain, vaginal bleeding, and timing of occurrence.

2. Bleeding during pregnancy is an emergency situation. List the steps you would take as emergency measures. Include both psychological and physiologic measures.

3. Observing for pregnancy-induced hypertension symptoms is a major responsibility in a prenatal setting. List common implementations you would provide to detect this in such a setting.

Laboratory Experiences

1. Ask a woman who experienced a bleeding complication of pregnancy or severe pregnancy-induced hypertension to come to a postconference and discuss how frightening this complication was for her. If she had a blood transfusion, did this increase her level of concern?

2. Few students can be assigned to care for women with bleeding complications of pregnancy or eclampsia as these women are immediately cared for by experienced emergency room personnel. Chart review or participation in medical rounds can be helpful as ways to supply insight into the emergency care undertaken.

3. Women who have had ectopic pregnancy and those with preeclampsia are hospitalized. Assign students to these women and stress that the student analyze the woman's blood values, particularly hemoglobin and hematocrit, to help the student appreciate the extent of the blood loss or shift of body fluid.

Care Study: A Woman With a Placenta Previa

Lynn Hollaman is a 19-year-old, G2P0, 38-week pregnant college sophomore admitted by ambulance to the maternity service with painless, profuse vaginal bleeding for the last hour.

Health History

- Chief Concern: "I'm bleeding bad."

- History of Present Illness: Client was showering when she suddenly began "gushing" vaginal blood. She lay down and called the emergency number for help when it hadn't stopped after 15 minutes. Blood pressure was 95/60, pulse at 90/minute in the ambulance. "Soaked" three towels during 20 minute transport period. She had a similar episode 1 week ago while at an amusement park. Client didn't notify health care providers of that episode because bleeding had stopped by the time she returned home.

- History of Past Illnesses: Chickenpox at age 4 years. Ovarian cyst and right ovary removed at 16 years. "Accidentally" swallowed an overdose of aspirin 2 years ago after a boyfriend left her.

- Gynecologic History: Menarche at 9 years; cycle duration: 30 days; duration of menstrual flow: 5 days. Moderate dysmenorrhea. Treated for herpes genitalis 1 year ago. No recent lesions noticed. Has been sexually active since 15; usually insists on partner using condom but had stopped insisting because she and partner had established a monogamous relationship.

- Obstetric History. Therapeutic abortion at 15 years; this pregnancy was planned, although since sexual partner left school 4 months ago, client admits she is not as pleased with pregnancy as she was originally. Has attended hospital clinic for prenatal care since 4th month and kept all appointments. Sonogram at 20 weeks reported adequate fetal growth and that placenta was low-lying. Has few supplies purchased for baby as she was waiting for semester to end before she did this.

- Personal/Social History: Client smokes one-half pack cigarettes daily (couldn't stop for pregnancy because of pressure of school); only occasional alcohol during pregnancy; no recreational drugs. Lives in college dormitory; eats in college cafeteria. Sexual partner deserted her at 25 weeks of pregnancy; states her parents are supportive and will help her raise child. Works as a TA in psychology department; job is not tiring; mostly correcting papers or other paper work.

- Review of Systems: Negative except for urinary tract: urinary tract infection at 15 years.

Physical Examination

- General Appearance: Pale appearing white pregnant female. Height: 5' 8''; weight: 140. Blood pressure: 90/50.

- HEENT: Two "shotty" lymph glands palpable on left posterior cervical chain; throat slightly reddened. Nose: mucous membrane swollen but not reddened.

- Chest: Heart rate at 86/minute. No murmurs. Respiratory rate: 24/minute. No adventitious sounds on auscultation.

- Abdomen: Fundal height 34 cm; Linea nigra present on abdomen. Fetus palpated to be in left anterior position; head not engaged. No uterine contractions noted. FHR: 90/minute.

- Pelvic Exam: Deferred. Vaginal bleeding, bright red in amount and profuse, still continuing.

- Extremities: Full range of motion in joints; patellar tendon 2+.

Laboratory Reports

- Hemoglobin: 10.7 g
- Hematocrit: 37%
- Urinalysis: Negative for protein and glucose; specific gravity: 1.030

Care Study Questions

1. This woman has a history of "accidentally" swallowing aspirin following a demeaning experience 2 years ago. Could this really have been a deliberate act? Could an event such as losing a pregnancy or giving birth to a low-birthweight infant create a similar circumstance?

2. Lynn lives in a college dormitory and eats her meals in the college cafeteria. What kind of problems can you anticipate this may have caused during pregnancy?

3. Lynn is bleeding heavily and her vital signs are falling because of placenta previa bleeding. Complete a nursing care plan that will identify and meet Lynn's immediate care needs.

Home Care of the Pregnant Client

*C*hapter 16 discusses care of the woman with preterm labor or preterm premature rupture of the membranes who will be cared for at home. The techniques of home visiting and uterine and fetal heart rate monitoring in the home are also discussed.

This is an area of care that is expanding in importance as it is a cost-effective method of care. Nurses have major roles in arranging for home care and keeping this safe for pregnant women.

Chapter Objectives

After mastering the contents of this chapter, the student should be able to:

1. Describe the usual health concerns that require home care nursing during pregnancy.

2. Assess the pregnant woman who is being cared for at home for both physical and psychosocial aspects of care.

3. Formulate nursing diagnoses related to care of the pregnant client at home.

4. Plan home nursing care interventions such as teaching a woman the signs of preterm labor.

5. Implement nursing care such as attaching and using a home uterine monitor to detect uterine contractions.

6. Evaluate outcome criteria to be certain that home care is a satisfying and effective experience for the woman and her family.

7. Identify national health goals related to home care during pregnancy that nurses can be instrumental in helping the nation to achieve.

8. Identify areas of home care nursing that could benefit from additional nursing research.

9. Use critical thinking to analyze how home care influences family functioning and develop ways to make nursing care more family centered.

10. Synthesize knowledge of home care with nursing process to achieve quality maternal and child health nursing care.

Key Points

- Home care is more cost effective than hospital care. Women with preterm labor or preterm premature rupture of the membranes can be monitored on bedrest at home.

- Home care requires careful planning and a combined effort between home care and hospital personnel so there is collaboration and continuity between the two types of care.

- Labor is preterm if it occurs after 20 weeks and before the end of the 37th week of pregnancy. A woman is said to be in preterm labor when she has had uterine contractions every 10 minutes for 1 hour.

- Tocolytics are drugs that can halt labor. The most frequent ones used are magnesium sulfate and beta-adrenergic agents such as ritodrine (Yutopar) and terbutaline (Brethine). All these drugs have toxic effects. Magnesium sulfate should not be administered unless the maternal respiratory rate is more than 12/min, urine output is more than 30 mL/h, and a patellar reflex is present. Beta-adrenergic drugs (ritodrine and terbutaline) should not be administered if the maternal pulse is more than 120 bpm.

- Once preterm labor is halted, women can be discharged to home care. They need instructions in uterine monitoring and the importance of taking their tocolytic consistently and on time.

- Preterm premature rupture of the membranes is tearing of the fetal membranes with loss of amniotic fluid before the pregnancy is at term. Preterm premature rupture is a serious complication because following rupture, there is a high risk of fetal and uterine infection (chorioamnionitis).

- If a fetus is not yet at a point of viability, following preterm premature rupture of the membranes the woman may be discharged to home care. Important aspects of care are bedrest and assessment of maternal temperature, white blood count, and fetal well being.

Definitions of Key Terms

chorioamnionitis: infection and inflammation of fetal membranes and amniotic fluid

home care: nursing care conducted in a client's place of residence

preterm premature rupture of membranes: rupture of the membranes before term preterm labor: labor occurring before the 37th week of gestation

tocolytic agent: a drug used to suppress preterm labor

Nursing Process Overview

The Nursing Process Overview in this chapter concentrates on helping students adapt nursing diagnoses and planning of care to the home setting.

Study Aids

Boxes

Box 16-1:   Symptoms of Preterm Labor That Women Can Self Assess

Box 16-2:   Tocolytic Therapy

Tables

Table 16-1:   Preterm Labor Risk Assessment Scale

Displays

Focus on National Health Goals

Focus on Family Teaching

Focus on Nursing Research

Focus on Cultural Awareness

Critical Thinking Exercises

1. Amy is an 18-year-old on bedrest at home following preterm premature rupture of membranes at 32 weeks of pregnancy. Amy belonged to a competitive synchronized swimming team before she became pregnant. She is concerned that she will miss too much school to be able to graduate and will be so weak from lack of exercise by the time she delivers that she won't be able to take care of a newborn.

    a. What physical examination and health history questions would you want to ask Amy to assure yourself that she is not developing chorioamnionitis? What questions would you want to ask to be certain that she is maintaining bedrest?

    b. How would you answer her concern about lack of exercise?

    c. Amy is home alone most of the day because her parents work. Her boyfriend visits between 9 AM and 10 AM and school friends visit in the afternoon. What time of the day would be best to schedule a home visit for Amy? What signs and symptoms of preterm labor would you want her to know?

2. Mary Beth is a woman who has started preterm labor at 32 weeks of pregnancy.

    a. What are conditions you would want to assess before Mary Beth is begun on a tocolytic to halt labor?

    b. What if Mary Beth states that she doesn't want the baby? How would this influence care?

    c. Mary Beth's contractions are effectively halted and she is being cared for at home. What measures would you instruct her to take if she should start to feel contractions?

Discussion Questions

1. Having a very small preterm baby because of preterm labor is almost the same as having the baby die because the long hospitalization—3 to 4 months—means the parents will not have a baby to care for. What is the best way to help parents feel more like parents while their newborn is hospitalized for a long period of time?

2. The fetus of a woman who has had preterm premature rupture of the membranes is at risk for developing an infection. On the other hand, if the baby is born early, all the risks of low birthweight will be present. What are the factors that cause some women to be cared for at home and some to have labor induced so the baby is born immediately? How would you explain these different circumstances to women?

3. Preterm labor, if it can't be halted, leads to the birth of low birthweight infants. What is the impact of a low birthweight baby on a family? On a community? On the cost of health care?

Written Assignments

1. Preterm labor can be different from term labor. List at least five differences. Are these differences advantageous for the mother? For the fetus?

2. If a woman begins preterm labor there are some emergency steps she should take to try and halt labor. List these steps.

3. Caring for a woman in her home has substantial differences from care in a hospital setting. What are these differences? What are the ways care needs to be modified because of these?

Laboratory Experiences

1. Women who are in labor with preterm labor often have no idea how small a 24 or 28 week gestation infant will be. Arranging for an experience in a Level III Neonatal Intensive Care Nursery offers an opportunity for students to learn the size and ability of such infants.

2. Arranging for a home visit with a community or home care nurse can offer students the opportunity to see first hand the difficulty that women have in maintaining bedrest while at home and the strain that women who threaten to begin preterm birth live with until their pregnancy reaches term.

3. Ask a woman who began preterm labor which was then halted to come to a clinical conference and describe how the weeks she spent waiting for the pregnancy to come to term were for her and what she would have liked health care personnel to do to improve the time period for her.

Care Study: A Woman in Preterm Labor

Darling Breaker is a 32-year-old woman who is on home care for preterm labor. You visit her at home for a health maintenance visit.

Health History

- Chief Concern: "I'm bored. How much longer will I have to stay at home?"

- History of Chief Concern: Ms. Breaker began preterm labor at 22 weeks of pregnancy. She was hospitalized, well hydrated, and given intravenous magnesium sulfate for 3 days until uterine contractions halted, then discharged to home care and bedrest with oral terbutaline 4 times a day. She is now $23\frac{1}{2}$ weeks pregnant. She is supposed to monitor fetal heart rate as well as for uterine contractions four times a day but admits she has done it only once a day the last 2 days.

- Past Medical History: History of lactose intolerance since early childhood. Chronic sinusitis during winter time. Slight hypertension at beginning of pregnancy (160/82).

- Family Medical History: Both parents alive and well. Maternal grandfather died of colon cancer. A cousin had a child born with "something wrong with genes."

- Personal/Social History: Client lives in two-bedroom apartment with stepfather who is the parent who raised her. Stepfather does the cooking and cleaning. Stepfather has a pension from a war-related injury. Ms. Breaker worked as a clerk at a fast food restaurant before required bedrest. Has used up sick leave so has no further income. Used to exercising daily at a health club to "keep her weight controlled." Prepregnancy weight: 166.

- Pregnancy History: Pregnancy unplanned but not unwelcome. Father of baby is "interested" in pregnancy but has not offered any financial support. When he heard of early labor, he said it was "nature's way of getting rid of a bad thing" and encouraged her not to do anything to prolong the pregnancy. Attended prenatal care since 16 weeks of pregnancy; no apparent complications before onset of labor.

- Gynecologic History: Menarche at 14 years; usual pattern: 7 days duration; 30 day cycle. Mild dysmenorrhea.

Not sexually active until present relationship. Did not use contraceptive because she was certain if she did become pregnant her partner would welcome a pregnancy and marry her.

- Review of Systems: Negative but for sinusitis recorded above.

Physical Examination

- General Appearance: Obese, energetic appearing woman resting on couch. Weight: 185 lbs. BP: 164/86.

- HEENT: Normocephalic. Eyes: Red reflex present; follows into six fields of vision. Ears: hearing equal to examiner's. Neck: subtle; no nodes palpable.

- Chest: Lungs clear to auscultation. Breasts tender to palpation; no lumps palpable.

- Heart: Heart rate: 78 bpm; grade 2 early systolic murmur present.

- Abdomen: Soft. Fundal height: 24 cm. No contractions present on monitor. Fetal heart rate: 154 bpm.

- Extremities: No varicosities noted. Slight edema in both ankles.

Care Study Questions

1. Home care of a woman with threatened preterm labor calls for all family members to cooperate so a woman can rest. Because Ms. Breaker lives with another adult, she has no responsibility for care of others. Does living in a home with few people make home care easier or harder?

2. Suppose Ms. Breaker lived in a family in which her grown children or her husband were not cooperative? What would be your role?

3. Ms. Breaker has only been on home care 7 days and already reports she is bored and has decreased her level of monitoring. Complete a nursing care plan that would meet the needs of Ms. Breaker.

High-Risk Pregnancy: The Woman With Special Needs

Chapter 17 discusses the family who needs special considerations in care during pregnancy due to special circumstances. The adolescent, the woman over age 35, and the woman with a spinal cord injury, cerebral palsy, mental retardation, vision or hearing impairment, cystic fibrosis, or drug dependency are discussed. Special considerations that need to be taken during pregnancy, at birth, and during the postpartal period are discussed. Ways to promote healthy parent-child bonding are stressed.

All of the situations discussed in this chapter are increasing in frequency in the United States and so have increasing relevance to the student in nursing as she or he prepares to nurse in the future. Practicing how to modify care for women with special needs has the added advantage of enlarging the student's ability to modify care for all clients and so improves overall competence in nursing.

Chapter Objectives

After mastering the contents of this chapter, students should be able to:

1. Describe the risks of pregnancy in the woman with special needs, such as the adolescent, the woman over age 35, the woman with a drug dependency, and the woman with a disability.

2. Assess the woman with special needs for safe health practices during pregnancy.

3. State nursing diagnoses for the woman with special needs.

4. Plan nursing care to respect the special growth and development needs of the adolescent and the woman over age 35 and the specific strengths and weaknesses of the woman with a physical disability or drug dependency.

5. Implement nursing care that is effective with a woman with special needs, such as education about the importance of exercise.

6. Evaluate outcome criteria to be certain that goals for care have been achieved.

7. Identify national health goals related to the woman with a special need that nurses can be instrumental in helping the nation to achieve.

8. Identify areas related to care of the woman with special needs during pregnancy that would benefit from additional nursing research.

9. Use critical thinking to analyze ways that nursing care of the pregnant woman with a special need can be optimally family centered.

10. Synthesize knowledge of risks of pregnancy and age extremes, drug use, and disability with nursing process to achieve quality maternal and child health nursing care.

Key Points

- As many as 7% of births in the United States are to teenagers. Adolescent pregnancy is a major problem not only because it occurs at such a high rate but because it can interfere with the development of both the adolescent and the fetus. Nursing care needs to be individualized to meet the prenatal needs of this age group. Helping adolescents to view a pregnancy as a growth experience can help them mature in their ability to parent.

- Women who delay childbearing until age 35 may have some needs during pregnancy that require special consideration by health care providers. They may need additional discussion time at prenatal visits to help them incorporate a pregnancy into their lifestyle. They may need reminding to save time during a day for rest, particularly if they have a degree of hypertension before pregnancy.

- Women who have physical disabilities such as vision and hearing impairment or spinal cord injury are apt to have special needs during pregnancy that must be addressed by health care providers. Providing time for discussion early in pregnancy so these needs can be identified and anticipated is an important role for nurses.

- Women with a physical disability may need help in adjusting their usual medical regimen to pregnancy. Be certain they are aware of how to contact help in an emergency. Assess that all medications they are taking for their primary disorder are safe during pregnancy.

- Women with mental retardation may need help in planning ways to follow prenatal instructions. As with all women with special needs, be certain they have support people around them so you can feel confident the baby will receive safe care.

- The woman who is drug dependent presents a unique challenge during pregnancy. Short-term goals must be directed toward encouraging the woman to decrease or halt her drug intake in order to safeguard the health of the fetus. Long-term goals must address the need for the woman to decrease drug intake for the remainder of her life so she can be a quality parent for her child.

- The fetus of a woman with drug dependency is at high risk because of the direct effects of the drug and the indirect effects of an unhealthy lifestyle. Women addicted to narcotics should be encouraged to join methadone maintenance programs if possible.

Definitions of Key Terms

autonomic dysreflexia: a syndrome that occurs as a result of impaired autonomic nervous system dysfunction. Simultaneous sympathetic and parasympathetic activity occurs leading to severe hypertension.

drug dependence: psychological craving for a drug

drug tolerance: the state in which cell adaptation to a drug occurs so increasingly larger doses are necessary to produce the usual effect

elderly primipara: a woman having her first pregnancy over age 35

Nursing Process Overview

The Nursing Process Overview for this chapter concentrates on helping the student appreciate that nursing care must be modified if it is to meet the needs of the woman with special circumstances such as drug use or a physical disability. The importance of planning ways to strengthen confidence and self-esteem levels are included. Helping to modify care in special circumstances improves the student's overall ability to modify care and to adapt to changing client circumstances.

Study Aids

Tables

Table 17-1: Areas of Planning With Physically Disabled Women During Pregnancy

Table 17-2: Level of Ambulatory Function Anticipated Following Spinal Injury

Displays

Focus on National Health Goals

Focus on Family Teaching

Focus on Nursing Research

Focus on Cultural Awareness

Critical Thinking Exercises

1. Mindy is a 14-year-old you meet in a prenatal clinic. She is 20 weeks pregnant. She lives with her mother and two younger sisters. She tells you she is old enough to be a responsible parent so plans on keeping her baby. What are specific measures you would want to teach Mindy to help her be ready for parenting? What clues would you look for in Mindy to see if her evaluation of herself is correct?

2. Chelsa is a 40-year-old woman who was recently married and is pregnant following in vitro fertilization. She works out at a health spa daily and flies 3 days every week to out-of-state locations for work. What advice would you want to give Chelsa to help her avoid complications of pregnancy? Suppose she had a very sedentary lifestyle? Would your advice be different?

3. Terry is a 22-year-old who is drug dependent on heroin. You suspect she supports her drug habit by prostitution. She refuses to be seen in clinic if she has to wait over 15 minutes. How could you arrange Terry's prenatal care to better help her? What specific advice would you want to stress with Terry to avoid complications of pregnancy?

Media Resources

Pregnancy After 35 (19 minute video)

A description of the risks of pregnancy after 35. Three women over this age are followed through their pregnancies. Medical technologies being used to decrease risks are stressed.

Source: Films for the Humanities and Sciences

Adolescent Parenting (30 minute video)

Critical tasks of parenting that are completed during pregnancy are reviewed. Nursing approaches to support development of early parenting skills by adolescents who are working with their own developmental tasks are stressed. Attachment and bonding processes significant to adolescent parenthood are included.

Source: Health Sciences Consortium

Women, Drugs and the Unborn Child (54 minute video)

Discusses how drugs reach and affect the pregnant woman and her unborn child. Includes two parts: "Treating the Chemically Dependent Woman" and "Innocent Addicts."

Source: Pyramid Film and Video

Drugs, Smoking and Alcohol During Pregnancy (12 minute film/video)

Clear information about how these substances affect the growing baby is presented. Simple animation illustrates the dangers of substance abuse. Caution in the use of all medication is stressed.

Source: Polymorph Films

Preventing Low Birth Weight: A Nurse's Guide (28 minute video)

The risk factors that increase a woman's chances of going into preterm labor and appropriate prenatal care for high-risk clients is discussed. Teaching clients early warning signs of preterm labor, hospital assessment and care of the client in preterm labor, and the effect of low birthweight on infants and their families are shown. The important role nurses play in assessment, client education, and support is stressed.

Source: Polymorph Films

Substance Abuse and Pregnancy: A Health Professional's Guide (30 minute video)

The scope of the problem and an overview of the nurse's role are provided. Techniques for risk assessment, good communication skills, and ways of offering effective ongoing support are demonstrated. Pregnancy is presented as an opportunity to change a client's long-term life behavior and effective ways of encouraging clients to effect these changes are shown.

Source: Polymorph Films

Discussion Questions

1. What societal reasons account for the fact that more women over age 35 and women with disabilities are planning pregnancies than previously? Can this trend be expected to continue into the future?

2. A very young woman and a woman over 35 have many similarities both psychologically and physiologically in their response to pregnancy. In what ways are their needs are similar? Different?

3. Adolescents and women over 35 both attend preparation for parenthood courses. How would you modify a class if the couples attending were mostly adolescents? Mostly over age 35?

Written Assignments

1. Helping adolescents to be responsible for their own health care aids achievement of a sense of identity. List things that even a very young girl could be responsible for during pregnancy.

2. Because many women with physical disabilities do not drive, they must rely on provided transportation. Investigate what resources are available in your community to such women. Write a paragraph describing these facilities and whether they are adequate to encourage women to attend prenatal care.

3. The ability to secure help in an emergency varies from community to community. Compile and describe ways in which a woman who cannot speak clearly could contact emergency help in your community.

Laboratory Experiences

1. Ask a woman with special needs to attend a postconference and discuss the special problems she encountered during a pregnancy. Ask her to stress how health care personnel could have been more helpful to her.

2. Assign students to inner city antepartal clinics so they have exposure to clients with drug dependency. Encourage them to adopt a "let me help you at the point you are at" philosophy of care rather than a critical one.

3. Have students role-play being a woman confined to a wheelchair so they can better appreciate the difficulty such a woman would encounter during pregnancy or giving care to a newborn.

Care Study: A Woman With Drug Abuse During Pregnancy

Andrea Drew is a 26-year-old, G3P2, 36-week pregnant woman admitted to the maternity service because of vaginal bleeding.

Health History

- Chief Concern: "I've had pain for over an hour."

- History of Present Illness: Client states that an hour ago she and her boyfriend were smoking "crack." Suddenly she noticed hard fundal pain followed by dark red vaginal bleeding. Her boyfriend immediately transported her to the hospital.

- History of Past Illnesses: Chickenpox at age 6; scarlet fever at 9 years. Viral pneumonia treated on an ambulatory basis at 18 years. No other major illnesses; no hospitalizations.

- Gynecologic History: Menarche at 10 years; cycle duration: 30 days; menstrual flow duration: 7 days. Severe premenstrual symptoms for 2 days prior to menstrual flow.

- Obstetric History: Boy, 5'13" born 4 years ago. This pregnancy was planned and wanted. Client signed up for prenatal care at hospital clinic but only kept two appointments.

- Personal/Social: Lives with boyfriend and one other couple in two-bedroom apartment; client does not work; boyfriend works as a truck driver. States finances are "all right." Smokes 1 pack of cigarettes daily; no alcohol since pregnancy began. Admits to using cocaine at least weekly.

- Nutrition: 24-hour nutritional recall history:

    Breakfast: 1 cup coffee; 1 bowl Cheerios with milk and sugar.

    Lunch: 1 cup strawberry yogurt; 1 glass cola beverage

    Dinner: 1 serving chicken with Chinese vegetables (take-out); 1 glass milk.

    Snack: Chocolate candy; 1 dish ice cream.

- Review of Systems: Essentially negative.

Physical Examination

- General Appearance: Pale appearing young adult pregnant woman with swollen face, hands, and ankles. Height: 7'6"; weight: 145. BP: 160/100.

- HEENT: Edema present on face; otherwise negative.

- Chest: Faint systolic heart murmur heard at left sternal border; heart rate: 82. Lungs clear to auscultation.
- Abdomen: Fundal height 34 cm and rigid. Very tender to touch. Abdominal contractions present on external monitor about every 6 minutes. Fetus palpated to be in breech position at -1 station. No fetal heart rate discernible by Doppler.
- Pelvic Examination: Cervix thick and dilated 2 cm; dark red blood observed flowing from cervix.
- Extremities: 3+ edema present in both hands and ankles. Full range of motion in body joints. Needle injection marks on arms and behind knees.

Laboratory Results

- Hemoglobin: 9 g
- Hematocrit: 33.5%
- Urinalysis: Negative for glucose; 2+ for protein; positive for blood

Care Study Questions

1. Andrea has taken some actions (no prenatal care; smoking cigarettes, cocaine use) that have led directly to birth of a low birthweight infant. How does it influence nursing care when you know a woman has been noncompliant with instructions in the past?

2. Andrea's baby may need extensive care because of low birthweight and probable premature separation of the placenta. Does Andrea have a firm support system in place to help her with child care?

3. Andrea has socioeconomic concerns that have interfered with pregnancy health and could interfere with childrearing as well as the immediate concern of early labor. Complete a nursing care plan that would identify and meet Andrea's needs.

The Labor Process

Chapter 18 discusses care of the woman and family during labor and delivery. The physiology of labor from the aspects of the passage, the passenger, and the power are discussed and illustrated. Both psychological and physiologic aspects of labor and the nursing care required to meet these needs are included. Stress is placed on making labor and delivery a family centered event in order to lay a firm foundation for family-child bonding.

Labor and delivery is a process that few students will have knowledge about prior to studying the content area. Because it does involve conceptual visualization, some visually oriented learners may need to view a delivery before they are able to understand and discuss the full scope of the content.

Chapter Objectives

After mastering the contents of this chapter, students should be able to:

1. Describe the common theories explaining the onset and continuation of labor as well as the role of the passenger, the passage, and the force in the labor process.

2. Assess a woman for stages and progress of labor.

3. Formulate nursing diagnoses related to both the physiologic and psychological aspects of labor.

4. Assist the woman in labor to establish realistic goals and criteria for progress in labor.

5. Implement nursing care for the family during labor such as providing for comfort and educating them about the process of labor.

6. Evaluate outcome criteria to be certain that nursing goals for care have been achieved.

7. Identify national health goals related to safe labor and birth that nurses can be instrumental in helping the nation to achieve.

8. Identify areas related to labor and birth that could benefit from additional nursing research.

9. Use critical thinking to analyze whether current nursing care measures truly meet the needs of women and their families in labor.

10. Synthesize knowledge of nursing care in labor with nursing process to achieve quality maternal and child health nursing care.

Key Points

- Labor is the series of events by which uterine contractions expel the fetus and placenta from the woman's body.

- The exact reason why labor begins is unknown. It most likely occurs because of an interplay between fetal and uterine factors.

- Effective labor depends on interactions between the passage, the passenger, and the power of contractions.

- Labor is an almost overwhelming experience because it involves sensations and emotions of such an intense level. Women need support people with them to help them cope with this level of experience.

- Fetal presentation (the fetal body part that will initially contact the cervix) and position (the relationship of the fetal presenting part to a specific quadrant of the woman's pelvis) are both important in determining the success of labor.

- The first stage of labor is the time span between beginning dilatation and the time the cervix is fully dilated. The second stage is from the time of full dilatation until the infant is born. A third or placental stage is from the time the infant is born until after the delivery of the placenta. A fourth stage (the first few hours following birth) is also currently identified.

- Cervical changes that occur are effacement (shortening and thinning of the cervix) and dilatation (enlargement of the cervical canal from 1 to 2 cm to 8 to 10 cm).

- Important nursing assessments to make in labor are health history, length and intensity of contractions, fetal assessment, and maternal vital signs.

- Monitoring uterine contractions and fetal heart rate are nursing responsibilities. Recognizing fetal bradycardia, tachycardia, and late and variable decelerations are important observations. Interventions to help prevent fetal distress are keeping the woman on her left side and promoting voiding. Offering psychological support is important to maternal well being.

- Pushing during the second stage of labor should be guided by the woman's felt need to push. Urge her not to hold her breath while doing this to prevent a valsalva maneuver.

- The placental stage follows birth and consists of placental separation and expulsion. Observe for excessive bleeding during this time. Do not pull on the cord to hasten separation as this can lead to uterine inversion.

- Danger signs of labor are abnormal fetal heart rate, meconium staining of amniotic fluid, abnormal maternal pulse or blood pressure, inadequate or prolonged contractions, formation of a pathologic retraction ring, development of an abnormal lower abdomen contour, and increasing apprehension.

- A fetus is in potential danger when membranes rupture because of the possibility of cord prolapse. Always assess FHR at this point to safeguard the fetus.

- A woman is at potential threat all during labor for hemorrhage because of the possibility the placenta could be dislodged. Assess for vaginal bleeding and vital signs to verify that this is not occurring.

Definitions of Key Terms

attitude: a reference to the relationship of the fetal parts to each other or the degree of flexion of the fetal head

breech presentation: a fetal position in which the buttocks present to the cervix

cardinal movements of labor: the typical sequence of positions assumed by the fetus as it descends through the pelvis during labor and delivery

cephalic presentation: a fetal position in which the head presents to the cervix

crowning: the appearance of the presenting part of the fetus at the vaginal orifice

dilatation: stretching of the external os of the cervix large enough to allow the passage of the fetus

effacement: thinning and shortening of the cervix that occurs just prior to dilatation

engagement: the entrance of the fetal presenting part into the superior pelvic strait

episiotomy: a surgical incision in the perineum to enlarge the vaginal introitus for childbirth

fetal descent: the maneuver of delivery in which the fetus passes beyond the ischial spines

Leopold's maneuver: a technique of manual palpation to discover the position and lie of the fetus

lie: the relationship between the long axis of the fetus and the long axis of the mother

lightening: descent of the fetus into the pelvis at about 2 weeks prior to delivery; also engagement

molding: overlapping of cranial bones or shaping of the fetal head that occurs to accommodate the head to the birth canal during labor

passage: the internal pelvic rim through which a fetus must pass in order to be born

passenger: the fetus during labor and delivery

pathologic retraction ring: an indentation horizontally across the uterus which denotes extreme stress on the divisions of the organ

physiologic retraction ring: the junction of the upper and lower uterine segments during labor

position: relationship of a chosen fetal reference point to its location in the front, back, or sides of the maternal pelvis

ripening: softening of the cervix that occurs just prior to labor

station: relationship of the presenting fetal part to an imaginary line drawn between the ischial spines of the pelvis

transition: the last phase of the first stage of labor when cervical dilation reaches 8 to 10 cm.

Nursing Process Overview

The Nursing Process Overview for this chapter concentrates on helping the students to view labor as a total process and to establish nursing diagnoses that are broad enough to meet the total needs of the laboring family. "Pain" for example, is a narrow focus. The effect of the pain, or "situational low self-esteem related to inability to use a prepared childbirth method," is a broader diagnosis. Labor is such a unique process that students may find it difficult to generalize from other nursing circumstances to labor care without this type of guidance.

Study Aids

Boxes

Box 18-1:   Possible Fetal Positions

Box 18-2:   Delivery Equipment and Supplies

Tables

Table 18-1:   Differentiation Between True and False Labor Contractions

Table 18-2:   Diameters of Fetal Skull Compared with Maternal Pelvic Diameters

Table 18-3:   Types of Cephalic Presentations

Table 18-4:   Types of Breech Presentations

Table 18-5:   Principal Clinical Features of the Divisions of Labor

Table 18-6:   Abnormal Phases of Labor Detectable by Graphing

Table 18-7:   Time Intervals for Nursing Interventions During First Stage of Labor

Table 18-8:   Time Intervals for Nursing Interventions During Second Stage of Labor

Procedures

Procedure 18-1:   Vaginal Examination in Labor

Displays

Focus on National Health Goals

Focus on Family Teaching

Focus on Nursing Research

Focus on Cultural Awareness

Critical Thinking Exercises

1. Mrs. Travillato is a woman in active labor you admit to a birthing room. She admits she has read nothing during her pregnancy about labor so has little idea of what to

expect. Would it be better to educate her about labor or let her follow her practice of not knowing? If you decide to teach her, what would you tell her early in labor? Midway in labor? Why would a woman enter labor not having read about it?

2. Mrs. Travillato's fetus is in a vertex presentation and an occipitoposterior position, and has a military attitude. Is this an optimum birth presentation and position? Is Mrs. Travillato's labor apt to be longer or shorter than normal because of this?

3. Most women today accept fetal monitoring equipment as an expected part of labor care. How would you manage a woman who states she absolutely does not want this type of monitoring?

Leopold's Maneuvers (15 minute video)

Leopold's maneuvers are described and demonstrated. Ways the maneuvers can be used to assess the physical adaptations between mother and fetus are discussed.

Source: Health Sciences Consortium

Birth in the Squatting Position (10 minute film/video)

This traditional form of childbirth is illustrated.

Source: Polymorph Films

Labor and Delivery: The LDR (26 minute video)

A couple is admitted to an LDR and followed through the early postpartum period. Determination of fetal lie, presentation, and position are described as are the four stages of labor. Coping strategies, analgesics, and anesthesia are discussed.

Source: Medcom, Inc.

Managing the Experience of Labor and Delivery (30 minute plus IAV-IVD IBM Info Window)

Clinical simulation focused on normal labor and delivery process. From the point of view of the student nurse, learner is allowed to progress through the menu-driven program engaging in the learning activities of choice.

Source: Health Sciences Consortium

Mrs. Weed, a Multipara Patient in Early Labor (CAI)

A clinical simulation focusing on nursing care during labor, delivery, and immediate recovery. Nursing assessments and interventions for the newborn are included.

Source: J.B. Lippincott Company

Human Birth (23 minute film, video)

Different types of deliveries such as vertex delivery with forceps; vertex delivery spontaneous; breech delivery assisted; breech delivery with forceps; breech delivery, extraction; multiple birth; and twins are depicted.

Source: J.B. Lippincott Company

Clinical Simulations in Nursing: Maternity Nursing Simulation (CAI)

Four simulations (pregnancy; labor, delivery, and postpartum; a complicated delivery; and assessment of a newborn) are provided. The simulations emphasize information gathering, decision making, and the use of therapeutic communication.

Source: Medi-Sim, Inc.

Essentials of Electronic Fetal Monitoring (60 minute video)

Three videotapes of 20 minutes each that present the principles of instrumentation, pattern interpretations, and guidelines for appropriate nursing interventions and documentation. Two workbooks included in package.

Source: NAACOG

Intrapartum Fetal Monitoring (video)

Currently employed instrumentation in fetal monitoring is demonstrated. Concepts of pathophysiologic effects of labor on the fetus and the clinical implications of a variety of fetal heart rate patterns are discussed.

Source: ACOG Distribution Center

FM Interpreture (CAI)

Computer-aided instruction for fetal monitoring interpretation. Components: fetal monitoring tutorial, draw a tracing, practice tracing interpretation, client management problems.

Source: Williams and Wilkins Electronic Media

Discussion Questions

1. A woman is often afraid to be alone while in labor. What are ways in which you could convey a caring attitude if you could not physically remain with her during every minute of labor?

2. In many settings, a woman's older children may watch a birth of a younger sibling. How might the presence of other children affect a woman during labor?

3. Most women will have fetal heart rate monitoring done early in labor and possibly all through labor. What are ways that fetal monitoring can be viewed as a positive experience for the woman?

Written Assignments

1. Most women think of labor as a local process, but it also involves systemic changes. List the changes that occur in the cardiovascular system and the respiratory system.

2. The terms effacement and dilatation are often confusing to women in labor. Write a paragraph explaining the difference in these terms.

3. A fetus must make positional changes in order to navigate a birth canal. List the positional changes that must be accomplished and the rationale for these position changes.

Laboratory Experiences

1. Using a simulated model, allow students the opportunity to have "hands on" practice in turning the model fetus through the cardinal positions of labor. Use a care study such as the one that follows to allow students to demonstrate nursing care planning for the woman in labor.

2. Assign students to a clinical setting where there is an option for couples to use a birthing (labor-delivery-recovery) room or a regular labor and delivery service. Ask students to evaluate the advantages and disadvantages and satisfaction to parents of both systems.

3. Set up a display in the laboratory area using a Mrs. Chase model. Lay the mannequin on her back, wrinkle the sheets, set a food tray next to her, etc. Announce she is a patient in labor and hold a contest to see how many things students can list that are right or wrong about her care. Offer a prize donated by a local fast food restaurant.

Care Study: A Woman in Labor

Sally Hudson is a 28-year-old, G1P0, 41 week pregnant woman admitted to the maternity service in labor.

Health History

- Chief Concern: ''I'm in labor.''

- History of Present Illness: Sally has been in labor for 8 hours; contractions have progressed from 30 minute intervals to 3 minute intervals; from 10 second duration to 60 second duration. Last ate: 8 hours ago.

- History of Past Illnesses: Chickenpox at 3 years. Dislocated knee at 14 years and again at 16 years. No major illnesses; no hospitalizations.

- Gynecologic History: Menarche at 11 years; duration of cycle: 32 days. Length of menstrual flow: 7 days. Was treated for trichomoniasis X 2 last year. No other STDs.

- Obstetric History: No previous pregnancies. This pregnancy was not planned but is wanted. Had prenatal care with private obstetrician since second month; was found to be anemic early in pregnancy; this was treated with extra iron supplement. Attended preparation for labor classes.

- Personal/Social: Separated from father of baby for 7 months. Sister is with her to be support person in labor. Client works as French teacher at State University; is taking courses part-time toward her doctorate. Lives in one-bedroom condo by self. Has supplies prepared for infant.

- Nutritional: 24-hour recall nutritional history reveals adequate pregnancy diet. Took prenatal diet and extra iron supplement.

- Review of Systems: Neuropsych: had febrile convulsions two times as preschooler; maintained on phenobarbital until she was 6. No further difficulty.

Physical Examination

- General Appearance: Composed, well-groomed, young adult pregnant woman breathing without apparent great distress with contractions. Height: 5'5''; weight: 142. Temperature: 38°C; BP: 112/70.

- HEENT: Normocephalic; Nose: profuse clear watery discharge present; mucous membrane red and swollen; Throat: reddened; geographic tongue; coughing periodically. Ears: tympanic membrane slightly inflamed; good motility.

- Chest: Breasts full and soft; no masses palpable. Lungs: rhonchi heard in all lobes. Respiratory rate: 20/minute. Heart rate is at 62/minute. No murmur.

- Abdomen: Fundal height at 35 cm; fetus palpable in LOA position; linea nigra and striae present. FHR = 150/minute.

- Pelvic Exam: Cervix 6 cm dilated; 100% effaced. Station +1.

- Extremities: negative

Care Study Questions

1. Sally appears to have an upper respiratory infection. How will this influence her care during labor? Her care of her newborn?

2. The father of Sally's baby will not be with her in labor but her sister will be. Does having a sister rather than a husband for a support person change your role? Would it be important to determine if Sally has continuing support after she returns home?

3. Complete a nursing care plan that will identify and meet Sally's needs.

Providing Comfort During Labor and Delivery

*C*hapter 19 discusses the nursing role in helping provide both formal and informal comfort measures during labor and delivery. The physiologic basis for pain is reviewed. Transcutaneous electrical nerve stimulation, administration of narcotic analgesics, and the administration of regional and general anesthetics are discussed. Nursing interventions such as positioning, supporting breathing exercises, and teaching are stressed.

What type of analgesia or anesthesia is used with women in labor differs a great deal among settings and regions of the country. Discussing all of the options available allows students to enlarge their knowledge of what options are available and to be better health teachers in this area.

Chapter Objectives

After mastering the contents of this chapter, students should be able to:

1. Describe the physiologic basis of pain in labor and birth and related theories of pain relief.

2. Compare and contrast the action of local, regional, and general anesthesia as used in labor and birth.

3. Assess the degree and type of pain a woman is experiencing and her ability to cope with it effectively during labor and birth.

4. State nursing diagnoses related to the effect of pain in labor.

5. Plan nursing interventions to relieve pain in labor.

6. List common measures used for pain relief in labor such as teaching breathing techniques or relaxation.

7. Evaluate goal criteria to be certain labor is a satisfying experience for the woman and her family.

8. Identify national health goals related to anesthesia and childbirth that nurses can be instrumental in helping the nation to achieve.

9. Identify areas related to comfort in labor that could benefit from additional nursing research.

10. Use critical thinking to analyze ways to maintain family centered care when analgesia and anesthesia are used in childbirth.

11. Synthesize knowledge of pain relief measures during labor and birth with nursing process to achieve quality maternal and child health nursing care.

Key Points

- Pain in labor occurs because of anoxia to uterine cells, stretching of the cervix and perineum, and pressure of the presenting part of the fetus on tissues.

- Gating theory proposes that pain can be reduced by stimulation of large-diameter nerve fibers, distraction, and misinterpretation of sensations.

- Pain is perceived differently by everyone. Only the woman herself can describe the extent of her pain.

- The better prepared a woman is for childbirth, the less amount of analgesia and anesthesia is necessary. Methods such as reducing anxiety, providing changes in position, increasing knowledge, and supporting prepared childbirth exercises should be used in conjunction with prescribed analgesics.

- Be certain to ask about allergy to medication before administering it in labor. Women under stress may omit mentioning this unless directly asked.

- Record a baseline FHR and maternal BP and pulse before administering medication; reassess 15 minutes later for fetal and maternal safety.

- Women may lose their ability to use controlled breathing following narcotic administration because of a ''lightheaded'' feeling. They may need additional support during this time to be able to continue with a breathing technique until the analgesic begins to have an effect.

- Regional anesthesia such as epidural anesthesia can be extremely effective in relieving labor pain. Be certain the woman is well hydrated with intravenous fluid and that blood pressure is within normal limits prior to administration.

- During regional or general anesthesia administration, if the woman must lie supine, she should have a wedge positioned under her right buttock to help prevent supine hypotension syndrome. If hypotension should occur following anesthesia administration, elevating the woman's legs is an emergency measure to help relieve the condition.

- Analgesics or anesthetics may interfere with labor progress if given too early in labor. As a rule of thumb, medication is not given until a primipara is 5 to 6 cm dilated; a multipara, 3 to 4 cm.

- If a narcotic analgesic is used, naloxone (Narcan) must be available for possible newborn resuscitation.

- General anesthesia is rarely administered for an uncomplicated labor as it has risks for both the mother and infant.

Definitions of Key Terms

analgesia: a lack of pain without loss of consciousness

anesthesia: the absence of pain and sensation

endorphin: a neuropeptide elaborated by the pituitary gland and acting on the central and peripheral nervous systems to reduce pain

epidural anesthesia: injection of a regional anesthetic outside the dura mater to reduce the pain of labor contractions

pressure anesthesia: anesthesia achieved by pressure to nerve endings

pudendal nerve block: injection of an anesthetic agent into the perineum to achieve anesthesia of the pudendal nerve

pain: a subjective symptom of physical or mental suffering

transcutaneous electrical nerve stimulation (TENS): a method of pain control by the application of electric impulses to nerve endings

pressure anesthesia: anesthesia achieved by pressure to nerve endings

Nursing Process Overview

The Nursing Process Overview for this chapter concentrates on helping the students not to be trapped into the belief that "pain" is the only nursing diagnosis relevant to this area. In many instances, diagnoses addressing the effect of pain, such as "powerlessness" or "disturbance in self-esteem," identify not only the actual problem but suggest concrete interventions that can be successful where relieving pain may not be possible. Planning to make childbirth a growth experience is stressed.

Study Aids

Tables

Table 19-1: Analgesics and Anesthetics Commonly Used in Labor and Birth

Table 19-2: Nursing Responsibilities With Epidural Anesthetic Administration During Labor

Displays

Focus on National Health Goals

Focus on Family Teaching

Focus on Nursing Research

Focus on Cultural Awareness

Critical Thinking Exercises

1. Heather is a P0G1 who is admitted to your birthing service. She did not attend a preparation for childbirth class and has no concept of how to use breathing exercises to reduce labor pain. What would be the best method to teach her to help her relieve pain in early labor? Later in labor?

2. Mrs. Batten is also admitted to your birthing service. She states she wants a general anesthetic for labor or she will leave the hospital. Her physician has said he cannot justify a general anesthetic for uncomplicated labor. What is your role? Would you advocate for a general anesthetic for her?

3. Carla is a woman who seemed well prepared for labor but, after an injection of meperidine early in labor, grew angry with her coach and refused to use breathing exercises as she felt "light-headedness and pain worse than before." How would you help her at this point?

Media Resources

Pharmacological Interventions in Obstetrical Care (CAI)

A simulation requiring application of pharmacologic knowledge to a woman during pregnancy through postpartal discharge.

Source: J.B. Lippincott Company

Spinal/Epidural Anesthesia (illustrations)

Posters showing sites and techniques and level of anesthesia achieved with spinal and epidural anesthesia.

Source: Childbirth Graphics Ltd.

Lisa and Billy—Birth #8 (10 minute video)

Lisa is 18 and single and although she has good support during labor, her pain tolerance is low and she is administered an epidural before delivery.

Source: Polymorph Films

Discussion Questions

1. Nursing interventions for regional block anesthesia administration are important to know because they can be life-saving for a mother or fetus. What are the important actions to take preceding and following epidural anesthetic administration?

2. Many women expect to receive something for pain immediately on admission to a hospital or birthing center. What is the reason that medication is not administered in early labor?

3. Hold a class debate on the pros and cons of the various forms of comfort promotion in labor. Ask a class panel to judge the presentations.

Written Assignments

1. Complete medication cards for those medications commonly used in labor. Include drug name (generic and trade), action, side effects, usual dosage, routes of administration, nursing implications, and contraindications.

2. Many couples do not know enough anatomy to understand readily the difference between a spinal and an epidural anesthetic. Write a short paragraph of the explanation you would give to a couple to help them differentiate between these two types of anesthesia.

3. A number of women still ask for a general anesthetic in labor. What would you want to teach a woman who says she "wants to be asleep for the whole thing?"

Laboratory Experiences

1. Assign students to a labor service where regional anesthesia, such as epidural blocks, is administered. Ask them to interview clients afterward as to their satisfaction with the pain control method.

2. Ask women who received various forms of discomfort relief in labor to come to a postconference and discuss their satisfaction with the methods. Would they ask for something different the next time? Did they feel as if they really had a choice of method or was something suggested so forcefully they felt they should select that method?

3. Ask students to interview postpartal clients who received no medication during labor as to how much pain they experienced in labor. Would they elect to have a medication-free labor again?

Care Study: A Woman Who Needs Pain Relief for Labor

Malvern Mazjewski is a 34-year-old woman, G2P1, 40 weeks pregnant, admitted to the maternity unit in active labor.

Health History

- Chief Concern: "I'm having terrible pain."

- History of Present Illness: Client woke this a.m. 10 hours ago with labor contractions. Contractions have progressed from 20 minute intervals to 5 minute frequency; from 20 second duration to 60 second duration. At first were mild; are now sharp and "biting" at peak. Slight pink show present. EDC: 2 days ago. Last ate: a piece of chocolate cake 2 hours ago. States she wants an epidural immediately for pain.

- History of Past Illnesses: No childhood communicable diseases; tonsillectomy at age 5 years. Fractured tibia at 10 years in fall from toboggan.

- Gynecologic History: Menarche at 12 years; cycle 35 days; menstrual flow duration: 6 days. Moderate dysmenorrhea; no STDs. Used birth control pills for 2 years prior to present pregnancy.

- Obstetric History: Girl, 7'12" born 4 years ago. Labor lasted a total of 4 hours; no analgesia or anesthesia used. Vaginal delivery; no complications.

This pregnancy was planned; client is concerned because labor seems so much longer and more painful than previous one. Also concerned because sister had a child born with a cleft lip last month. Husband voiced concern that malformed head of this baby could be possible reason for what they perceive as long labor. Couple didn't attend preparation for labor classes as client barely used them last time since her labor was so short.

- Personal/Social: Married for 6 years; client works as first grade teacher; husband works as accountant at Chevrolet plant. Couple lives in 3-bedroom house. They have supplies ready for baby. Husband wants to view birth unless there is a possibility something will be wrong with baby.

- Review of Systems: Essentially negative.

Physical Examination

- General Appearance: Distressed appearing, young African American woman, alternately crying and screaming with contractions. Height: 5'4"; weight: 156; BP: 130/80.

- HEENT: Negative

- Chest: Breasts full and soft; areolae dark; veins prominent. Heart rate: 78/minute; no murmurs heard. Lungs clear to auscultation. Respiratory rate: 20/minute.

- Abdomen: Fundal height: 36 cm; fetus palpable in LOA position; FHR: 134/minute. Contractions every 3 minutes by external monitor; 60 second duration. Moderate in intensity.

- Pelvic Examination: Cervix dilated 5 cm; effacement: 80%. Station: -1. Pink cervical discharge present.

- Extremities: Full range of motion in body joints; no edema

Care Study Questions

1. Because every labor is different, it is not unusual for people to read any difference in labor as abnormal labor. Would these parents have benefited from a preparation for childbirth class? Are there reasons for attending such classes other than learning a method for pain relief?

Parents who are worried during labor that a child may be abnormal may experience a greater than usual amount of pain in labor because they cannot relax. Could that be adding to this patient's discomfort?

3. Mrs. Mazjewski has asked for pain relief in early labor. Complete a nursing care plan that will identify and meet the Mazjewski family's needs.

Cesarean Birth

Chapter 20 discusses the nursing role in caring for the woman undergoing both planned and unplanned cesarean birth. The types of surgery and incisions used, establishment of surgical risk, necessary preoperative procedures and teaching, and postoperative interventions including patient-controlled analgesia are discussed. The role of the nurse in promoting family-child interactions is stressed.

Caring for a cesarean birth client may be a beginning student's first introduction to caring for a surgical patient. Extra time needs to be spent with students to help them appreciate that the woman is not only a surgical client but a postpartum woman with special needs.

Chapter Objectives

After mastering the contents of this chapter, students should be able to:

1. Describe the indications for cesarean birth.
2. Assess a woman in terms of surgical risk for cesarean birth in order to plan nursing care preoperatively, intraoperatively, and postoperatively.
3. Formulate nursing diagnoses related to cesarean birth.
4. Plan nursing care such as preoperative teaching measures for cesarean birth or ways to maintain family-centered care.
5. Implement common preoperative and postoperative care measures for cesarean birth such as providing relief for pain.
6. Evaluate outcome criteria to be certain that goals for nursing care were achieved.
7. Identify national health goals related to cesarean birth that nurses can be instrumental in helping the nation to achieve.
8. Identify areas related to cesarean birth that could benefit from additional nursing research.
9. Use critical thinking to analyze common complications of cesarean birth and ways they can be prevented.
10. Synthesize knowledge of cesarean birth with nursing process to achieve quality maternal and child health nursing care.

Key Points

- The term cesarean "birth" is preferred to cesarean "section" because of the focus on the childbirth rather than surgery elements of the procedure.

- Cesarean birth may be either planned or unplanned. Cesarean birth is more hazardous to the infant than vaginal birth and is undertaken only when medically necessary.

- Establishing surgical risk should include assessment of nutritional status, age, general health, fluid and electrolyte balance, and psychological condition.

- Measures prior to surgery should include vital sign determination, urinalysis, blood studies such as complete blood count, electrolytes, blood typing and cross-matching, and sonography.

- Skin preparation for a cesarean incision is generally from under the breasts to the midthigh, including the pubic hair. The skin incision may be vertical (a classical incision), although it is usually a horizontal one just above the pubic hair. The internal incision into the uterus is also usually a horizontal incision into the lower uterine segment.

- The old saying "once a cesarean, always a cesarean" is no longer true, providing that a cephalopelvic disproportion does not exist and the previous incision was a low transverse one.

- When women have epidural or spinal anesthesia for cesarean birth, a support person can share the experience with them.

- Support people can lose a great deal of their ability to support if they feel intimidated and out of place in an operating room; offer support as needed to make this a positive experience for them as well.

- Cesarean birth is one of the safest types of surgery performed. To keep the woman safe following the procedure, remember that she is both a surgical and a postpartum client after the surgery. Make assessments to ensure neither postpartum nor postsurgical complications occur.

- Women are physically exhausted after cesarean birth and may be psychologically exhausted because of the emergency nature of the experience. Provide rest time to relieve the physical strain and a chance to verbalize the experience to help relieve the psychological strain.

- A major intervention after cesarean birth is early ambulation. The woman has incisional pain, making this difficult, and will require strong nursing support.
- Patient-controlled anesthesia (PCA) is an ideal method for providing pain relief after cesarean birth, because it allows a woman a sense of control as well as effective pain relief.

Definitions of Key Terms

cesarean birth: birth through an abdominal incision

classic cesarean incision: a vertical midline incision of the upper segment of the uterus

low cervical incision: a transverse incision in the supracervical portion of the uterus

patient-controlled analgesia: a medication delivery system whereby a client dispenses his/her own doses of IV narcotic analgesia

transcutaneous electrical nerve stimulation: a method of pain control by the application of electric impulses to nerve endings

Nursing Process Overview

The Nursing Process Overview for this chapter concentrates on helping students to focus on the overall goal of maternity care—a healthy mother and a healthy infant—and not solely on the unfortunate circumstances that necessitated a cesarean birth. Planning that includes anticipatory guidance and allows the family to grow from the experience is stressed.

Study Aids

Boxes

Box 20-1: Indications for Cesarean Birth
Box 20-2: Postoperative Vital Sign Parameters

Tables

Table 20-1: Drugs That May Result in Complications of Surgery

Procedures

Procedure 20-1: Preoperative Skin Preparation

Displays

Focus on National Health Goals

Focus on Family Teaching

Focus on Nursing Research

Focus on Cultural Awareness

Critical Thinking Exercises

1. Margorie is a woman you admit to a birthing room. When she is told that she will need to have a cesarean birth because her fetus is presenting breech, she begins to scream hysterically. What would be your best action?

2. Beth is a woman who has patient-controlled anesthesia ordered after a cesarean birth. She tells you she is not interested in this and would rather have injections for pain. What would be your action? Would you advocate

for use of PCA or advocate with her physician for a changed order?

3. Mr. Trevino tells you he cannot possibly stay with his wife in the operating room while she has a cesarean birth. He states he will feel nauseous and probably faint. His wife wants very badly to have him come with her. What would be your action?

Media Resources

Cesarean Delivery (30 minute video)

Nursing care interventions for the family experiencing a cesarean delivery are demonstrated.

Source: Medcom

Jan West, a 26-year-old Multipara Undergoing a C-section (CAI)

A simulation of a G3P2 at 38 weeks gestation who has an emergency cesarean birth due to fetal distress. Interactions span from time of birth to postpartum follow-up.

Source: J.B. Lippincott Company

Deliverance: A Family's Cesarean Experience (15 minute film/video)

A cesarean birth which is family oriented, shared, and moving, is shown. Emphasis is placed on adequate preparation, knowledge, and proper attitude as the key ingredients to a successful, enjoyable birth.

Source: Polymorph Films

If by Cesarean (20 minute video)

A video designed to encourage women to ask questions of their physicians well before labor. Reasons that cesareans are performed are presented. A cesarean being performed is shown. To contrast, a successful vaginal birth after cesarean (VBAC) is also shown.

Source: Polymorph Films

Discussion Questions

1. Discuss the advantages and disadvantages of referring to a cesarean procedure as a cesarean birth rather than a cesarean section.

2. Many women today have a second child by vaginal birth after cesarean birth (VBAC). How would you explain the risks and advantages of this to a pregnant woman trying to make an informed choice in this area?

3. What postpartal complications are most apt to occur following a cesarean birth? How can these be prevented?

Written Assignments

1. Preparing a woman for a cesarean birth differs in a number of ways from preparing a woman for other abdominal surgery. List and discuss these differences.

2. Investigate the incidence of cesarean birth at your practice setting. Analyze whether this is higher or lower than the national average. What factors are influencing this rate?

3. If a woman is awake for a cesarean birth, her support person is asked to observe. Describe the pros and cons of the support person observing if the woman will have a general anesthetic and so will not be awake.

Laboratory Experiences

1. Assign students to care for women who have experienced cesarean birth so they can better appreciate the increased level of pain and concern that occurs postpartally.

2. Ask a woman who underwent a planned cesarean birth and one who had an unplanned one to discuss their reactions to the procedures. Ask them to elaborate on how health care personnel could have been more helpful to them in alleviating their concerns.

3. Assign students to observe cesarean births not only so they can better understand the procedure to use in health teaching but for the opportunity to enlarge their own knowledge of pelvic anatomy.

Care Study: A Woman Needing a Cesarean Birth

Amy Steiner is a 30-year-old, G5P2, 38 week pregnant woman admitted to the maternity unit in active labor.

Health History

- Chief Concern: "I'm in labor."

- History of Present Illness: Labor began 6 hours ago with spontaneous rupture of membranes. Pattern has progressed from contractions 45 minutes apart and 20 seconds in duration to 3 minutes apart and 60 seconds in duration. Moderate amount of pink vaginal discharge present.

- History of Past Illnesses: Appendectomy at 14 years. Black mole removed from left shoulder at 26 years; no malignancy found on biopsy.

- Family Medical History: Mother died of cervical cancer when Amy was 20; grandfather and father have both had cerebral vascular accidents; sister has skin cancer.

- Gynecologic History: Menarche at 12; cycle duration is 28 days; length of flow: 5 days. No STDs. Used natural family planning to space children.

- Obstetric History: Early spontaneous abortion 6 years ago.

  Boy, 7'2" born 4 years ago; vaginal delivery, alive and well.

  Girl, 8'1" born 3 years ago; vaginal delivery, congenital hip dysplasia, corrected; alive and well.

Early spontaneous abortion 2 years ago.

This pregnancy was planned and wanted. Had prenatal care from private obstetrician/midwife practice since 2nd month. No complications or concerns. Sonogram at 20 weeks showed good fetal and placental growth. Alphafetoprotein level normal. Attended preparation for labor classes. States she "is a veteran" at labor.

- Personal/Social: Client works as buyer for department store, part-time. Husband, 36 years old, is an assistant district attorney. Finances are "good." Couple owns an older home in a restored section of the inner city. Is aware of the danger of lead paint in older homes.

- Nutrition: 24-hour nutrition recall reveals adequate pregnancy diet. Prenatal vitamin taken daily.

- Review of Systems: Skin: concerned about developing skin cancer as she used to spend entire summers exposed to sun as a life guard. Genitourinary: frequent yeast infections she treats herself with over-the-counter fungicide suppositories.

- Extremities: swelling of ankles since 30th week of pregnancy.

Physical Examination

- General Appearance: Relaxed appearing pregnant woman with marked swelling of ankles present. Height: 5'3". Weight: 144 lbs. BP: 117/70.

- HEENT: Slight swelling of gumline noted.

- Chest: Heart rate: 72; no murmur present. Lungs sounds clear to auscultation; rate: 22/minute.

- Abdomen: Fundal height: 36 cm; fetus palpated to be in left occiput position by Leopold's maneuver's; head not engaged. FHR: 190/minute. Contractions occurring at 3 to 7 minute frequency, 60 second duration; moderate intensity.

- Pelvic Exam: Varicosity of left labia noted. Cervical dilation approximately 5 cm with little effacement. Station: -1. Umbilical cord palpated in vagina.

- Extremities: Prominent varicosity present on medial aspect of left thigh.

Care Study Questions

1. Prolapsed cord is always a serious complication during labor. What emergency steps would you want to take when this occurs?

2. This is an emergency situation. Complete a nursing care plan for this family that would identify and meet their immediate care needs.

The Woman Who Develops a Complication During Labor and Delivery

Chapter 21 discusses care of the woman and family when a complication of labor and delivery occurs. Problems that occur as the result of the force of labor such as hypotonic and hypertonic contractions, precipitate labor, uterine rupture, inversion of the uterus, and amniotic fluid embolism; problems with the passenger such as prolapse of the cord, multiple gestation, occipitoposterior position, and malformation of the placenta; and problems with the passage such as pelvic contraction are discussed. The nursing role when augmentation by oxytocin and vacuum or forceps extraction are used is included. Promotion of family-child bonding in the face of a complication of labor is stressed.

Not all students have the opportunity to care for a woman who develops a complication in labor because the incidence of these complications is low. Such content is important, however, as it helps the student to appreciate what problems can occur and encourages students to complete careful, meaningful assessment on all clients in labor.

Chapter Objectives

After mastering the contents of this chapter, students should be able to:

1. Define the general term "dystocia" and the common deviations in the force of labor, the passage, or passenger that can cause dystocia.

2. Assess the woman in labor and during birth for deviations from the usual labor process.

3. Formulate nursing diagnoses related to deviations from normal in labor and delivery.

4. Plan nursing interventions such as helping a woman prepare for a cesarean birth or augmentation of labor that will help the family meet established goals.

5. Implement care related to potential complications in labor or birth, such as those caused by breech presentation, multiple gestation, fetal distress, and prolapsed cord.

6. Evaluate outcome criteria to ensure that nursing goals related to deviations from the normal in labor and birth were achieved.

7. Identify national health goals related to complications of labor that nurses can be instrumental in helping the nation to achieve.

8. Identify areas related to complications of labor that could benefit from additional nursing research.

9. Use critical thinking to analyze ways that nursing care can be kept family centered when deviations from the normal in labor and birth occur.

10. Synthesize the knowledge of deviations from normal in labor and delivery with nursing process to achieve quality maternal and child health nursing care.

Key Points

- Complications of labor arise from problems with the force of labor, the passage, or the passenger. Hypotonic, hypertonic, and uncoordinated contractions all can occur resulting in ineffective first or second stages of labor.

- Precipitate labor is delivery that is completed in less than 3 hours. It can be responsible for subdural hemorrhage in the fetus and cervical lacerations in the mother.

- Uterine rupture is a rare occurrence that is suggested by a pathologic retraction or constriction ring (an indentation across the abdomen over the uterus).

- Uterine inversion is a grave complication. If the situation is not immediately corrected, emergency hysterectomy is necessary to save the woman's life. Almost all occurrences of uterine inversion can be avoided by two axioms of care: __do not put pressure on an uncontracted fundus immediately postpartum__ (massage first to cause it to contract); and **do not exert pressure on an umbilical cord to achieve placental delivery**. Patience will achieve the same result in most instances and do it safely.

- Amniotic fluid embolism occurs when amniotic fluid is forced into an open maternal uterine blood sinus. The woman notices chest pain and dyspnea. Administer oxygen and notify the woman's primary care provider of this emergency.

- Prolapse of the umbilical cord is an emergency situation that requires prompt action. Often, the nurse is the person with the woman when this occurs. Position the woman quickly into either a trendelenburg or knee-chest position to relieve cord compression; cover the cord with sterile, saline-soaked pads; and notify the woman's physician of the emergency. With cord prolapse, there are fewer than 5 minutes to institute relief measures to prevent irreparable central nervous system damage to the infant.

- Multiple gestation can complicate delivery. Many infants of multiple gestations are delivered by cesarean birth.

- Abnormal position, presentation, or size of the fetus, including occipitoposterior position, breech, face, or brow presentation and transverse lie, as well as problems of the passage such as inlet and outlet contraction can lead to labor complications.

- Be certain that a woman meets the criteria for labor induction before preparing an oxytocin solution: no cephalopelvic disproportion is suspected; the fetal head is engaged and the cervix is "ripe." Question an order if the above criteria are not present.

- Always prepare oxytocin as a "piggyback" solution, being extremely careful of the dose used. Both a uterine and FHR monitor should be used continuously during labor induction. Observe that contractions occur no more than 2 minutes apart and are no longer than 70 seconds in duration.

- Increase oxytocin flow rate only in increments of 2 to 4 mU to avoid causing hypertonic contractions or uterine tetany. Urge and support the woman to use breathing exercises and to remain on her left side during a labor induction to offer a good blood supply to the uterine muscle.

- If uterine contractions should become too strong or too frequent or fetal bradycardia, tachycardia, or abnormal decelerations should occur, discontinue an oxytocin solution immediately. Do not increase the rate of oxytocin more than 16 mU/min without specific directions to do so because this high a rate invariably leads to tonic uterine contractions.

- Anomalies of the placenta and cord such as placenta succenturiata, placenta circumvallata, battledore placenta, or a two-vessel cord can lead to delivery complications.

- Vacuum extraction and forceps delivery are methods to assist delivery. Both mother and infant need special observation following these procedures.

Definitions of Key Terms

amniotic fluid embolism: a substance causing blockage in a maternal blood vessel caused by passage of amniotic fluid into the maternal blood stream

augmentation of labor: strengthening labor contractions by the use of a technique such as intravenous oxytocin

battledore placenta: a placenta with the umbilical cord inserted on the periphery rather than the center

cephalopelvic disproportion: a delivery condition in which the mother's pelvis is too small or too misshaped to allow the infant's head to pass through; the most common reason for which cesarean birth is performed

constriction ring: an indentation horizontally across the uterus which denotes extreme stress on the divisions of the organ

dysfunctional labor: labor that progresses slower than usual due to ineffective contractions

dystocia: difficult delivery

external cephalic version: rotating a fetus into a cephalic lie by external maneuvers against the mother's abdomen

forceps birth: birth by the means of forceps to extract the fetus

hypertonic uterine contractions: contractions that maintain a high resting tone

hypotonic uterine contractions: contractions that are infrequent and ineffective

induction of labor: artificial stimulation of labor by a technique such as intravenous oxytocin

oxytocin: a hormone secreted by the posterior pituitary; acts to maintain and strengthen uterine contractions

pathologic retraction ring: an indentation horizontally across the uterus which denotes extreme stress on the divisions of the organ

placenta accreta: abnormal adherence of the placenta to the uterine wall, making placental delivery very difficult

placenta circumvallata: a placenta with the fetal surface covered by chorion

placenta marginata: a placenta with the edge of the fetal surface covered by chorion

placenta succenturiata: a placenta with one or more accessory lobes

precipitate labor: labor with uterine contractions so strong that the woman delivers with only a few rapidly occurring contractions

umbilical cord prolapse: an umbilical cord that is presenting at the cervix prior to birth of the fetus

uterine inversion: turning inside out of the uterus; could occur following childbirth from an action such as pulling on the umbilical cord before the placenta separates

vacuum extraction: delivery of a fetus by suction applied to the presenting part

Nursing Process Overview

The Nursing Process Overview for this chapter concentrates on helping students to use nursing process in emergency situations. Developing short-term goals for the length of the emergency are stressed. Including parents in planning to the extent possible so they can retain a sense of control over their situation is included.

Study Aids

Boxes

Box 21-1:   Common Causes of Dysfunctional Labor

Box 21-2:   Conditions High Risk for Prolapsed Cord

Box 21-3:   Causes of Breech Presentation

Box 21-4:   Apt Test

Tables

Table 21-1:   Comparison of Hypotonic and Hypertonic Contractions

Table 21-2:   Length of Phases of Stages of Normal Labor in Hours

Table 21-3:   Classification of Breech Presentations

Table 21-4:   Scoring of Cervix for Readiness for Elective Induction

Table 21-5:   Solution Concentration of Oxytocin with Various Dilutions

Table 21-6:   Common Types of Delivery Forceps

Displays

Focus on National Health Goals

Focus on Family Teaching

Focus on Nursing Research

Critical Thinking Exercises

1. Josiah and Eva are a young couple having their first child. After rupture of membranes, you notice that the fetal monitor shows variable decelerations. On inspection, you are able to see the cord at the vaginal opening. You are aware that this is a fetal emergency. List the steps you would take in order of their priority.

2. Brenda is a 23-year-old having her first child. Her obstetrician has told her that her baby is in a posterior position. She asks you what this means in terms of the length and type of her labor. How would you answer her?

3. Mrs. Cranley began labor spontaneously at 10 AM. Mrs. Bellow had an oxytocin infusion for induction of labor at 10 AM because her pregnancy has extended 2 weeks beyond her expected due date. Which woman would you anticipate will deliver first? Will both women be able to use breathing exercises with contractions? What are the priority observations to make with Mrs. Cranley? With Mrs. Bellow?

Media Resources

Labor and Delivery Augmentation (30 minute video)

Nursing care indicated for the woman during labor stimulation with oxytocin is demonstrated.

Source: Medcom

Mirna and Mario—Birth #3 (10 minute video)

Mirna and Mario are shown having their fourth child. Mirna is induced with pitocin because she has a history of precipitous labors and is already at 42 weeks.

Source: Polymorph Films

A Complicated Delivery in Maternity Nursing (CAI)

A simulation of a complicated delivery of a client. Objectives are to identify nursing diagnoses based on analysis of data and to select appropriate nursing interventions.

Source: Medi-Sim, Inc.

To Touch Today (24 minute video)

Discusses how parental love and bonding develop and the dimensions of mourning that bereaved parents experience. Offers supportive suggestions to the parents during their period of mourning.

Source: Health Sciences Consortium

Some Babies Die (54 minute film)

A documentary following a family coping with the death of their newborn and the counseling process that encourages them to acknowledge their baby's life and death and allows grieving to begin. Narrated by Dr. Elizabeth Kubler-Ross.

Source: University of California Extension Media

Discussion Questions

1. Mrs. Taylor is a woman whose fetus is found to be in a breech presentation and thus will be delivered by a cesarean birth. What are the reasons that cesarean birth is most often the choice for a breech presentation today?

2. A lengthy labor is both a physical and psychological stress to a woman and her support person. What measures could you take to lessen a couple's stress?

3. A woman with a complication of labor will have continual external and possibly internal fetal monitoring throughout labor. What are measures you would use to keep her from feeling overwhelmed by the technology applied so she still remains in control of what is happening to her?

Written Assignments

1. While caring for Mrs. Herman in labor, you notice a prolapsed cord has occurred. List the emergency care actions you would take.

2. Graph the process of a woman's labor using a Friedman graph. Analyze whether it falls into the usual pattern or not. At what point would you notify the physician that you are concerned with the woman's progress?

3. Fetal scalp blood sampling is a technique often used to assess fetal well being when a complication of labor occurs. List the nursing responsibilities concerned with this procedure.

Laboratory Experiences

1. Assign students to a clinical setting where high-risk women are cared for. As not all students will be able to participate in these experiences, have students share perceptions of the experience at postconference, particularly in reference to how to prepare women for all the technical procedures that may be necessary.

2. Ask a woman who had a complication of labor and delivery but had a satisfactory outcome to come to a postconference and discuss her feelings during the time of labor and delivery. Could she have been better prepared for this? How could health care personnel have been more helpful to her?

3. Complications of labor and delivery produce emergency situations. Hold a contest where students draw a slip of paper listing a complication of labor and delivery and write on the blackboard the steps of care and the rationale for these they would initiate. Compare the responses to see which students best understand the correct steps.

Care Study: A Woman With a Complication of Labor

Barbara Deska is a 24-year-old, G2P1, 41 week pregnant woman admitted to the maternity service in active labor.

Health History

- Chief Concern: "I'm in labor and there's something wrong."

- History of Present Illness: Client was alerted at last prenatal visit that her fetus was in a posterior position so labor might be long. Contractions began 8 hours ago; pattern has never become regular. Contractions 5 to 30 minutes apart; duration about 30 seconds. Having back pain with contractions and asking to have something for pain relief.

- History of Past Illnesses: Near-drowning accident in neighbor's pool at 2 years; revived by paramedics with no apparent sequelae; tonsillectomy at 7 years. No major illnesses or hospitalizations except for previous childbirth.

- Family Medical History: Maternal aunt has child with Down syndrome; client's father died of liver failure from alcoholism at 45. Husband's family has "many" people with peptic ulcers.

- Gynecologic History: Menarche at 14 years; cycle duration 28 days; length of menstrual flow: 7 days. Treated for exposure to syphilis at 18 years. Uses vaginal foam as contraceptive.

- Obstetric History: Spontaneous abortion 4 years ago. Boy, 8'4'', vaginal delivery, born 3 years ago with Down syndrome. This pregnancy was planned and welcomed. Attended late for prenatal care (6th month)

because of finances. No amniocentesis or CVS for chromosomal studies done because of lateness of care. No preparation for labor class attended. "Not interested in being brave" given as reason.

- Personal/Social: Client not employed as she volunteers days at center for retarded children where son attends preschool. Husband works as a garage mechanic. Finances are "tight." Couple lives in a furnished apartment in paternal grandmother's house. Marriage is "shaky" due to strain of finances, family disagreements, and "getting married before we knew each other very well."

- Nutrition: 24-hour nutrition recall reveals diet high in carbohydrate and low in protein. Prenatal vitamin not taken.

Physical Examination

- General Appearance: Distressed and exhausted appearing obese, young adult pregnant woman. Height: 5'3''; weight: 170 lbs; BP: 135/86.

- HEENT: negative.

- Chest: Heart rate: 76/minute; physiologic splitting marked. Lungs: clear to auscultation; respiratory rate: 20/minute.

- Abdomen: Fundal height: 38 cm. Fetus palpated to be in left occiput posterior position and large by Leopold's movements. Head fixed in pelvis. FHR: 150/minute.

- Pelvic Examination: Diagonal conjugate measured at 12 cm. Pubic arch wide; ischial diameter: 12 cm; coccyx movable. Cervical dilation: 4 cm; effacement: 20%. Station: 0.

- Extremities: unremarkable.

Care Study Questions

1. Mrs. Deska did not attend either prenatal care or a preparation for labor class because of finances. If finances were this tight, could there have been other things that she omitted during pregnancy?

2. Mrs. Deska has an oxytocin infusion prescribed for her to augment labor. How would you explain this to her? How would you physically prepare her for it?

3. Complete a nursing care plan that would identify and meet the needs of the Deska family.

Nursing Care of the Postpartal Woman and Family

Chapter 22 discusses care of the woman and family during the 6 weeks of the postpartal period. Psychological and physiologic changes, physical assessment, and nursing care to promote comfort and healing are included. The importance of promoting early and consistent family-child interaction is stressed.

As many woman read extensively about pregnancy, they are well informed about what to expect during this time. In contrast, women may read very little about changes expected after birth. Students in nursing, therefore, almost immediately begin to use the information they learn about the period in client teaching. This helps them grasp concepts quickly as they appreciate its importance and usefulness.

Chapter Objectives

After mastering the contents of this chapter, students should be able to:

1. Describe the psychological and physiologic changes that occur in the postpartal woman.

2. Assess a woman and her family for physiologic and psychological changes following childbirth.

3. State nursing diagnoses related to physiologic and psychological changes of the postpartal period.

4. Plan nursing care such as measures to aid uterine involution or encourage bonding.

5. Implement nursing care such as helping aide the progression of physiologic changes or psychological family changes.

6. Evaluate outcome criteria to be certain that goals for nursing care were achieved.

7. Identify national health goals related to the postpartal period that nurses can be instrumental in helping the nation to achieve.

8. Identify areas related to care of the postpartal family that could benefit from additional nursing research.

9. Use critical thinking to analyze ways that postpartum nursing care can be more family centered.

10. Synthesize knowledge of the physiologic and psychological changes of the postpartal period with the nursing process to achieve quality maternal and child health nursing care.

Key Points

- The postpartal period or the puerperium is the 6-week period following childbirth.

- The postpartal period is an important one for a family as it marks the beginning of the child's introduction to the family. Women can be seen to move through an initial "taking-in" phase in which they are dependent, a "taking-hold" phase in which they manifest independence, and a "letting-go" phase in which the mother role is finally defined.

- Rooming-in is the preferred health care agency arrangement for postpartal families as it allows the new family the best chance for quality interaction. The more time new parents spend with a newborn, the more likely it is that effective bonding will occur. Help parents to feel comfortable with their newborn by offering anticipatory guidance and role modeling of infant care.

- "Postpartal blues" are a normal accompaniment to childbirth. Women need assurance that this is normal and supportive care until the emotion passes.

- Uterine involution is the process whereby the uterus returns to its prepregnant state. A uterus decreases in size 1 fingerbreadth a day until it disappears under the pelvic bone at about day 10. Lochia is the name of the vaginal flow following childbirth. This is lochia rubra (red) for the first 3 to 4 days; lochia serosa (pink to brown) until day 7 to 10; and lochia alba (white) until 2 to 6 weeks.

- A woman is at great risk for hemorrhage in the postpartal period, so assessments done during this time are some of the most critical assessments made in nursing. Don't discount the importance of these assessments because the overall content of the postpartal period is so focused on wellness.

- Lactation is the production of breast milk. Colostrum is present immediately after birth; milk forms on the 3rd to 4th postpartal day. A feeling of warmth and tension on this day is termed engorgement.

- Women may need various comfort measures to alleviate pain from sutures, uterine pain (afterpains), and breast tenderness. Application of warmth and administration of analgesics are important nursing interventions.
- Women need teaching about self care before health care agency discharge so they can maintain self care at home. Follow-up by a telephone call or home visit is helpful. All women should conscientiously return for a 6-week visit to be certain that their reproductive organs have returned to normal. A menstrual flow should return 6 to 10 weeks following birth in the nonbreastfeeding mother, and 3 to 4 months in the breastfeeding mother.

Definitions of Key Terms

afterpains: alternating contracting and relaxation of the uterine muscle following birth to accomplish involution. Most noticeable in women who are multigravida and nursing

diastasis recti: a separation of the rectus abdominis muscle

en face position: a position in which one person looks at another with his or her face in the same vertical plane as the other; the typical position in which a mother holds her newborn

engorgement: local congestion of the breasts associated with lactation

Homans' sign: pain in the calf of the leg on dorsiflexion of the foot; an indication of a thrombophlebitis in a vein in the calf

involution: the return of the uterus to its nonpregnant state.

letting-go phase: Rubin's last stage of postpartal adjustment during which the mother redefines her new role as a mother

lochia alba: a whitish vaginal discharge during the postpartal period

lochia rubra: a red vaginal discharge similar to a menstrual flow during the postpartal period

lochia serosa: a pinkish-brown vaginal discharge during the postpartal period

rooming-in: a postpartal care pattern in which the neonate stays in the mother's room rather than a separate nursery in order to encourage maternal-infant bonding

sitz bath: a bath in which only the hips and buttocks are submerged

taking-hold phase: the second phase of postpartal adjustment according to Rubin in which the mother begins to take an active role in child care

taking-in phase: the first phase of postpartal adjustment according to Rubin in which the mother is chiefly interested in her own care

uterine atony: lack of uterine tone that leads to hemorrhage

Nursing Process Overview

The Nursing Process Overview for this chapter concentrates on helping students to formulate nursing diagnoses that can be realistically measured within the short time frame that postpartal families remain in hospitals or birthing centers. The importance for establishing care that is family centered and allows parent-child interaction to begin is included. The responsibility for teaching women evaluation criteria so they can continue to monitor their health after they return home is stressed.

Study Aids

Boxes

Box 22-1:   Signs of Good Parent-Child Adaptation

Tables

Table 22-1:   Characteristics of Lochia

Table 22-2:   Timetable for Nursing Interventions: Postpartum

Table 22-3:   Muscle-Strengthening Exercises

Table 22-4:   Postpartal Discharge Instructions

Table 22-5:   Six-Week Physical Assessment

Procedures

Procedure 22-1:   Sitz Baths

Displays

Focus on National Health Goals

Focus on Family Teaching

Focus on Nursing Research

Focus on Cultural Awareness

Critical Thinking Exercises

1. Liz is a 25-year-old woman 1 day postpartal. She delivered an 8 lb girl without an episiotomy incision. You thought she would have little perineal discomfort because she does not have stitches. Instead, she states her perineal pain is excruciating. You notice she has hemorrhoids. What could you suggest to Liz to make her more comfortable?

2. Marsha Taylor is an 18-year-old woman 1 day postpartal. You hear her telling her husband that he is acting selfishly for paying more attention to their new son than her. You notice that she hands her baby roughly to her husband. Would you be concerned about the Taylor family? What additional information would you want to know before you reached a firm conclusion of the new family's health?

3. Mrs. Acker is a woman you see at a 6 week postpartal checkup. What are the specific assessments you would want to make to feel confident that Mrs. Acker has physically and emotionally adjusted well to childbirth?

Media Resources

Postpartum Nursing Assessment (22 minute video)

Techniques of assessment for physiologic and psychosocial changes that occur during the first 7 to 10 days postpartum are presented. Identification of specific areas for nursing interventions is stressed.

Source: Health Sciences Consortium

Postpartum Physical Assessment (20 minute video)

Systematic assessment of the postpartum client is presented.

Source: AVC Nursing Series

The Twelve-Point Check (CAI)

A clinical simulation that guides the learner through a 12-point postpartum assessment. Can be used as tutorial, clinical simulation, or competency testing at the instructor's or learner's discretion.

Source: J.B. Lippincott Company

Right From the Start (55 minute video)

The importance of early contact between mother, father, and newborn is explored. The research of various experts—Harlow, Spitz, Bowlby, and Brazelton, for example—are cited to prove the importance of bonding. Klaus and Kennell's research is described in detail.

Source: Prime Time School Television

Discussion Questions

1. Many women remain in a health care facility only 24 hours following delivery. What is important health-teaching information prior to discharge for such women?

2. What is the advantage of asking a woman to fill out a standardized form such as the neonatal-perception inventory to evaluate her relationship with her newborn rather than just observing her?

3. Sibling visitation is allowing older children to visit a new baby in the hospital or birthing center. What would you teach a mother in regard to how to prepare children for this experience?

Written Assignments

1. Write a paragraph describing the phases of taking in, taking hold, and letting go, of Rubin's theory on adjustment to parenting.

2. List the normal parameters of a lochia flow.

3. Assessing a woman for bladder filling postpartally is a major nursing responsibility. List and describe the measures you would use to do this.

Laboratory Experiences

1. Assign students to postpartal hospital units so they can care for women and their infants during the postpartal period.

2. Ask a postpartal client to come to postconference and describe how little she knew about what to expect postpartally and in what ways she would like to have been better prepared.

3. Ask students to make a home visit on a postpartal client they care for. Ask them to compare how the woman's concepts of what problems she expected after she returned home coincided with problems that actually occurred.

Care Study: A Postpartal Woman

Faye Chang is a 28-year-old, G4P3 woman cared for in a labor-delivery-recovery room following delivery of a 6'13'' girl.

Health History

- Chief Concern: "Pain. Lots of it. And I'm worried about taking a baby so small home because we own two cats. Don't cats suck the breath out of small babies?"

- History of Present Concern: Client delivered a 6'13'' infant girl, 37 weeks gestation, at 1:05 PM with no analgesia other than local xylocaine for episiotomy repair. Now at 3:00 PM she reports "sharp and pulling" perineal pain. Is concerned that new baby is abnormally small because other children both were over 8 pounds at birth.

- History of Past Illnesses: Venomous snake bite at age 15 years while on a camping trip. Antivenin given immediately; no sequelae. Hospitalized for three previous childbirths. Was followed for 1 year for hydatidiform mole 8 years ago.

- Gynecologic History: Menarche at age 17; cycle duration: 30 days. Menstrual flow duration: 7 days. Both she and sexual partner were treated for chlamydia X 1 last year. Was relying on sexual partner to use condoms as method of reproductive life planning prior to last pregnancy.

- Obstetric History: Hydatidiform mole pregnancy, 8 years ago. Followed for 1 year with HCG levels. Never any elevation in levels.

  Boy, 8'6'', vaginal delivery, alive and well, 4 years ago.

  Boy, 8'8'', vaginal delivery, alive and well, 3 years ago.

  Girl, 6'13'', vaginal delivery, 2 hours ago, no anomalies at birth. Pregnancy was not planned but not unwelcome.

- Personal/Social: Client was married at 20 years but marriage ended after trophoblast proliferation pregnancy. Currently living with a boyfriend in a 2-bedroom house; works as a clerk in a mail catalog house part-time. Boyfriend works as a taxi driver. Finances are reported as "okay." Boyfriend appeared supportive throughout labor. Voiced pleasure at sex and appearance of new child.

- Review of Systems: Essentially negative.

Physical Examination

- General Appearance: Distressed appearing, Asian heritage, young adult woman.

- HEENT: Hair: unwashed; oily. Some postpartal hair loss beginning.

- Chest: Heart rate: 70/minute; no murmurs present. Lungs: no adventitious sounds present; respiratory rate: 22/minute.

- Abdomen: Soft; fundal height 1 F under umbilicus and firm and midline. Linea nigra and striae present.

- Perineum: Edematous; mediolateral episiotomy line intact. Lochia: rubra, moderate, no clots. A 4 cm wide purple colored, warm to touch elevated lesion is present at distal end of episiotomy incision.

- Extremities: Homans' sign negative; no edema over tibia

Care Study Questions

1. Ms. Chang voices a common superstition, that cats suck the breath out of babies. How do you imagine such a superstition originated? Is it related to sudden infant death syndrome? In light of this worry, what position would you want to tell Ms. Chang to always place her infant when she puts him down to sleep?

2. Ms. Chang is going to be very busy after she returns home with three children under four to care for. What suggestions would you want to give her regarding rest and nutrition? Jealousy can be a major problem with preschool children. What would you advise her about this?

3. Complete a care plan that would identify and meet the needs of the Chang family.

Nursing Care of the Newborn and Family

Chapter 23 discusses nursing care of the newborn and family immediately following birth and in the first few weeks at home. Physiologic adjustment to birth, physical characteristics of newborns including gestational age assessment, and birthing room care are discussed. Suggestions for encouraging family-child interaction are stressed. The controversy of circumcision and newer techniques of administering analgesia are presented.

Nursing care of the newborn is a specialty area so many students in nursing are not aware prior to studying the content how much specific care and assessment is given to newborns. Such content forms the foundation for teaching families about newborn care and beginning family-child interaction. Practicing Apgar, Dubowitz, and behavioral assessments on newborns helps students appreciate the advantages of standardized measures or improves their understanding of nursing research.

Chapter Objectives

After mastering the contents of this chapter, students should be able to:

1. Describe characteristics of the term newborn.
2. Assess a newborn for normal growth and development.
3. Formulate nursing diagnoses related to the newborn and/or family of the newborn.
4. Plan nursing care to enhance normal development of the newborn, such as ways to aid parent-child bonding.
5. Implement nursing care of the normal newborn such as administering the first bath or instructing parents on how to care for their newborn.
6. Evaluate outcome criteria to be certain that goals of nursing care have been achieved.
7. Identify national health goals related to newborns that nurses can be instrumental in helping the nation to achieve.

8. Identify areas related to newborn assessment and care that could benefit from additional nursing research.
9. Use critical thinking to analyze ways in which the care of the term newborn can be more family centered.
10. Synthesize knowledge of newborn growth and development and immediate care needs with nursing process to achieve quality maternal and child health nursing care.

Key Points

- Converting from fetal to adult respiratory function is a major step in adaptation to extrauterine life. Newborns need particularly close observation during the first few hours of life to determine that this adaptation has been made adequately.

- Monitoring body heat is a second major problem of newborns. The temperature of the baby's environment should be about 75°F (24°C). When procedures that require undressing the infant for an extended period of time are being done (eg, circumcision), a radiant heat source should be used.

- Newborns may suffer hypoglycemia in the first few hours of life because they use energy to establish respirations and maintain heat. Signs of jitteriness or a serum glucose under 45 mg by Dextrostix help to identify hypoglycemia.

- Identification bands should be attached securely; careful assessment of these bands should be carried out before hospital discharge. To help prevent the possibility of kidnapping on a newborn unit be certain of the identification of anyone to whom you give a newborn.

- So that parents can feel confident with newborn care, they need to hold and give care to newborns in the hospital. Encouraging them to spend as much time as possible with the newborn and to give care is a major nursing role.

- The best method of care for newborns and their mothers is rooming-in, as this allows women to have maximum contact with their new baby.

Definitions of Key Terms

acrocyanosis: mottled cyanosis of hands and feet; a normal finding in newborns

caput succedaneum: a localized edematous area on the scalp of a newborn caused by pressure on the presenting part of the head against the cervix during labor

cavernous hemangioma: dilated vascular spaces

cephalhematoma: an elevated area on a newborn's head caused by the extravasation of blood between the skull bone and its periosteum from the pressure of birth

conduction: the transfer of body heat to a cooler solid object in contact with a newborn

convection: the flow of heat from the body surface to cooler surrounding air

Crede treatment: the application of antibacterial therapy to a newborn's eyes

erythema toxicum: rash of the newborn marked by minute papules on an erythematous base caused from the first exposure to environmental contaminants

evaporation: the loss of heat through conversion of a liquid to a vapor

hemangioma: a collection of blood vessels forming a birth mark

jaundice: a yellow color of the skin or mucous membrane caused by an increase in bilirubin

kernicterus: accumulation of indirect bilirubin in brain cells causing cell destruction

lanugo: the fine, downy hair formed on the shoulders and back of the fetus

meconium: the first stool of the newborn, dark green or black in color

milia: minute, white papules commonly found on the nose and cheeks of neonates; unopened sebaceous glands

mongolian spot: a slate gray area of pigment on the skin of the neonate

natal teeth: erupted teeth in the newborn.

neonate: an infant during the first 28 days of life

neonatal period: the first 28 days of life

nevus flammeus: a permanent, port-wine colored birthmark

physiologic jaundice: yellowing of the skin that occurs from the normal breakdown of red blood cells at birth in the newborn

radiation: loss of heat to a distant cold surface

strawberry hemangioma: a benign tumor of newly formed blood vessels

subconjunctival hemorrhage: blood visible on the sclera from a ruptured conjunctival vessel

thrush: candidiasis of the mouth

transitional stool: green-colored stool that occurs in newborns following meconium and prior to yellow breastfed or formula-fed infant stools

vernix caseosa: the cream——cheese——like covering of the fetus to protect it from water maceration

Nursing Process Overview

The Nursing Process Overview for this chapter concentrates on helping students to formulate nursing diagnoses and set goals when their client is unable to participate actively in decision making. The importance of assessing for adaptation to extrauterine life is stressed. Techniques for planning with parents (family-centered care) is stressed.

Study Aids

Boxes

Box 23-1: Behavioral Items Assessed on the Brazelton Neonatal Behavioral Assessment Scale

Tables

Table 23-1: Changes in the Cardiovascular System at Birth

Table 23-2: Periods of Reactivity: Normal Adjustment to Extrauterine Life

Table 23-3: Apgar Scoring Chart

Table 23-4: Congenital Anomaly Appraisal

Table 23-5: Clinical Criteria for Gestational Assessment

Table 23-6: Categories on Brazelton's Neonatal Behavioral Assessment

Displays

Focus on National Health Goals

Focus on Family Teaching

Focus on Nursing Research

Critical Thinking Exercises

1. Baby Dowe is a newborn you examine at birth. What newborn reflexes would you assess with him? Suppose it is cold in the room so you only have time to test one reflex. Which one would you test? Why?

2. Baby Okasuki is a newborn with a macular purple (port-wine) lesion on her left thigh. Her parents tell you they are not concerned because they know all birthmarks fade by the time children are school-age. Do you agree with their statement? Suppose this type of lesion is one that doesn't fade? Would it be better to tell the parents this or not?

3. The Towers family is getting ready to go home from the hospital with their newborn when you discover that they have no car seat to transport the baby. What would you do? Ask them to stay until they arrange to rent or borrow one? Suppose they insist on putting the baby in the car without a car seat? Do you have a legal obligation to detain them in the health care agency?

Media Resources

The Sensational Baby (30 minute slide-tape, video, film)

Fetal reactions to sensory stimuli are explored. Effects of labor on a fetus and infants reacting to their parents at birth are shown.

Source: Polymorph Films

Immediate Assessment and Care of the Newborn (CAI)

A simulation focusing on the assessment and related nursing interventions which are needed to support the neonate's initial adaptation to extrauterine life. The learner interacts with newborn Tim and his parents from the moment of birth to Tim's transfer to the newborn nursery.

Source: J.B. Lippincott Company

Newborn (28 minute film)

Three neonatal researchers—T. Berry Brazelton, Lewis Lipsitt, and Louis Sander—are shown testing newborns. An impressive array of newborn reflexes, sensory abilities, and learning potential is demonstrated.

Source: Filmmakers Library

Dubowitz Assessment of the Newborn Gestational Age (44 minute film, video)

The examination and scoring of a term baby and two preterm infants of 30 and 36 weeks gestation for gestational age are shown.

Source: Polymorph Film

Physical Assessment of the Normal Newborn (30 minute video)

A systematic assessment of the normal newborn is presented. Stimuli to elicit and newborn reflexes are included.

Source: J.B. Lippincott Company

Physical Examination of the Newborn (18 minute video)

A nurse performing a complete physical examination of the newborn is shown. Included is general appearance and assessment of all body systems.

Source: Health Sciences Consortium

Appraisal of the Newborn (26 minute video)

Physical examination of a normal newborn infant is demonstrated. Existing abnormalities are identified and a basis upon which changes can be assessed is provided.

Source: AJN Company Educational Services Division

Perinatal Assessment of Maturity (20 minute video)

Three steps necessary to assess a newborn's maturity are described: determining the gestational age with a physical and neurologic exam, plotting the infant's weight on an intrauterine growth chart to determine size for gestational age, and analysis of this information.

Source: Health Sciences Consortium

LaNewborn Baby (simulated model)

A model of a lifelike baby only one day old with umbilical cord still visible and a ''soft spot'' on sculptured head. Soft vinyl body with jointed arms and legs. Anatomically correct. 20'' long.

Source: Nasco Health Care Educational Materials

Baby Care Demonstration Kit (simulated models)

A kit including a doll and articles for demonstrating infant bathing and feeding, plus a book of infant care instructions.

Source: Nasco Health Care Educational Materials

Discussion Questions

1. It is important when doing physical assessment of newborns to prevent them from becoming chilled during the process. How would you control this in a birthing room? A hospital nursery?

2. Performing a newborn assessment by a mother's bedside helps her get acquainted with her infant. What findings in a newborn would be most important to discuss with her?

3. Deciding whether to have an infant circumcised or not is a decision new parents must make. What are the pros and cons of circumcision?

Written Assignments

1. Determining an Apgar score can be a nursing responsibility. List what observations you would complete and how you would rate them for this score.

2. Newborns are administered vitamin K at birth. Write a paragraph explaining the rationale for this.

3. Assessing newborn reflexes is a vital part of newborn assessment. List and describe how to elicit common newborn reflexes.

Laboratory Experiences

1. Assign students to newborn nurseries and ask them to complete a newborn examination including newborn reflexes.

2. Ask students to complete a Dubowitz examination and rate the infant as to gestational age.

3. Assign students to newborns born 12 hours apart from each other. Ask students to compare the infants as to their stage of reactivity.

4. Assign students to labor and delivery settings so they can see Apgar scoring being recorded. Ask them to score an infant and compare their findings with the official score given.

Care Study: An Infant Born Breech

Jordina Farmer is a 1-day-old female who was born from a frank breech position.

Health History

- Chief Concern: ''She looks funny and maybe has some brain damage.''

- History of Chief Concern: Labor began with ruptured membranes; amniotic fluid was stained ''dark green.'' When Mrs. Farmer arrived at hospital, a sonogram was done and she was told that fetus was presenting breech; as dilatation was already at 8 cm, she was allowed to give birth vaginally. Infant was born with aid of Piper forceps; was intubated immediately to assess for meconium. None visualized beyond vocal cords. Apgars 9 and 9. Retains intrauterine position (legs extended at knee; sharply bent at hip).

- Pregnancy History: Mother is G2P1. Pregnancy was unplanned as older child is only 1 year old (mother had not begun on a contraceptive as yet following first birth). No complications with pregnancy other than breech presentation. Mother states as long as children are so close together, she would have preferred a second boy, not a girl.

- Personal/Social History: Parents are married; father works as a Park Ranger at state park; mother works part-time as a paralegal in lawyer's office. Finances are "adequate." Family lives in a two-bedroom condominium on lake front. Mother concerned that something is wrong with baby because she was born breech; points to stiffness of legs as indication that some neurologic problem must be present.

Physical Examination

- General Appearance: Well proportioned, alert female newborn who assumed a frank breech position. Weight: 6lb, 5oz. Height: 19.5 inches. Head circumference: 34cm.

- Head: Normocephalic. No molding. Ant. fontanelle: 3 X 3 cm; post. fontanelle: 1 cm.

- Eyes: Red reflex present; follows to midline without difficulty. Ears: Normal alignment; canal patent.

- Nose: Midline septum; no drainage.

- Mouth: No teeth; palate intact; midline uvula.

- Neck: No lymph nodes palpable. Midline trachea.

- Chest: Occasional rhonchi present; no rales. Respiratory rate: 20/min.

- Heart: No murmurs; heart rate: 145 bpm.

- Abdomen: Soft; no masses; liver palpable 1 cm.

- Genitalia: Normal female; slight blood-tinged discharge from vagina.

- Extremities: Full range of motion in upper extremities. Lower extremities are positioned sharply bent at the hip with extended knees. Knees flex but with difficulty. No fractures in long bones palpable. Unable to flex and abduct hips to assess for subluxated hip.

- Neurologic: Moro, sucking, and rooting reflexes present. Step-in-place, crossed extension, tonic neck poorly demonstrated because of stiffness of legs.

Care Study Questions

1. From the physical exam listed above, would you be able to assure her that the infant has normal leg function?

2. A second reason that Jordina's mother is concerned is because amniotic fluid was heavily meconium stained. How would you explain why this occurred with Jordina's birth?

3. Complete a nursing care plan that would identify and meet the Farmer family's needs.

Nutritional Needs of the Newborn

Chapter 24 discusses nutritional needs of the newborn and how both breastfeeding and formula methods can meet newborn needs. The advantages of breastfeeding for both mother and infant are stressed. Techniques of breast and formula feeding, composition and calculation of infant formulas, and common problems of infant feeding are included.

Infant nutrition is not covered as content in many nutrition courses so it is an area of nutrition information that students need to spend additional time learning at this point in their nursing program. The many questions that clients ask them about infant feeding help them to appreciate how valuable is this area of information for health teaching.

Chapter Objectives

After mastering the contents of this chapter, students should be able to:

1. Describe nutritional requirements of the term newborn.
2. Assess nutritional intake of a newborn to determine if he or she is receiving adequate nutrition.
3. State nursing diagnoses related to newborn nutrition.
4. Plan with a mother a method of infant feeding that will be satisfying for both her and the infant.
5. Implement feeding procedures with newborn infants such as giving a first feeding.
6. Evaluate goal outcomes in relation to nutrition to be certain nursing goals were achieved.
7. Identify national health goals related to newborn nutrition that nurses can be instrumental in helping the nation to achieve.
8. Identify areas related to nutrition and newborns that could benefit from additional nursing research.
9. Use critical thinking to analyze ways that nurses can help mothers problem-solve feeding difficulties and make newborn nutrition more family centered.
10. Synthesize knowledge of normal newborn nutrition with nursing process to achieve quality maternal and child health nursing care.

Key Points

- Breastfeeding is the preferred feeding method for newborn infants as it can supply antibodies to the newborn. Urge all women to at least try breastfeeding unless they are taking some drug that would interfere with this or there is a potential for spread of microorganisms through breast milk.

- Almost all drugs pass in breast milk. The breastfeeding mother must be certain not to take any medication without contacting her primary care provider for safety with breastfeeding.

- Both breast milk and commercial formulas have 20 Kcal/oz. A term newborn requires 120 Kcal/kg/day; 160 to 200 mL/kg of fluid.

- Breastfeeding mothers should be encouraged to drink fluoridated water; formula should be prepared using fluoridated water. If a newborn will not have exposure to sunlight, the breastfeeding mother may need to take a supplement of vitamin D.

- If a baby will be bottle fed, be certain the parents understand the potential danger of warming bottles using a microwave oven (the inner core of milk may be very hot).

- Caution parents not to prop bottles. An infant may aspirate from this, and it also deprives him or her of the pleasure of being held for feedings.

- To avoid bottle syndrome (cavitied teeth), infants should not be put to bed with a bottle.

- Linoleic acid is an essential fatty acid necessary for growth and skin integrity that cannot be manufactured by the body. It is supplied by both cow's and human milk but not by skim milk.

Definitions of Key Terms

areola: the pigmented circle of epidermis that surrounds the nipple of the breast

bifidus factor: a growth-producing factor that the bacteria lactobacillus bifidus needs to grow

colostrum: the light yellow fluid secreted as the first milk following delivery

engorgement: local congestion of the breasts associated with lactation

foremilk: breast milk formed prior to the let-down reflex

hind milk: breast milk formed following the let-down reflex

interferon: a protein formed when cells are exposed to a virus that prohibits the growth of viruses

lactiferous sinuses: the glands of the breasts where breast milk is stored

lactoferrin: an iron-binding protein found in breast milk that interferes with the growth of bacteria

let-down reflex: a reflex initiated by an infant's suckling that releases oxytocin from the posterior pituitary, contracts the myoepithelial cells surrounding milk glands, and brings hindmilk forward to the nipple

lysosome: a cytoplasmic particle capable of dissolving cells

prolactin: a hormone produced by the anterior pituitary gland that stimulates milk production in the mammary glands

Nursing Process Overview

The Nursing Process Overview for this chapter concentrates on helping students to identify their role as a teacher rather than a provider of newborn nutrition. The importance of establishing goals that will be realistic for specific families (whether they choose to breastfeed or not, for example) is stressed. The importance of being certain that families have identified a health care provider for the infant and are planning on maintaining regular first-year assessment visits is included.

Study Aids

Boxes

Box 24-1:   Terminal Sterilization of Formula

Tables

Table 24-1:   Common Problems of Breastfeeding

Table 24-2:   Recommended Daily Allowances During Lactation

Table 24-3.   Quantities of Food Necessary for Lactating Women

Table 24-4:   Common Problems of Formula Feeding

Displays

Focus on National Health Goals

Focus on Family Teaching

Focus on Nursing Research

Focus on Cultural Awareness

Critical Thinking Exercises

1. Jackie is a 1-day-old newborn who is being breastfed. Her mother tells you she is unsure Jackie is receiving enough milk. How could you assure the mother that the baby is receiving enough milk?

2. Mrs. Wheeler has chosen to bottle feed her newborn. Her mother tells you she used to prepare formula using evaporated milk and corn syrup, a form that was cheaper than commercial formula. She asks you why this type of formula isn't recommended today. She also says that at 3 months, babies were changed to skim milk to keep them from gaining too much weight. Why is this no longer recommended?

3. Mrs. Curtis is a woman who is breastfeeding and will be returning to work in a busy office. What suggestions for maintaining breastfeeding would you make to her?

Media Resources

Breastfeeding (46 color illustrations)

Color illustrations describing common terms such as engorgement, manual expression of milk, and the rooting reflex.

Source: Childbirth Graphics

Infant Nutrition: Newborn to Two Years (CAI)

A program to help the learner expand a basic knowledge of infant nutritional requirements and feeding practices.

Source: Medi-Sim, Inc.

Unfinished Child (30 minute film)

Narrated by Patricia Neal, this film discusses the impact of maternal, fetal, and infant nutrition on physical and mental development. Poor nutrition is identified as a factor in the perpetuation of the poverty cycle.

Source: March of Dimes Birth Defects Foundation

Breastfeeding: A Practical Guide (30 minute video)

A two-part program that includes an overview of breast milk production, maternal preparation, breastfeeding positions, the let-down reflex, common problems and interventions, methods of expressing and storing milk, nursing in public, and attitudes toward breastfeeding.

Source: AJN Educational Division

Discussion Questions

1. Many women stop breastfeeding after they leave the hospital because they do not believe they can return to work and continue breastfeeding. What are suggestions you could make to help a woman integrate breastfeeding and return to work?

2. Choosing a commercial formula is difficult today because of the many brands and types available. What type of preparation would you recommend for a woman who must economize? For a woman who is more concerned with convenience than cost?

3. Debate the pros and cons of breastfeeding versus formula feeding for the "typical" mother. Does this differ for the woman who is physically disabled? The adolescent? The woman over age 35? The drug dependent woman?

Written Assignments

1. Engorgement with breastfeeding causes pain. List suggestions you could make to lessen this discomfort.

2. Interview a mother of a young infant who is formula fed as to the amount of formula taken daily. Calculate whether the amount is adequate or excessive. List suggestions for improving the infant's nutritional intake.

3. Terminal sterilization is little used today but is still necessary for the woman who does not use a chlorinated water supply. List the steps necessary for terminal sterilization.

Laboratory Experiences

1. Ask students to investigate the price of different brands of infant formula at different locations and communities and then analyze how much a woman could save by breastfeeding in various communities.

2. Assign students to both breastfeeding and formula-feeding women so they can become skilled in caring for both. Stress that encouraging breastfeeding is an important nursing role.

3. Assign students to an antenatal clinic where they have the opportunity to teach the advantages of breastfeeding and influence women to make this choice.

4. Ask both a breastfeeding and a formula-feeding mother to come to a postconference and discuss why they chose the method of feeding that they did. Are they happy with their choice?

Care Study: An Infant Who Is Breastfed

Harris Dupont is a 2-day-old, 8'2'' boy born by cesarean birth following placement of cerclage sutures in his mother. His mother planned on breastfeeding him since the 4th month of pregnancy; now that he is born and she is experiencing a great deal of pain from surgery, she is not as certain that she wants to breastfeed.

Health History

• Chief Concern: ''My breasts are too sore to breastfeed.''

• History of Present Concern: Client has breastfed for 2 days every 3 to 4 hours for 10 minutes each breast. Breasts are firm and filling; nipples protuberant. Infant alert and sucks well. Weight today 8'0''.

Mother did no preparation for breastfeeding during pregnancy such as nipple rolling because of danger of initiating preterm labor.

• Obstetric History: Girl born at 28 weeks because of incompetent cervix. Died at 2 days of age. Cerclage sutures placed at 14th week of this pregnancy. No complications or threatened labor during pregnancy. Membranes did not rupture.

• Personal/Social: Married. Husband is member of large family; states he feels comfortable in caring for newborn although is not certain breastfeeding is necessary. Mother is only child; admits to lacking experience with newborns. Her mother-in-law will be coming to stay with her for a week to help with infant; is aware that mother-in-law never breastfed any of her children.

Care Study Questions

1. Harris has lost 2 oz in the last 2 days. How much could he lose before you would be concerned?

2. Some women continue to breastfeed for a full year; others stop almost immediately after they return home. Which of these is apt to happen with Mrs. Dupont? How important are support people toward encouraging women to continue breastfeeding?

3. Complete a nursing care plan that will identify and meet the needs of the Dupont family.

Nursing Care of the Woman and Family Experiencing a Postpartal Complication

*C*hapter 25 discusses common complications of the 6-week period following childbirth. The chapter begins with an overview of nursing process specific to the woman with a postpartal complication. Postpartum hemorrhage, infection, thrombophlebitis, postpartal pregnancy-induced hypertension, reproductive tract displacements, postpartal depression, and psychosis are discussed. The care of the woman whose infant is ill or who dies is also included. The concept that almost all postpartal complications can be prevented is presented. Efforts to keep care family-centered even with a complication present is stressed.

Because postpartal complications are rare, not all students have the opportunity to care for women with these disorders. Being familiar with these complications, however, encourages students to make careful observations to prevent hemorrhage and to use aseptic techniques in giving postpartal care so they can play an active role in prevention of infection.

Chapter Objectives

After mastering the contents of this chapter, students should be able to:

1. Describe common deviations from the normal that can occur during the puerperium.
2. Assess the woman and her family for deviations from the normal during the puerperium.
3. State nursing diagnoses related to deviations from the normal during the puerperium.

4. Plan implementations that meet the special needs of the postpartum family with a postpartal complication such as planning for an extended hospitalization.
5. Implement nursing care when a postpartal complication such as hemorrhage, infection, hypertension of pregnancy, or postpartal psychosis develops.
6. Evaluate outcome criteria to be certain that nursing goals established were achieved.
7. Identify national health goals related to postpartal complications that nurses could be instrumental in helping the nation to achieve.
8. Identify areas related to care of women with postpartal complications that could benefit from additional nursing research.
9. Use critical thinking to analyze ways that nursing care can remain family centered when a postpartal complication occurs.
10. Synthesize knowledge of puerperium complications with nursing process to achieve quality maternal and child health nursing care.

Key Points

*   Establishing a firm family-newborn relationship is difficult when a woman has a postpartal complication. Investigate ways that will allow the woman to care for her baby or offer necessary support to family members so they can fulfill this role.

*   Hemorrhage is a major danger in the immediate postpartal period. It is defined as a loss of blood over 500 mL within a 24-hour period. The most frequent cause of postpartal hemorrhage is uterine atony. Remember that continuous limited blood loss can be as important over time as sudden, intense bleeding. With hemorrhage, administration of an oxytocin may be necessary to initiate uterine tone and halt hemorrhage.

*   Other causes of hemorrhage are lacerations (vaginal, cervical, or perineal) and retained placental fragments. Lacerations are most apt to occur with forceps birth or with birth of a large infant.

*   Puerperal infection is a potential complication following any birth until the denuded placental surface has healed. Retained placental fragments and the use of internal fetal heart monitoring leads are potential sources of this.

*   Thrombophlebitis is inflammation of the lining of a blood vessel and is a grave complication of the postpartal period. It occurs most often in the postpartal period

as an extension of an endometrial infection. Therapy is bedrest with heat applications and anticoagulation administration. Never massage the leg of a woman with a phlebitis or thrombophlebitis or the clot may move and become a pulmonary embolus, a possibly fatal complication.

- Mastitis is infection of the breast. The symptoms are pain, swelling, and redness in a breast.

- A woman whose child is born with a disability or special need requires special consideration following the birth. This is obviously a time of stress for the woman that calls for supportive nursing care.

- Postpartal "blues" are a normal accompaniment to birth. Postpartal depression (a feeling of extreme sadness) and postpartal psychosis (an actual separation from reality) are not normal and need accurate assessment so women can receive adequate therapy.

Definitions of Key Terms

endometritis: inflammation of the inner uterine lining

mastitis: inflammation of breast tissue

peritonitis: inflammation of the serous lining of the abdominal cavity

postpartal depression: faulty coping that occurs in the postpartal period

postpartal psychosis: a psychiatric disorder that occurs in the postpartal period

Sheehan's syndrome: pituitary necrosis and hypopituitarism occurring from circulatory collapse as a result of uterine hemorrhage

thrombophlebitis: inflammation of a vein with accompanying thrombus formation

Nursing Process Overview

The Nursing Process Overview in this chapter concentrates on helping the student promote parent-infant bonding in the face of a postpartal complication. Examples of nursing diagnoses that speak to this are given. The importance of including the entire family in planning is stressed. The possibility is suggested that long-term follow-up, perhaps from a community health nurse, may be required.

Study Aids

Boxes

Box 25-1:   Conditions That Make Women High Risk for Postpartal Hemorrhage

Box 25-2:   Conditions That Make Women High Risk for Postpartal Infection

Box 25-3:   Common Isolation Guidelines for the Woman With a Postpartal Infection

Tables

Table 25-1:   Classification of Perineal Lacerations

Displays

Focus on National Health Goals

Critical Thinking Exercises

1. Mona is a 29-year-old woman who delivered an 8-lb boy yesterday. When you left work yesterday she was rooming-in with the baby and beginning breastfeeding without apparent difficulty. Today, you find her sitting on the side of her hospital bed crying and stating she has to kill her baby because the voices inside her head have told her he is an interplanetary spy. What would be your first action? Suppose Mona said she needed to kill herself as well? Would your first action be different?

2. Mary Ann is a 39-year-old who entered her pregnancy with marked varicose veins. One day postpartum, you notice red streaks on both legs along the course of the veins. In addition, she has pain on dorsiflexion of her foot. You are concerned she is developing a thrombophlebitis. Are there measures Mary Ann should have taken during pregnancy to decrease the risk of thrombophlebitis? Are there preventive measures that could have been suggested during labor? In the immediate postpartal period?

3. Postpartal hemorrhage can lead to extensive hypovolemia if allowed to continue undetected. If you entered a postpartal room and discovered a woman with active vaginal bleeding, what would be your first action? How would you teach women to assess vaginal bleeding so they can self assess when they are home?

Media Resources

After Childbirth: The Postpartum Experience (14 minute video).

Physical and emotional adjustment women must make immediately following birth are shown.

Source: Professional Research

The Depressed Client (30 minute video, film).

Depressed behavior from mild to severe is illustrated through vignettes that deal with postpartum depression, a postoperative mastecomy patient, and a depressed psychiatric patient. Identification of depression and guidelines for nursing interventions are given.

Source: AJN Company Educational Services

Discussion Questions

1. Hemorrhage is a serious complication following childbirth. What steps would you take if you discovered a woman with vaginal hemorrhage at the first hour following childbirth?

2. Symptoms of postpartal depression may be subtle. What specific observations would you make to detect this?

3. Parent-child bonding must be encouraged in the family when a complication of the postpartal period occurs. What are concrete ways to encourage bonding?

Written Assignments

1. Make a series of flash cards or a word game that would encourage a family to use extra days of required hospitalization to increase their knowledge of newborn care.

2. Write a paragraph tracing the process whereby a pulmonary embolus occurs, beginning with an endometritis.

3. Infection in the postpartal period generally occurs because of contamination during delivery. What precautions should you always observe during delivery to prevent postpartal infection?

Laboratory Experiences

1. Assign students to women with any degree of postpartal complication. Ask students to share their experiences at postconferences.

2. Ask a woman who had a complication of the postpartal period to come to class to discuss how devastating this was for her in trying to establish breastfeeding or bonding with her infant.

3. Have students role-play how they would comfort a woman whose infant has died. Practice the technique of showing a deceased baby to a couple in order to allow grieving to begin.

Care Study

Pamela Barth is a 17-year-old, GIPO woman transferred to the postpartal service following the birth of a 9 lb 4 oz infant boy.

Health History

- Chief Concern: "Should I be bleeding this much?"

- History of Present Concern: Client delivered a 9 lb 4 oz boy under epidural anesthesia at 7:25 AM. A modified Crede's maneuver was used to deliver placenta. Fifteen u pitocin in 500 mL of 5% dextrose was administered intravenously following delivery. Blood loss from delivery estimated at 750 mL. At present, client reports vaginal bleeding is so heavy she is saturating a perineal pad every 20 minutes.

- History of Past Illness: Chickenpox at 5 years: acne since she was twelve. No major illnesses; no hospitalizations.

- Gynecologic History: Menarche at 10 years; cycle duration, 29 days; menstrual flow duration. 5 days. No STDs. Not using a contraceptive before present pregnancy.

- Obstetric History: No previous pregnancies. This pregnancy was not planned but not unwelcome. No complications during pregnancy except for minimal edema formation. Proteinuria of 2+ and blood pressure increase to 140/98 for last 2 weeks.

- Personal/Social: Lives with mother, two older sisters, five nieces and nephews in a three-bedroom house. Has "borrowed" supplies for baby from sisters. Father of child is said to be supportive but did not come to be with her in labor.

- Review of Systems: Neurologic: Treated for five years when younger for "small seizures." No longer takes medication for this. Mouth: Severe malocclusion treated with oral braces since age 14.

Physical Examination

- General Appearance: Apprehensive-appearing, slender black woman. T: 98.6°F., BP: 100/60.

- HEENT: Integument: approximately five black comedones present on forehead.

- Mouth: Full upper and lower metal braces present. No ulcerations or abrasions on gumlines.

- Chest: Heart rate: 100/minute. No murmurs present. Lungs: rhonchi present in upper lobes. Respiratory rate; 22/minute.

- Abdomen: Soft. Fundus palpated at 2F above umbilicus and boggy. Massaged and large firm clot 5 cm in diameter was expelled vaginally. Fundus somewhat firmer following massage but height did not change.

- Perineum: Midline episiotomy line intact; no hemorrhoids, Lochia: continuous bright red vaginal flow present; no clots.

Laboratory Results

- Hemoglobin: 8.9 g/dL.

Care Study Questions

1. Pamela is bleeding heavily following birth of her baby. Does she have risk factors that would make her particularly prone to postpartal hemorrhage?

2. Pamela is saturating a perineal pad about every 20 minutes. Is this excessive? What do her vital signs reveal about the extent of bleeding?

3. Complete a nursing care plan that would identify and meet Pamela's needs.

Nursing Care of the High-Risk Newborn and Family

*C*hapter 26 discusses care of the newborn who is born with an altered gestational age or low weight or who experiences difficulty with the adjustment to extrauterine life. The chapter begins with a Nursing Process Overview to help the student adapt nursing process to the needs of infants. Problems and concerns of the low-birthweight, small-for-gestational age, large-for-gestational age, and postmature infant, and those infants ill at birth with such disorders as respiratory distress syndrome, meconium aspiration, blood incompatibility, necrotizing enterocolitis, retinopathy of prematurity, or complications resulting from a maternal infection are discussed.

Chapter Objectives

After mastering the contents of this chapter, students should be able to:

1. Define the terms small-for-gestational-age infant, term infant, large-for-gestational-age infant, preterm infant, and postterm infant and describe common illnesses that occur in these high-risk newborns.

2. Assess a high-risk newborn in the early neonatal period to determine if the infant has completed a safe transition to extrauterine life.

3. List nursing diagnoses concerned with the high-risk newborn.

4. Establish plans for care, respecting priorities of the newborn (ie, establishing respiratory function, cardiovascular adjustment, temperature regulation, nutrition, bonding, and developmental care), to help a high-risk newborn stabilize body systems.

5. Implement nursing care for the high-risk infant, such as providing an intravenous or gavage-feeding.

6. Evaluate outcome criteria to assure that nursing goals for care have been achieved.

7. Identify national health goals related to high-risk newborns that nurses could be instrumental in helping the nation to achieve.

8. Identify areas related to the care of high-risk newborns that could benefit from additional nursing research.

9. Use critical thinking to analyze the special crisis imposed on families when alterations of newborn development, length of pregnancy, or neonatal illness occur.

10. Synthesize knowledge of the needs of the high-risk infant with nursing process to achieve quality maternal and child health nursing care.

Key Points

- Priorities for care of infants born with special needs, such as the preterm or postterm infant, are the same as with term infants: initiation and maintenance of respirations, establishment of extrauterine circulation, control of body temperature, intake of adequate nourishment, establishment of waste elimination and an infant-parent relationship, prevention of infection, and provision of developmental care for mental and social development.

- Many high-risk infants need resuscitation at birth. Prompt action with such measures as suctioning, intubation, oxygen, and warmth are needed.

- A small-for-gestational-age (SGA) infant is one whose birth weight is below the 10th percentile on an intrauterine growth curve for that age infant. The infant could be preterm, term, or postterm.

- Small-for-gestational-age infants have particular difficulty maintaining body warmth because of low fat stores and developing hypoglycemia from low nutritional stores. Common nursing diagnoses identified for them are "High-risk for altered respiratory function related to underdeveloped body systems at birth," "High-risk for ineffective thermoregulation related to lack of subcutaneous fat," and "High-risk for altered parenting related to high-risk status and child's possible cognitive impairment from lack of nutrients in utero."

- A large-for-gestational-age (LGA) infant is one whose birth weight is above the 90th percentile on an intrauterine growth chart for that gestational age. The infant could be born preterm, term, or postterm.

- Large-for-gestational-age infants tend to be infants of diabetic mothers; they are particularly prone to hypoglycemia or birth trauma. Common nursing diagnoses identified for them are "High-risk for altered respiratory function related to possible birth trauma," "High-risk for altered nutrition, less than body requirements related to additional nutrients needed to maintain weight or prevent hypoglycemia,'' and ''High-risk for altered parenting related to infant's high-risk status.''

- A preterm infant is one born before 37 weeks of gestation. Preterm birth occurs in as many as 7% of live births. Preterm infants have particular problems of respiratory function, anemia, persistent jaundice, persistent patent ductus arteriosus, and intracranial hemorrhage. Infants who are born between weeks 30 and 36 of gestation (weighing 1500 to 2500 g) are also termed low-birth-weight (LBW) infants; those born between 26 and 30 weeks gestation (1000-1500 g) are very-low-birth-weight (VLBW); those born between 24 and 26 weeks gestation (500 to 1000 g) are extremely-very-low-birth-weight (EVLBW)infants. All such infants need level III (neonatal intensive) care from the moment of birth to give them their best chance of survival without neurologic after-effects due to their being so critically close to the age of viability.

- A postterm infant is one who has remained in utero past week 42 of pregnancy. Postterm infants have particular problems with establishing respirations, meconium aspiration, hypoglycemia, temperature regulation, and polycythemia.

- Respiratory distress syndrome (RDS) occurs in preterm infants from lack of surfactant in alveoli. Without surfactant, alveoli collapse on expiration and require extreme force for reinflation. Primary therapy is synthetic surfactant replacement at birth by endotracheal tube insufflation followed by oxygen and ventilatory support.

- Transient tachypnea of the newborn is a temporary condition caused by slow absorption of lung fluid at birth. Close observation of the infant is necessary until the fluid is absorbed and respirations slow to a normal rate.

- Meconium aspiration syndrome occurs from the infant inhaling meconium-stained amniotic fluid during birth. Meconium is irritating to the airway so may lead to both airway spasm or pneumonia. Infants need oxygen, ventilatory support, and possibly an antibiotic until the effects of the insult to the airway subside. It is important that they are suctioned before oxygen administration under pressure to prevent meconium being forced further into their lungs.

- Apnea is a pause in respirations longer than 20 seconds with accompanying bradycardia. This tends to occur in preterm infants who have secondary stresses such as infection, hyperbilirubinemia, hypoglycemia, or hypothermia. Apnea monitors are placed to detect the incidence. Infants who are high-risk for this return home on a home-monitoring apnea program.

- Sudden infant death syndrome (SIDS) is the sudden, unexplained death of an infant. It is associated with infants sleeping on their stomachs (prone) and infants who were born preterm. An important preventive measure may be advising parents to position their infant on the side or back for sleeping.

- Hemolytic disease of the newborn is destruction of red blood cells from Rh or ABO incompatibility. The administration of RhIG (Rh antibodies) to Rh-negative mothers during pregnancy and following birth of an Rh-positive infant to an Rh-negative mother has greatly reduced the incidence of the condition. Affected infants are jaundiced from release of bilirubin from injured red blood cells. Therapy is phototherapy or exchange transfusion to prevent kernicterus or deposition of bilirubin in brain cells with destruction of the cells.

- Hemorrhagic disease of the newborn is a lack of clotting ability resulting from a deficiency of vitamin K at birth. Prevention is by injection of vitamin K to all infants at birth.

- Retinopathy of prematurity is destruction of the retina due to exposure of immature retinal capillaries to oxygen. Monitoring arterial blood gases is an important preventive measure.

- Severe infections that may be seen in newborns are streptococcal group B pneumonia, hepatitis B infection, gonococcal conjunctivitis, and herpes virus infection. Assessing newborns for symptoms of these infections is an important nursing responsibility.

- Infants of diabetic women and those of drug-abusing women are both examples of infants who are high-risk at birth for further complications. Both need careful assessment for respiratory distress and hypoglycemia.

Definitions of Key Terms

apnea: cessation of respirations

apparent life-threatening event: a phenomenon where an infant stops breathing; commonly called ''near-miss'' sudden infant death syndrome

azotemia: excess nitrogenous wastes in the blood stream

brown fat: unique fat located between the scapula; around the neck, kidneys, and adrenals; and behind the sternum that has a rich nerve and blood supply and generates heat in the neonate

cephalopelvic disproportion: a delivery condition in which the mother's pelvis is too small or too misshaped to allow the infant's head to pass through. The most common reason for which cesarean birth is performed

extremely-very-low-birthweight infant: a newborn weighing less than 1000 g or between 24 and 26 weeks gestation age

gestational age: the number of weeks of fetal development calculated from the first day of the last menstrual cycle

hemorrhagic disease of the newborn: decreased clotting ability in a newborn caused by a deficiency of vitamin K

hyperbilirubinemia: excessive bilirubin in the blood stream

hyperglycemia: a greater than normal amount of glucose in the blood stream

hypocalcemia: a lessened amount of calcium present in the blood stream hydrops fetalis: a fatal state caused by blood incompatibility evidenced by edema, anemia, and congestive heart failure

hypoglycemia: a lessened amount of glucose present in the blood stream

intrauterine growth retardation: an infant born or in utero with a weight below the 10th percentile for gestational age

kernicterus: accumulation of indirect bilirubin in brain cells causing cell destruction

large-for-gestational-age infant: an infant above the 90th percentile for weight for gestational age

low-birth-weight infant: an infant born weighing less than 2500 grams

macrosomia: large body size

ophthalmia neonatorum: infection of the conjunctiva within the first 30 days of life; commonly used to describe gonorrheal infection of the conjunctiva

periodic respirations: a respiratory pattern of premature infants in which short periods of apnea occur

periventricular leukomalacia: abnormal formation of the white matter of the brain caused by an ischemic episode in utero

postterm infant: an infant born after 42 weeks of pregnancy

postterm syndrome: an infant born after 42 weeks of pregnancy with signs of nutritional deficiency

preterm infant: an infant who weighs 2500 grams or less at birth or is less than 38 weeks gestation age.

primary apnea: the state when respiratory function was never established in a newborn

retinopathy of prematurity: the formation of fibrotic tissue behind the lens of the eye causing blindness; occurs in immature infants from hyperoxemia

secondary apnea: cessation of respirations after they were initially established

shoulder dystocia: difficulty with delivery of a newborn's shoulder or shoulders

small-for-gestational-age infant: an infant whose weight is below the 10th percentile for gestational age

term infant: an infant born between 38 and 42 weeks of pregnancy

very-low-birthweight infant: a newborn weighing between 1000 and 1500 gram or between 26 and 30 weeks gestation

Nursing Process Overview

The Nursing Process Overview in this chapter concentrates on the importance of assessing newborns for difficulty in initiating and sustaining respiratory function and for gestational age and weight. Nursing diagnoses that accentuate a newborn problem as a family-centered problem are given. Implementations that speak to long-term follow-up are discussed.

Study Aids

Boxes

Box 26-1: Factors That Make Infants High-Risk for Respiratory Difficulty in the First Few Days of Life

Box 26-2: Factors Associated With Low Birthweight

Tables

Table 26-1: Important Assessment Criteria for a Large-for-Gestational-Age Infant

Table 26-2: Differences Between Small-for-Gestational-Age and Low-Birthweight Infants

Table 26-3: Formulas Commonly Used With Low-Birthweight Infants

Displays

Focus on National Health Goals

Focus on Family Teaching

Focus on Nursing Research

Focus on Cultural Awareness

Critical Thinking Exercises

1. Mrs. Terry is in preterm labor; her child will be high-risk for the development of respiratory distress syndrome. How would you explain to her why her baby will be high-risk for this? Mrs. Terry is asked to make a decision as to whether she wants surfactant administered prophylactically to her baby at birth or to wait and allow the baby to receive it only after (and if) symptoms of respiratory distress begin. Mrs. Terry asks your advice in helping her decide what to do. How would you advise her?

2. Retinopathy of prematurity is an example of a disease that is caused by the therapy given the infant. How can nurses help safeguard infants against this disorder?

3. Infants who are cared for in neonatal nurseries may need either reduced stimulation because they fatigue so easily or increased stimulation because their stay in the nursery will be so extended. What are measures to reduce stimulation in such a nursery? How could you increase stimulation?

Media Resources

Neonatal Problems: The Low-Birth-Weight Infant (slide/audiocassette)

Recommended procedures for recognizing and treating the low-birthweight infant are presented. The problems of and therapy for respiratory distress, heat maintenance, asphyxia, hydration, and hyperbilirubinemia are explored.

Source: Health Sciences Consortium

Vulnerabilities of the Premature Infant (12 minute video)

The major problems associated with premature birth and methods for monitoring and caring for such infants are presented. Care studies are integrated to demonstrate specific content.

Source: Health Sciences Consortium

The Handicapped Child: Infancy Through Preschool (film-strip)

An eight-part program presents an overview of the child with developmental alterations during infancy and early childhood. Family crisis and risk factors are identified, followed by initial assessment and intervention criteria. Specific guidelines for encouraging development and promoting self-help skills are stressed.

Source: Concept Media

Introduction to an Intensive-Care Nursery (10 minute video)

A basic introduction to an intensive-care nursery is presented. Protective procedures used to enter the nursery, the steps involved in transporting and admitting a child, special equipment used, and the contribution of parents to their infant's care and well being are included.

Source: Health Sciences Consortium

Neonatal Problems: Respiratory Distress (slide/audiocassette)

Issues pertinent to the stabilization of the infant with respiratory distress are presented. Factors associated with respiratory distress, immediate interventions required, diagnostic methods, therapy, and the means for assessing the effects of excessive or deficient oxygen level are included.

Source: Health Sciences Consortium

Neonatal Problems: Apnea (slide/audiocassette)

A detailed description of the recommended procedures for recognizing and treating the infant with apnea is presented. Procedures for resuscitating and stabilizing infants and identifying the cause of apnea are included.

Source: Health Sciences Consortium

Discussions With Parents of a Premature Infant (32 minute film)

The concerns of parents of premature infants are presented. Two couples reveal their concerns, sense of helplessness, fear of holding the infant, and jealousy of nurses. The changes in lifestyle that parents must undergo in order to be ready for discharge care is explored.

Source: Polymorph Films

The Respiratory Distress Syndrome (slide/audiocassette)

A self-instruction unit covering the major aspects of respiratory distress syndrome is presented. The clinical manifestations of the disease, major maturational changes in the fetal lung, effects of hypoxia, and biochemical changes are included.

Source: National Medical Audiovisual Center

Gestational Age Assessment (30 minute video)

Introduction to the Ballard scale for gestational age and the techniques used for performing gestational age assessment are shown.

Source: J.B. Lippincott Company

Discussion Questions

1. Mrs. Bryan visits the intensive care nursery daily where her low-birthweight infant is cared for but states she does not want to touch him for fear of hurting him. What measures would you initiate to encourage better bonding between Mrs. Bryan and her son?

2. Infants may be small, average, or large for gestational age. What specific measures would you need to plan for at the births of these three types of infants to ensure their safe care?

3. Keeping a low-birthweight infant warm is a primary nursing responsibility. What are specific measures you would take to conserve heat in an immature infant?

Written Assignments

1. Some infants have difficulty initiating respirations at birth. List the steps you would take with an infant who does not breathe spontaneously.

2. Many immature infants are gavage-fed because they cannot suck as yet. List the steps you would take to complete a gavage feeding successfully.

3. Children with elevated indirect bilirubin levels are cared for under bilirubin lights. What are special measures you would take with such infants to safeguard them against dehydration and retinal damage?

Laboratory Experiences

1. Assign students to observe in a neonatal intensive care unit so they can become familiar with the extensive care needed for infants who are ill at birth.

2. Assign students to experience in an ambulatory clinic where NICU ''graduates'' come for care so they can better appreciate the long-term difficulties some of these children will have in development.

3. Assign students to a nursery school or preschool program for children with physical disabilities so students can better appreciate the long-term consequences of anoxia at birth.

Care Study: A Preterm Infant With Necrotizing Enterocolitis

Merry Anorak is a 4-day-old, 34 week, low-birthweight infant cared for in a neonatal intensive care unit.

Health History

- Chief Concern: ''She isn't digesting anything.''

- History of Present Concern: Baby has been gavage-fed since birth. Before last feeding, infant's stomach was noted to be distended. 3 mL of fluid was aspirated from stomach. His nurse held his feeding and notified the physician.

- Family Profile: Family intact. Father is State Assemblyman; mother is homemaker. Mother volunteers for Junior League and Homeless Mission 3 days a week. Finances are ''generous.'' Family lives in 4-bedroom house; father is in state capital on business 4 days a week. Mother visits infant daily. Father visits when in town.

- Pregnancy History: Pregnancy planned; mother had upper respiratory infection followed by premature rupture of membranes at 32 weeks of pregnancy. Mother was admitted to the hospital and placed on complete bedrest. At 34 weeks, her white blood count rose to 18,000 and labor began. Infant was born after 4 hours of labor. No spontaneous respirations noted; infant was intubated and administered 100% oxygen. Has been maintained on ventilation with positive end pressure at 89% oxygen.

- Past Medical History: Immaturity; infant rated as average for gestational age.

- Review of Systems: Head: Severe bruising on vertex.

- Respiratory: Infant maintained on ventilator since birth.

- GI: Symptoms as in chief concern.

Physical Examination

- General Appearance: Listless, frail appearing immature infant with distended abdomen; nasogastric tube in place in right nostril. Oral intubation tube inserted.

- Head: Circumference: Anterior fontanelle: 2 cm X 2 cm; posterior fontanelle: $\frac{1}{2}$ cm X 1 cm. Sagittal suture line overriding and freely movable. Small abraded area on left cheek. Ecchymotic bruising 2 cm X 1 cm on vertex of head.

- Eyes: Red reflex present; no discharge.

- Ears: Normal alignment; pinna soft; external ear meatus present.

- Nose: Nares patent; midline septum.

- Mouth and Throat: Mucous membrane dry; midline uvula.

- Neck: Full range of motion; midline trachea.

- Lungs and Chest: Rhonchi in all lobes; respirations maintained by ventilator at 20/minute; no palpable breast tissue present.

- Heart: Rate: 142/minute. Continuous murmur auscultated.

- Abdomen: Distended; firm to palpation. Cord still present; drying; no discharge. Neither liver nor spleen able to be palpated.

- Genitalia: Immature female; prominent labia minora.

- Extremities: Full range of motion; poor muscle tone; foot creases $\frac{1}{8}$ sole only. Intravenous site in dorsum of left hand; no erythema. Pulse oximeter in place on right hand.

- Neurologic: Poor sucking reflex; no rooting reflex. No tonic neck. No moro.

Care Study Questions

1. Merry was diagnosed as having necrotizing enterocolitis. She was born after membranes had been ruptured for 2 weeks and had difficulty breathing at birth. How did these incidences add to the present problems?

2. A secondary problem that Merry has is extensive ecchymosis from birth trauma. What is apt to be the effect of this?

3. Complete a nursing care plan that would identify and meet the needs of Merry and her family.

Principles of Growth and Development

Chapter 27 discusses principles of childhood growth and development. The chapter begins with an overview of the nursing process specific to assessing growth and development of children. Factors that influence growth and development, the developmental theories of Freud and Erikson, the cognitive theory of Piaget, the moral development theory of Kohlberg, and the temperament theory of Church and Thomas are discussed. The importance of knowing growth and development in health promotion and in individualizing nursing care is stressed.

Most students have had exposure to growth and development theories from previous course work. Their task before they can become adept at caring for children is learning to apply this knowledge to everyday situations and specific children. To this end, in addition to class discussion, they need experience in caring for a variety of children from different age groups.

Chapter Objectives

After mastering the contents of this chapter, students should be able to:

1. Describe principles of growth and development and developmental stages according to major theorists.
2. Assess a child to determine the stage of development the child has reached.
3. Formulate nursing diagnoses regarding both a potential for and an actual delay in growth and development.
4. Plan nursing care to assist a child in achieving and maintaining normal growth and development.
5. Implement nursing care, such as providing age-appropriate play materials, to support normal growth and development patterns.
6. Evaluate outcome criteria to be certain that nursing goals related to growth and development have been achieved.

7. Identify national health goals related to growth and development in which nurses can be instrumental in helping the nation to achieve.
8. Identify areas related to growth and development that could benefit from additional nursing research.
9. Use critical thinking to analyze factors that influence growth and development and ways to strengthen paths to achieving a new developmental stage.
10. Synthesize knowledge of growth and development with nursing process to achieve quality maternal and child health nursing care.

Key Points

- Nurses use knowledge of growth and development to promote health and prevent illness through assessment and anticipatory guidance.

- Genetic factors that influence growth and development are gender, race and nationality, intelligence, and health. Environmental influences are quality of nutrition, socioeconomic level, parent-child relationship, ordinal position in the family, and environmental health.

- Common theories of development are Freud's psychoanalytic theory and Erikson's theory of psychosocial development. Both these theories describe specific tasks, which children complete at each stage of development in order to mature to a well-adapted adult.

- Piaget's theory of cognitive development describes ways that children learn. Kohlberg has advanced a theory of moral development or how children use moral reasoning to solve problems they face.

- Temperament is a child's characteristic manner of thinking, behaving, or reacting. Chess and Thomas have described an ''easy to care for child'' and a ''difficult child'' based on temperament. Helping parents understand the effect of temperament is a nursing role.

- Although growth and development occur in known patterns, their rate varies from child to child. Caution parents not to be concerned because two siblings are different as long as they both fit within usual parameters.

- Preschool-age and younger children do not perform well ''on command.'' A history of the child's usual play or language development may reveal more information than asking the child to perform set tasks.

- Adolescents can be as concerned about their development as their parents were about it when they were younger. Teaching them about usual development patterns prepares them for what is to come and helps them feel good about puberty and other changes that will soon occur.

Definitions of Key Terms

abstract thought: the ability to think in terms of possibility rather than what already exists

accommodation: the ability to adapt thought processes to fit what is perceived

adaptability: ability to change one's reaction to stimuli over time

approach: a child's response to initial contact with a new stimulus

assimilation: the ability to change how a set is perceived to coincide with beliefs

attention span: the length of time a child retains interest in an activity

autonomy versus shame: the developmental task of the toddler period according to Erikson

cognitive development: intellectual growth; the ability to learn from experience

concrete operational thought: form of cognitive thought of the 7- to 12-year-old.

conservation: the ability to discern truth even though physical properties change

conventional development: the stage of moral development by Kohlberg from 7 to 12 years of age

development: an increase in skill or ability to function; a qualitative change

developmental milestone: an important marker of developmental progress

developmental task: a skill responsibility arising at a particular time, the successful accomplishment of which will provide a foundation for the accomplishment of future tasks

distractibility: ability to have interest diverted to a new object

egocentrism: having all of one's ideas centered about oneself

formal operational thought: a cognitive stage in which abstract thought is possible

growth: an increase in physical size; a quantitative change

identity versus role confusion: the developmental task of the adolescent: learning what kind of person he or she is

industry versus inferiority: the developmental task of the school-age child; learning how to do things well

initiative versus guilt: the developmental task of the preschool child according to Erikson

intuitive thought: spontaneous thought or thought without reasoning

libido: sexual desire

maturation: mature development

mood quality: the overall degree of happiness or sadness a child exhibits

permanence: the knowledge that an object exists even when it is out of sight

postconventional development: the moral stage of development according to Kohlberg of the child older than 12 years

preoperational thought: form of cognitive thought of children from ages 2 to 7 years

pre-religious stage: the infant period of moral reasoning

reversibility: the cognitive ability to retrace steps

rhythmicity: the degree to which a child maintains a regular or predictable pattern of behavior and response

role fantasy: a type of thought in which the child is influenced by how he or she would like a situation to turn out

schema: a substage of cognitive development according to Piaget

sensorimotor stage: the form of cognitive thought of children from 1 month to 2 years

temperament: a person's innate emotional composition

threshold of response: the point at which a child will exhibit evidence of frustration

trust versus mistrust: the developmental task of the infant according to Erikson

Nursing Process Overview

The Nursing Process Overview in this chapter concentrates on helping the student to include growth and development parameters in assessment as a basis for formulating nursing diagnoses. Including growth and development milestones in planning enlarges the student's scope of understanding of the effect of childhood illness on families. Stress is placed on the importance of ongoing evaluation, whether goals or interventions are appropriate, because children continually change.

Study Aids

Tables

Table 27-1: Basic divisions of childhood

Table 27-2: Summary of Freud's and Erikson's theories of personality development

Table 27-3: Piaget's stages of cognitive development

Table 27-4: Kohlberg's stages of moral development

Displays

Focus on National Health Goals

Focus on Family Teaching

Focus on Nursing Research

Focus on Cultural Awareness

Critical Thinking Exercises

1. Mrs. Peters is a mother who describes her two children as "totally different". One is shy and quiet and agreeable and one is aggressive and persistent. What characteristic is Mrs. Peters describing? Which child does she probably view as easiest to care for? What anticipatory guidance could you give her to help her better understand these differences in her children?

2. Joey is a two-year-old from a family whose members tend to be underachievers. His parents want Joey to be able to achieve well. They ask you what specific steps they should take to foster high achievement in Joey. What advice would you give them?

3. Children who are hospitalized for long periods need their development tasks strengthened during this time. What specific measures could you take to aid a sense of autonomy in a hospitalized 2-year-old? To aid a sense of industry in a hospitalized 10-year-old?

Media Resources

Erikson on Erikson: On Development Stages (19-minute film)

A conversation between Erikson and students in which he explains his eight stages of man.

> Source: Parents Magazine Films

Everybody Rides the Carousel (72-minute film)

Erikson's eight psychosocial stages of development are portrayed in animation.

> Source: Michigan Media

Piaget's Developmental Theory (Three films: 17 minutes, 28 minutes, and 32 minutes)

Piaget's developmental theory, methods of classification, and stages in the development of intelligence are described. Many demonstrations of children's thinking at different stages of development are demonstrated.

> Source: Davidson Films

Child Development (CAI)

Nine tutorial computer software programs that cover growth and development from conception through adolescence. A general introduction is included that defines terms and research methods relevant to the study of development.

> Source: Career Aids

Whatever Happened to Childhood? (45-minute videocassette, film)

Changes in Western society that have contributed to the pressure placed on children today to become adults at a young age are explored. Young people and adults discuss their perceptions of the modern family, drug use, and sexual behavior and how these factors are making an impact on shortening childhood.

> Source: Churchill Films

Discussion Questions

1. Helping parents to understand normal growth and development is a major teaching role in health maintenance settings. What visual aids could you use to accomplish this?

2. A toddler is at an egocentric stage of development (sees himself as more important than others). How would this affect your nursing career?

3. In past years, Freud was considered the predominant developmental theorist. What are some reasons that Erikson's theory is more accepted today?

Written Assignments

1. Erikson's theory of developmental tasks explains much of the behavior of children. List the developmental tasks for each age group and a nursing action that would promote this.

2. Interview a child with the question, "Why is it wrong to steal from your neighbor?" and write a short paragraph evaluating what stage of moral development the child has reached.

3. Ask a child to observe you pouring water from a tall thin glass to a short wide one and to tell you which glass holds more water. Write a short paragraph describing the child's answer and whether he or she has grasped the concept of conservation or not.

Laboratory Experiences

1. Assign students to a nursery school and a grade school setting so they have interaction with well children. Ask them to assess a child from each setting for milestones of growth and development.

2. Ask students when they are caring for ill children in a hospital or ambulatory setting to include growth and development assessment and a nursing diagnosis pertinent to growth and development on all care plans so they can appreciate how growth and development influences children's physical care.

3. If students are exposed to only a narrow age range of children in clinical settings due to limitations of the setting, ask acquaintances who have children from other age groups to come to class. Have the class interview the parents as to each child's level of growth and development.

Child Health Assessment

Chapter 28 discusses techniques of health assessment of the child. The chapter begins with an overview of nursing process specific to the care of the child during health assessment. Techniques of interviewing, physical examination, and assessing vision, hearing, development, intelligence, and temperament are included. Differences that occur because of age are noted. The nursing role in assessment and the necessity to individualize assessment techniques to meet the needs of individual children and age groups are stressed.

Health assessment is an increasingly important role for nurses; it involves adapting procedures that may have been learned for use with adult clients. In order to do this well, students need not only to learn the theory but also to practice techniques until they become proficient and can develop judgment to evaluate findings.

Chapter Objectives

After mastering the contents of this chapter, students should be able to:

1. State the purposes for health assessment in children of all ages.
2. Assess a child and family by conducting a health interview, physical examination, and development screening.
3. Formulate nursing diagnoses based on health assessment findings.
4. Plan nursing care based on health assessment findings, such as informing parents of health deviations.
5. Implement nursing care such as conducting an age-appropriate health interview or physical examination by modifying techniques based on the child's age.
6. Evaluate outcome criteria to be certain that established goals were achieved.
7. Identify national health goals related to health assessment of children that nurses can be instrumental in in helping the nation to achieve.
8. Identify areas related to health assessment of children that could benefit from additional nursing research.
9. Use critical thinking to analyze ways that health assessment skills can be incorporated into nursing care procedures.
10. Synthesize nursing process with knowledge of health assessment to achieve quality maternal and child health nursing care.

Definitions of Key Terms

audiogram: a diagram showing the acuteness of an individual's hearing.

auscultation: assessment by the act of listening for sound

bruit: the sound of irregular blood flow through a vessel or organ

chief concern: the reason stated by a person as to why he or she is visiting a health care facility

cognitive learning: the development of problem-solving or intellectual ability

conjunctivitis: inflammation of the mucous membrane lining the surface of the sclera

deep tendon reflexes: contraction of muscles in response to a sharp stimulus; indicates spinal nerve integrity

diaphragmatic excursion: the distance the diaphragm descends or rises on inspiration and expiration

epispadias: a congenital defect in which the urinary meatus is on the dorsal surface of the penis

esotropia: inward deviation of an eye

exotropia: outward deviation of an eye

fasciculations: a fine tremor

general appearance: the overall appearance of a person prior to a physical examination

geographic tongue: a rough "maplike" appearance of the tongue from uneven papillae

gingivae: the gumline

hordeolum: an infection at the margin of the eyelid occurring in a sebaceous gland of an eyelash

hydrocele: an accumulation of fluid in the tunica vaginalis near the testis

hypospadias: a congenital defect in which the urinary meatus is on the ventral surface of the penis

inspection: observation

intelligence: the ability to learn from experience

intercostal spaces: the hollow spaces between the ribs

kwashiorkor: a malnutrition syndrome caused by protein deficiency

palpation: assessment by feeling with the hands

percussion: assessment by listening to the sound made by one finger striking another part

physiologic splitting: a delayed second heart sound made by delayed closure of the aortic valve

point of maximum impulse: the place on the chest where the impulse of the left ventricle can be felt

ptosis: an abnormal condition in which an upper eyelid does not fully open

retractions: inward movement of the chest wall on inspiration

review of systems: a summary of body systems obtained at the end of a health interview

sinus arrhythmia: irregularity of the heart beat influenced by inspiration and expiration

strabismus: deviation of an eye

superficial reflexes: a neural reflex initiated by stimulation of the skin

temperament: a person's innate emotional composition

tinea capitis: a fungal infection characterized by circular bald patches with erythema and scaling

turgor: elasticity of the skin implying adequate fluid content in subcutaneous tissue

varicocele: dilation of a blood vessel of the spermatic cord

Nursing Process Overview

The Nursing Process Overview for this chapter focuses on ways to integrate child health assessment into care. The importance of being able to conduct a thorough health assessment as well as to assess only specific health care areas at other times is stressed.

Study Aids

Boxes

Box 28-1:   Techniques of physical examination

Box 28-2:   Testicular self-examination

Box 28-2:   Goodenough-Harris Draw-a-Man Test

Tables

Table 28-1:   Techniques of physical examination based on child's age

Table 28-2:   Significant body odors

Table 28-3:   Skin findings in children that suggest illness

Table 28-4:   Breath sounds heard on auscultation

Table 28-5:   Heart sounds heard on auscultation

Table 28-6:   Description of accessory heart sounds

Table 28-7:   Grading of deep tendon reflexes

Table 28-8:   Common vision screening indicators and procedures

Table 28-9:   Levels of hearing impairment

Displays

Focus on National Health Goals

Focus on Family Teaching

Focus on Nursing Research

Focus on Cultural Awareness

Critical Thinking Exercises

1.   Mary is a 2-year old seen in a health maintenance clinic for well child care. She is very resistant to being examined. What are some techniques you could use to help Mary adjust better to a physical examination?

2.   Children may cheat on vision and hearing tests because they do not understand the importance of them. What are techniques to use to keep children from doing this with these assessments?

3.   Children should be completely undressed for physical examinations and all body surfaces inspected. What would be your response if a parent said she did not want to undress a child? What if she could not account for multiple bruises on the child?

Media Resources

Interviewing Children: The Initial Assessment (34-minute videocassette)

The special skills involved in interviewing children are shown. The purposes of an initial assessment interview are discussed and an interview is demonstrated.

Source: University of Michigan

Physical Assessment of a Child (33-minute videocassette)

The technique for performing a physical examination on a young child is demonstrated. Along with the techniques of inspection, palpation, percussion, and auscultation, techniques for establishing trust and a positive rapport with a child during the physical examination are also demonstrated.

Source: AJN Educational Services

Pediatrics: Physical Care Program 6: Using a Otoscope (filmstrip, videocassette)

The anatomy of the outer and middle ear and the procedure for viewing these structures with an otoscope. Normal and abnormal findings are described.

Source: Concept Media

Modifications of Examination Techniques: The Difficult-to-Handle Child (33-minute videocassette)

Specific ways to handle a child who is especially fearful or uncooperative during a physical examination. Methods to involve the child, ways to reassure the child and parent, various methods of restraint, sequencing procedures, and ways to promote rapport are included.

Source: Medical Electronic Education Services, Inc.

Physical Examination of the Preschool Child (32-minute videocassette)

Physical assessment techniques for the examination of the preschool child are shown.

Source: Career Aids

Search: The Art of Observation in Pediatrics (16-minute videocassette)

A quick systematic method of assessing illness in an infant, using only one's eyes and brain. The mnemonic SEARCH represents social stimulation, energy, appearance, reaction to parent, cry, and hydration.

Source: Health Sciences Consortium

Neurological Assessment of the Pediatric Patient (28-minute videocassette)

The basic neurological examination for infants and children, including level of consciousness, Glasgow Coma Score, and pupillary reflexes. Age-appropriate examination techniques and responses are shown, as well as those for the developmentally delayed or handicapped.

Source: AJN Educational Services

Breast Examination Stimulator (simulated model)

A life-size, lifelike model designed for teaching and practicing breast palpation techniques. Breast tissue has realistic feel; replacement breasts with abnormalities are available.

Source: Nasco Health Care Educational Materials

Partners With Your Doctor (7-minute videocassette)

A comprehensive, concise overview of breast self-examination techniques.

Source: Nasco Health Care Educational Materials

Teaching Breast Self-Examination (28-minute videocassette)

A nurse teaches a woman how to examine her breasts. Advice on how to motivate someone to overcome a fear of performing the examination. Other screening methods such as mammography, anatomy of the breast, and changes to expect during the menstrual cycle are included.

Source: AJN Educational Services

Testicle Self-Exam Model (simulated model)

A soft, simulated form of the scrotum and testicles has been embedded with five simulated tumors that can be discovered by palpation.

Source: Nasco Health Care Educational Materials{/DES}

Discussion Questions

1. History taking with children is not as easy as it first appears. How would you explore whether or not an adolescent is sexually active? How a preschool-age child swallowed poison?

2. Small children need to be restrained for parts of a physical examination. For what parts would you use restraint? Under what conditions would you ask the parents to do this?

3. Parents can overinterpret the results of a Denver Developmental Screening Test unless they understand the purpose of the test. How would you explain the purpose of a DDST to a parent?

Written Assignments

1. Vision testing is a major role for nurses. How would you explain a preschool E test to a preschooler? A Snellen test to a school-age child?

2. Inspecting for such aspects of health as whether a child is experiencing a high level of stress is difficult. What would you ask about in a history or inspect for on a physical examination to detect this?

3. Testing deep tendon reflexes requires practice and knowledge. What reflexes would you test or on a routine examination? How would you elicit these?

Laboratory Experiences

1. Assign students to ambulatory departments of hospitals or school settings where children are having physical examinations performed so the can participate in these assessments. Students need practice in all age groups before they become proficient at judging the importance of physical assessment findings.

2. Ask acquaintances to bring children to class so students can practice assessment procedures such as heart assessment, vision and hearing and DDST with children.

3. Show a film on physical assessment of a child. Ask students to comment on the examination technique and if it is age appropriate. How would they modify the procedure for another age child?

Care Study: A Toddler Who Is Light in Weight

Joey Diller is a 15-month-old male you see in an ambulatory care setting.

Health History

- Chief Concern: "Everyone says he seems short."

- History of Chief Concern: Infant weighed 9 lbs, 6 oz at birth. Mother was told he was "doing well" at 2-, 4-, and 6-month health check-ups. Father then lost job, so family no longer had health insurance and child received no further health maintenance care. Mother feels he has not grown or gained weight during last 6 months.

- Pregnancy History: This is the first pregnancy for 24-year-old mother. Mother had "slight" elevation of glucose during pregnancy; followed closely by obstetrician but no therapy initiated. Birth was at 40 weeks; infant breathed spontaneously. Parents were delighted with healthy boy.

- Past Medical History: "Occasional" colds; no major illnesses or hospitalizations. No poisonings or emergency room visits.

- Nutrition: Infant breast-fed for 3 months until mother returned to work. Took Similac with iron for 3 months, then changed to whole milk at 9 months; 2% milk at 12 months. Currently takes 16 oz milk daily by bottle, about 6 oz by glass. Eats table food. Typical day: Breakfast: scrambled eggs with cheese, 1 tbs. Lunch: pieces of baloney and cheese, chunks of watermelon. Dinner: $\frac{1}{2}$

toasted cheese sandwich, chunks of canned pears. Snacks: 1 pretzel, 1 cracker, few pieces popcorn.

- Personal/Social: Family intact. Father currently unemployed; receives unemployment compensation. Mother works as assistant in florist shop. Both parents have associate college degrees. Family lives in a 2nd floor, 2-bedroom apartment. Finances rated as ''not good'' because of large car payment and high monthly rent.

- Review of Systems: Occasional diaper rash; fell on porch steps yesterday and received ''brush burn'' on forehead. Bowel movements: two daily, yellow and ''baby-like''; voiding frequently.

Physical Examination

- General Appearance: Small but well proportioned and active 15-month-old Caucasian male. Height:.... Weight:.... Head Circumference:....

- Head: Normocephalic; fontanelles closed. Abrasion 11 cm on forehead.

- Eyes: Red reflex present; follows to 6 cardinal fields of gaze.

- Ears: TMs pink; light reflex present. Slight cerumen.

- Nose: Midline septum; no discharge; membrane pink.

- Mouth: 18 teeth; no cavities; palate intact; tonsillar tissue enlarged but not reddened. Midline uvula.

- Neck: Full range of motion; no nodes present; midline trachea.

- Chest: Lungs clear to auscultation; respiratory rate: 20/min.

- Heart: Rate 96/min. Grade I systolic murmur at left 4th intercostal space.

- Abdomen: Soft; no masses.

- Genitalia: Normal male; testes descended.

- Extremities: Slight genu valgum (bow legs); walks with wide-placed toddler gait. Full range of motion; one ecchymotic lesion 1 ½ cm over left tibia.

- Neurologic: Responsive; motor and sensory function grossly intact.

Care Study Questions

1. Plot Joey's height and weight on a standard growth chart. Is he small for his age?

2. Assess Joey's diet. Is he ingesting all five food groups? Is the type of milk he drinks right for him? Are his snacks appropriate for a 15-month-old?

3. Complete a nursing care plan that identifies and meets Joey's needs.

The Family With an Infant

Chapter 29 discusses growth and development from one month to one year. The chapter begins with an overview of the nursing process specific to care of the infant. Physical growth including development of the senses, development of new skills such as language and play, and emotional and cognitive development are discussed. Health promotion such as providing safety for the child and increasing family development are stressed. The chapter concludes by discussion of common problems of the infant year such as teething, thumb sucking, sleep problems, colic, and night-bottle syndrome. The unique concerns of a family with an infant who is physically disabled or chronically ill is included.

Many parents have questions about infant development. Because the child changes so rapidly parents need to change as well to keep up. Students are stimulated to learn the content in this area when they realize how effective they can be as health educators.

Chapter Objectives

After mastering the contents of this chapter, students should be able to:

1. Describe normal growth and development and associated parental concerns.

2. Assess an infant for normal growth and development milestones.

3. Formulate nursing diagnoses related to infant growth and development and associated parental concerns.

4. Plan nursing care to meet the infant's growth and development needs, such as planning anticipatory guidance to prevent problems such as diaper rash, sleep disturbances, and colic.

5. Implement nursing care related to normal growth and development of the infant such as helping parents plan stimulating activities.

6. Evaluate goal outcomes established for care to be certain goals associated with growth and development have been achieved.

7. Identify national health goals related to infant growth and development that nurses can be instrumental in in helping the nation to achieve.

8. Identify areas related to nursing care of the infant that could benefit from additional nursing research.

9. Use critical thinking to analyze methods of care for the infant to be certain care is family-centered.

10. Synthesize knowledge of infant growth and development with nursing process to achieve quality maternal and child health nursing care.

Key Points

- The infant period is from 1 month to 12 months. Children double their weight at 4 to 6 months and triple it at 1 year.

- Infants develop their first tooth at about 6 months; by 12 months they will have 6 to 8 teeth.

- Important gross motor milestones during the infant year are lifting chest off bed at 2 months; sitting at 6 to 8 months; creeping at 9 months; "cruising" at 10 to 11 months; and walking at 12 months.

- Important fine motor accomplishments are ability to pass an object from one hand to the other (7 months) and a pincer grasp (10 months).

- Important milestones of language development during the first year are differentiating a cry (2 months); making simple vowel sounds (5 to 6 months); and saying two words besides ma-ma and da-da (12 months). The more infants are spoken to, the easier for them to acquire language.

- Providing infants with proper toys for play helps development. All infant toys need to be checked that they are not small enough to be aspirated.

- Important milestones of vision development are ability to follow a moving object past the midline (3 months); and ability to focus securely without eyes crossing (6 months).

- The developmental task of the infant year according to Erikson is the development of a sense of trust versus mistrust.

- Infants must be protected from aspiration of small objects and falls. Be aware that a skill, such as crawling, which an infant cannot accomplish one day, may be accomplished the next.

- Remember that parent—infant attachment is critical to mental health. Urge parents to continue to give as much care as possible to sick infants to maintain this important relationship.

- Infants experience the world with their senses. Touching, smiling, and talking are important communication techniques.

- Common concerns related to infant development are teething, thumb sucking, use of pacifiers, sleep problems, constipation, colic, and diaper dermatitis. Night-bottle syndrome is a syndrome of decayed teeth from infants sucking on a bottle of formula while they sleep. Nurses can help prevent this by advising against this practice.

Definitions of Key Terms

baby-bottle syndrome: severe tooth decay in infants caused by being put to bed with a bottle

binocular vision: the use of both eyes simultaneously for vision

coordination of secondary schema: the cognitive development stage of late infancy

deciduous teeth: ''baby'' or first teeth

eighth-month anxiety: separation anxiety that peaks at the eighth month of life

extrusion reflex: a response that occurs when an object is placed on the newborn's tongue; fades at about 4 months of life

fine motor development: motor development concerned with small tasks such as writing

gross motor development: motor development concerned with large tasks such as walking

hand regard: the special fascination a 3-month-old has with his or her hands

Landau reflex: when held in a horizontal plane, an infant raises the head and flexes the arms and legs

natal teeth: erupted teeth in the newborn

neck-righting reflex: when the head of a newborn is turned right or left, the infant turns the shoulders as well

neonatal teeth: teeth present in a newborn

object permanence: the awareness that an object continues to exist even when out of sight

parachute reaction: when an infant is held horizontally and lowered toward a surface, he or she pushes out the arms as if to break a fall

pincer grasp: the ability to approximate the index finger and thumb to pick up an object

prehensile ability: the ability to use the hands and fingers to grasp objects

primary circular reaction: a stage of cognitive development in which the an infant does not yet differentiate between those actions he or she causes and those that occur independently

seborrhea: a skin condition in which there is an overproduction of sebum resulting in excessive oiliness

secondary circular reaction: the stage of cognitive development in which an infant learns that he or she can initiate pleasurable sensations

separation anxiety: fear and apprehension caused by separation from the primary caregiver

social smile: a smile in response to another's face; a developmental milestone of 2 months

thumb opposition: ability to approximate the thumb and fingers in order to grasp

ventral suspension: a position for examination; holding an infant lying in a prone position suspended horizontally{/GL}

Nursing Process Overview

The Nursing Process Overview in this chapter concentrates on helping the student adapt nursing care planning to the unique needs of the infant. Including the entire family in planning is stressed. Planning must allow for ongoing evaluation as to whether goals or interventions remain appropriate in the light of the infant's rapid growth.

Study Aids

Tables

Table 29-1: Health maintenance schedule, infant period

Table 29-2: Summary of infant growth and development

Table 29-3: Ways for nurses to help develop a sense of trust in an ill infant

Table 29-4: Common difficulties parents experience in evaluating the health of infants{/UL}

Displays

Focus on National Health Goals

Focus on Family Teaching

Focus on Nursing Research

Focus on Cultural Awareness

Critical Thinking Questions

1. Katie is a 3-month-old who will be hospitalized for several months in a hospital out of state because of severe burns. What steps could you take to foster a sense of trust in Katie in light of this extensive parental separation?

2. Marty is a 10-month old whose mother tells you is ''into everything.'' At a well child assessment, what specific questions would you want to ask in order to feel confident that Marty's house is safe for him?

3. Pattie is a 1-month-old who is going to be following in your health maintenance setting. What immunizations would you discuss with her father as those commonly recommended for the first year?

Media Resources

Human Development: A New Look at the Infant (videocassette)

Psychological development in early infancy is explored, including development of self, social cognition, communication, and attachment.

Source: Concept Media

Infant Care: Instructional Series for New Parents (videocassette)

A three-part series demonstrating infant care for parents: (1) breast- and bottle-feeding, (2) sleep, comfort, development, safety, and family needs, and (3) bathing and grooming.

Source: Mead Johnson Nutritionals

The Infant (38-minute videocassette)

A documentary film showing a nurse practitioner conducting well baby examinations during the first year in order to demonstrate the growth and development of an infant. The theories of Freud, Piaget, Erikson, Kohlberg, and Duval are reviewed. Both physical and psychosocial milestones are described. (Note: The recommendations for immunization described are outdated.)

Source: AJN Educational Services

Benjamin (42-minute film)

The development of Benjamin from birth to 6 months is shown. The emphasis is on his responsiveness to social interaction. Differences in the ways mothers and fathers play with their infants are demonstrated.

Source: Time/Life

Individual Differences (18-minute film)

The broad range of human behavior and human characteristics that are present even in infants is shown. Included is demonstration of a Denver Development Screening Test.

Source: CRM/McGraw-Hill

The Infant and the Toddler Years (21-minute videocassette)

An overview of assessment and nursing care for children during infancy and toddlerhood. Normal growth and development are highlighted, along with guidelines for planning care to enhance development in light of a childhood illness; emotional support for family members is stressed.

Source: Medcom/Trainex-Nasco Health Care Educational Materials

Discussion Questions

1. Colic is a common problem that parents encounter during the infant period. What are suggestions you would make to parents to help relieve the infant's distress?

2. Teaching parents ways to promote a sense of trust in their child during the first year is a major nursing responsibility. What measures would you suggest to parents to promote this?

3. Teething is a common concern of parents during the first year. What anticipatory guidance would you give parents?

Written Assignments

1. Whether or not parents should offer a pacifier is a controversial issue. List the pros and cons of pacifiers.

2. "Childproofing" is a major responsibility of parents and an important area for health education. What specific measures should parents take in the kitchen? the bathroom? their garage or yard?

3. Parents may be confused about what toys to select for babies. What would be the ideal toy for a newborn? A 6-month-old? A 12-month-old?

Laboratory Experiences

1. Assign students to a setting such as a day care center and ask them to assess an infant for growth and development parameters of the infant year. Compare with the standard for the age.

2. Ask an acquaintance with an infant to bring him or her to a postconference. Allow the class to interview the parent about growth and development and any problems encountered in care. See if the class can identify if a sense of trust is being promoted.

3. Ask students who are caring for ill infants in hospital or ambulatory settings to include assessment of growth and development and a nursing diagnosis in relationship to this on all nursing care plans. Requiring this helps students look at the child and not the illness and improves their ability to give comprehensive care.

Care Study: An Infant With a Feeding Problem

Tina Burrows, 4 months old, is seen for a well child check-up.

Health History

- Chief Concern: "She seems to be small and is sick all the time."

- History of Present Concern: Parents voice that they are worried that Tina is not growing as fast as she should. Child is breast-fed; parents started giving "occasional" supplemental baby fruit and cereal 2 weeks ago. Child has developed loose bowel movements and vomiting since then.

- History of Past Illnesses: Child has been attending well child conference for routine care since birth. Parents have kept all appointments. Immunizations up-to-date. No major illnesses or hospitalizations; no accidental poisoning. Home family lives in is pre-1950s. Infant never observed chewing on windowsills or other sources of paint.

- Personal/Social: Infant's parents live with grandparents in their home. Both parents smoke. Mother works at a fast food restaurant; father temporarily unemployed due to a motorcycle accident and back injury. Finances are reported as "not the best," but family has applied for welfare assistance.

- Pregnancy History: Pregnancy not planned but not un-welcome. Parents were married 1 month before infant was born. No complications during pregnancy except mother's weight gain was limited to 18 pounds. Birth weight: 6 lb 15 oz; length: 20 inches.

- Growth and Development: Child bears weight when placed in standing position. Makes cooing sounds as if trying to talk. Lifts arms to be picked up.

- Nutrition: Child is breast-fed four times during day. Mother began giving ½ jar infant cereal for breakfast, other half for dinner; 1 jar fruit for lunch 2 weeks ago to try and make child gain more weight. Two bottles (4 oz each) of Similac with iron given daily by husband while mother is at work.

- Review of Systems: Gastrointestinal: has had loose stools for past 2 weeks; has vomited once daily for last week.

Physical Examination

- General appearance: Well-proportioned, 4-month-old girl sitting on mother's lap. Temperature: 98.4gF axillary. Weight: 5.0 kg. Height: 58 cms.

- Head: Normocephalic; anterior fontanelle: 34 cm; posterior fontanelle: closed. Head circumference: 38 cms.

- Eyes: Red reflex; follows past midline to all fields of vision. PERLA.

- Ears: Normal alignment. Tympanic membrane pink; landmarks present. Mouth: No teeth as yet. Midline uvula present. Gag reflex intact.

- Throat: Midline trachea; two lymph nodes palpable in right posterior cervical chain.

- Chest: Rhonchi present in all lobes of lungs; respiratory rate 60/crying.

- Heart: Rate 110/min. No murmurs heard.

- Abdomen: Soft; liver palpable 2 cms; spleen not palpable. No masses.

- Genitourinary: Bright red rash present on diaper area. No open lesions.

- Neurologic: Moro reflex no longer present. Patellar reflex: 2.

Laboratory Results

- Hemoglobin: 13.6 g/dL
- Hematocrit: 40

Care Study Questions

1. Plot Tina's height and weight on a standard chart. Is she small as her parents fear or within normal parameters for her age?

2. Tina's mother began solid food at the same time that the diarrhea began. Could there be a connection between these two things?

3. Complete a nursing care plan that would identify and meet the needs of Tina.

The Family With a Toddler

Chapter 30 discusses growth and development of the toddler. The chapter begins with an overview of the nursing process specific to care of the toddler. Physical growth, language development, and emotional, cognitive, and moral growth are discussed. Ways to promote the developmental task of the toddler, to develop a sense of autonomy, are stressed. The nursing role in health promotion with this age group, including toddler safety, care, and interventions for parent's concerns, is discussed. Problems associated with the toddler period such as temper tantrums, negativism, toilet training, separation anxiety, and concerns of the family with a disabled or chronically ill child are included.

Most students have some understanding of childhood growth and development from previous course work. Their task, before caring for toddlers, is to individualize this knowledge to a specific child. Concrete examples of ways that care needs to be modified because of the child's developmental level help students to appreciate the importance of learning growth and development.

Chapter Objectives

After mastering the contents of this chapter, students should be able to:

1. Describe normal growth and development of the toddler period and common parental concerns.

2. Assess a toddler for normal growth and development milestones.

3. Formulate nursing diagnoses related to toddler growth and development of parental concerns regarding development.

4. Plan nursing care to meet the toddler's growth and development needs, such as anticipatory guidance to prevent problems such as sleep disturbances, temper tantrums, and inappropriate toilet-training practices.

5. Implement nursing care to promote normal growth and development of the toddler, such as discussing toddler developmental milestones with parents.

6. Evaluate goal outcomes established for care to be certain nursing goals associated with growth and development have been achieved.

7. Identify national health goals related to the toddler age group that nurses can be instrumental in in helping the nation to achieve.

8. Identify areas related to care of the toddler that could benefit from additional nursing research.

9. Use critical thinking to analyze methods of care for the toddler to be certain care is family centered.

10. Synthesize knowledge of toddler growth and development with the nursing process to achieve quality maternal and child health nursing care.

Key Points

- Toddlers make great strides forward in development but their physical growth slows.

- A critical milestone of toddler development is being able to form two-word sentences by 2 years of age.

- Erikson's developmental task for the toddler period is to form a sense of autonomy or independence.

- Toddlers are capable of preoperational thought or are able to deal much more constructively with symbols than they could while still an infant.

- Important aspects of care are promoting toddler safety, including screening for lead poisoning, promoting toddler development such as promoting daily activities and healthy family functioning.

- Common concerns of parents during the toddler period are toilet training, dawdling, ritualistic behavior, negativism, temper tantrums, discipline, and separation anxiety.

- Promoting autonomy in the child who is disabled or chronically ill calls for creative planning, sinces there may be many tasks that must be done for the child to be certain they are done safely.

Definitions of Key Terms

<u>assimilation:</u> the ability to change how a set is perceived to coincide with beliefs

<u>autonomy:</u> the ability to function independently

<u>deferred imitation:</u> the ability to remember an action and imitate it later

<u>discipline:</u> to enforce a set of rules that govern behavior

<u>lordosis:</u> an increased anterior concavity of the spine

<u>parallel play:</u> side-by-side play enjoyed by toddlers

preoperational thought: the form of cognitive thought before concrete thought is possible

punishment: the penalty for misbehavior

tertiary circular reaction stage: the cognitive stage of development in which the child explores with trial and error

Nursing Process Overview

The Nursing Process Overview in this chapter concentrates on helping the student adapt nursing care planning to the unique needs of the toddler. Including the entire family in planning is stressed. Planning must allow for ongoing evaluation as to whether goals or interventions remain appropriate in the light of the toddler's changing development.

Study Aids

Tables

Table 30-1:   Parental difficulties in evaluating illness in toddlers

Table 30-2:   Milestones of toddler growth and development

Table 30-3:   Cognitive and emotional development of the toddler

Table 30-4:   Health maintenance schedule: Toddler period

Table 30-5:   Differentiating temper tantrums, breath holding, and seizures

Table 30-6:   Nursing interventions to help the disabled or chronically ill child develop a sense of autonomy{/UL}

Displays

Focus on National Health Goals

Focus on Family Teaching

Focus on Nursing Research

Focus on Cultural Awareness

Critical Thinking Questions

1.   Bryan is a 2-year-old whose mother tells you has at least three temper tantrums a day. She asks you how to deal with these when they happen while shopping. What would you advise?

2.   People with a sense of autonomy are capable of independent function. Describe the actions of someone who does not have a good sense of autonomy. Would you enjoy working with this person as a fellow nurse?

3.   Many working mothers are concerned that toilet training will be especially difficult because their child has two or three caretakers every day. What suggestions could you offer to make toilet training easier\er when this occurs?

Media Resources

The Infant and Toddler Years (21-minute videocassette)

An overview of assessment and nursing care for children during infancy and toddlerhood. Normal growth and development are highlighted, along with guidelines for planning care to enhance development in light of a childhood illness and emotional support for family members.

Source: Medcom/Trainex-Nasco Health Care Educational Materials

The Toddler (40-minute videocassette)

A documentary describing the physical, cognitive, and psychosocial development of the child from age 1 to 3 years. Developmental theories are described with emphasis on fostering autonomy. Health promotion needs and accident prevention are stressed.

Source: AJN Educational Services

The Stress of Separation (20-minute film)

Children in a British day-care center are shown reacting to the departure of their parents, sometimes with tears, sometimes quite happily. Developmental changes in reaction to separation stressed.

Source: Filmmakers Library

Pediatrics: Physical Care: Safety (20-minute filmstrip, videocassette)

Factors in growth and development that make infants, toddlers, and preschool children prone to accidents and interventions to prevent accidents are discussed. Emphasis is placed on prevention of strangulation, aspiration, and falls.

Source: Concept Media

Discussion Questions

1.   Toddlers manifest autonomy in daily activities. How would you teach parents to handle this?

2.   Temper tantrums are the hallmark of the toddler. How would you teach parents to handle these? What action would you take if a toddler had a temper tantrum in the hallway of a busy nursing unit?

3.   The toys that parents choose for toddlers have to be different from those they chose when the child was an infant. What are ways that toys should differ? What are examples of good toddler toys?

Written Assignments

1.   Whether or not a toddler meets the speech milestone at age 2 years should be determined at assessment. What is this milestone and why is it so vital in assessment?

2.   Toddlers are such active children that keeping them safe is difficult. List specific ways that parents should "childproof" a house for a toddler. What are measures to take on a hospital unit? An ambulatory clinic?

3.   Caring for toddlers can be a challenge because of their use of the word "no." What are specific ways to avoid hearing this word during your care?

Laboratory Experiences

1.   Assign students to a setting such as a day-care center and ask them to assess a toddler for growth and development parameters. Compare with the standard for the age.

2. Ask an acquaintance with a toddler to bring him or her to a postconference. Allow the class to interview the parent about growth and development and any problems encountered in care. See if the class can identify if a sense of autonomy is being promoted.

3. Ask students who are caring for ill toddlers in hospital or ambulatory settings to include assessment of growth and development in nursing care plans. Requiring this helps students look at the child and not the illness and improves their ability to give comprehensive care.

Care Study: A Toddler With Delayed Language Development

Terry Wallace is a 2-year-old seen at a private pediatrician's office for a health maintenance visit.

Health History

- Chief Concern: "He doesn't speak in sentences yet."

- History of Previous Concern: Mother states she feels that child's development is behind typical milestones. Can speak clearly but frequently reverts to baby talk. The best sentence he can accomplish is "him go" (meaning he wants to go). Mother is presently pregnant with second child; appears exhausted and grew impatient and angry with Terry because he wouldn't talk for clinic personnel. States that she works in the chemical industry and is concerned that "chemicals affected Terry mentally." Concerned that same thing will happen to baby from present pregnancy.

- Family Profile: Mother has a PhD in chemistry and works as a researcher in local chemical plant; father is personnel manager at same company. Finances are "no problem." Family lives in large home in suburbs of city; Terry has own room; adequate play space. Attends daycare center from 7:00 to 5:00 daily.

- Past Medical Illnesses: Has had two episodes of bilateral otitis media, one at 4 months and one at 18 months. Both parents smoke and do not try to keep a "smoke-free" area for child. One episode of diarrhea at 12 months required overnight hospitalization. Routine health maintenance visits have been kept. Immunizations are up-to-date.

- Pregnancy History: Pregnancy was planned following 4 years of an infertility work-up. Mother was treated with Danazol and surgery for endometriosis. Is currently pregnant again as she was told to have a second child close to first before endometriosis returned.

  Prenatal care was begun at 2 months. Terry was a vaginal birth attended by a nurse-midwife; no complications known; breathed spontaneously; Apgars: 9 and 9. Both he and his mother were discharged from the birthing center at 12 hours postbirth.

- Growth and Development: 2 months, social smile; 4 months, rolled over; 6 months, first word (da-da); 7 months, sat alone; 12 months, toilet training started. Child dry during day at present; nocturnal enuresis every night. 14 months, walked steadily.

- Family Medical History: An uncle of child's father has sickle cell anemia. Both parents are negative for trait and disease. Maternal grandfather has lung cancer.

- Review of Systems: Genitourinary: slight hypospadias present; no surgery as yet.

Physical Examination

- General Appearance: Alert-appearing, black, well-proportioned two-year-old. Height: 36 in. Weight: 28 lbs. HC: 17.8 in.

- Head: Normocephalic; both fontanelles closed.

- Eyes: PERLA; red reflex present.

- Ears: Normal alignment. TMs; pink with cone of light present. Moderate amount of cerumen in left canal; drum not obstructed. Child turns toward whispered word; hearing comparable to examiner's.

- Nose: Nares patent; midline septum; no rhinitis.

- Mouth and Throat: Palate intact. 20 teeth present, no cavities; gag reflex active.

- Neck: Supple; no palpable lymph nodes. Midline trachea.

- Chest: No adventitious sounds on auscultation; respiratory rate: 22/minute.

- Heart: Rate 110/min; no murmurs.

- Abdomen: Bowel sounds present in all 4 quadrants; liver palpable 1 cm under right lower costal margin; spleen not palpable.

- Genitalia: Testes are descended bilaterally. Foreskin uncircumcised; easily retracted. Slight ventral displacement of meatus present.

- Neurologic: Patellar reflex 2; Fine motor: picks up raisin with pincer grasp. Gross motor: walks with toddler wide-placed steps.

- Language: not assessed; child refused to repeat words for examiner.

Care Study Questions

1. Plot Terry's height and weight on a standard growth chart and compare his growth and developmental milestones to normal. Is he developing normally? Is his language at the point it should be?

2. Terry was born with a hypospadias that has not yet been repaired. Is it usual for surgery to be delayed this long? Is it usual for boys not to be circumcised with this disorder?

3. Complete a nursing care plan that would identify and meet the needs of the Wallace family.

Chapter

31

The Family With a Preschooler

Chapter 31 discusses growth and development of the preschool-age child. The chapter begins with an overview of the nursing process specific to care of the preschool child. Physical growth, language skills, and emotional, cognitive, and moral growth are discussed. Methods to encourage development of a sense of initiative are stressed. The nursing roles in health promotion, such as promoting safety, care, and healthy family functioning, are included. Possible concerns over problems encountered during the period such as fear of the dark, imaginary friend, sibling rivalry, and the need for sex education are discussed. Techniques for preparing a child for a beginning school experience are presented. The chapter includes discussion of the unique concerns of a child who is disabled or has a chronic illness.

Most students have had exposure to growth and development of the preschool-age child from previous course work. The task to accomplish before they can become adept at caring for preschool children is to learn to apply this knowledge to everyday situations and specific children. To do this they need experience in caring for children of this age as well as class discussion.

Chapter Objectives

After mastering the contents of this chapter, students should be able to:

1. Describe normal growth and development and common parental concerns of the preschool period.
2. Assess a preschool child for normal growth and development milestones.
3. Formulate nursing diagnoses related to preschool growth and development and common parental concerns.
4. Plan nursing care to meet the preschool child's growth and development needs, such as planning age-appropriate play activities.
5. Implement nursing care related to normal growth and development of the preschool child, such as preparing the child for an invasive procedure.

6. Evaluate outcome criteria established for care to be certain normal growth and developmental goals have been achieved.
7. Identify national health goals related to the preschool period that nurses can be instrumental in in helping the nation to achieve.
8. Identify areas related to care of the preschool-age child that could benefit from additional nursing research.
9. Use critical thinking to analyze additional ways in which growth and development problems of the preschool child can be prevented and care can be family centered.
10. Synthesize knowledge of preschool growth and development with the nursing process to achieve quality maternal and child health nursing care.

Key Points

- Although preschool children grow only slightly and gain only slight weight, they seem much taller because their contour changes to a taller and slimmer one than the toddler's.
- Erikson's developmental task for the preschool period is to gain a sense of initiative or of learning how to do things. Play materials ideal for this age group are those that stimulate creativity such as modeling clay or colored markers.
- Promoting childhood safety is a major role, since the preschool child's active imagination can lead him or her into dangerous situations.
- Common parental concerns during the preschool period are ''broken fluency,'' imaginary friends, difficulty sharing, and sibling rivalry.
- Preschool is often the time when a new sibling is born. Good preparation for this is necessary to prevent intense sibling rivalry.
- Preschool children have a number of universal fears: fear of the dark, mutilation, and abandonment. All care provided for this age group must include active measures to reduce these fears as much as possible.
- Preschool children are still operating at a cognitive level that prevents them from understanding conservation (objects have not changed substance although they have changed appearance). This means they need an explanation of how they will be the same person postoperatively as they are preoperatively, for example.
- Preschool children are self-centered (egocentric). This makes it difficult for them to share or view another side

111

of a problem. They need good explanations of how a procedure will benefit them before they can agree to it.

- Many preschool children begin preschool programs or day care. Parents often appreciate some help in orienting children to these new experiences.

- Preschool children are at high risk for childhood poisoning because of their active imaginations. Be certain to remove any objects from their environment that could harm them following care.

- Preschool children who are disabled or who have chronic illnesses may have difficulty achieving a sense of initiative, because they may be limited in their ability to participate in activities that stimulate initiative. They may need special play times set aside for stimulation and learning.

Definitions of Key Terms

broken fluency: the inability of the preschool child to speak without repeating sounds or words

bruxism: grinding of the teeth

conservation: the ability to discern that although substances change their shape they do not change their basic composition

ectomorphic body build: a body build characterized by slenderness and fragility

Electra complex: Freudian concept that preschool girls fall in love with their fathers

endomorphic body build: a body build characterized by a soft round physique

genu valgus: inward curving of the knees (knock-knees)

intuitional thought: the cognitive developmental period in which children are first able to view themselves as others see them

Oedipus complex: Freudian belief that preschool boys fall in love with their mother

secondary stuttering: difficulty with stammering that occurs after the child has already spoken without the disorder

Nursing Process Overview

The Nursing Process Overview in this chapter concentrates on helping the student adapt nursing care planning to the unique needs of the preschool child. Including the entire family in planning is stressed. Discussion notes the need to plan ongoing evaluation as to whether goals or interventions remain appropriate in the light of the preschool child's changing development.

Study Aids

Boxes

Box 31-1:   Suggestions for parents on how to help limit stuttering in the preschool child

Tables

Table 31-1:   Summary of preschool growth and development

Table 31-2:   Health maintenance schedule, preschool period

Table 31-3:   Parental difficulties evaluating illness in the preschool child

Table 31-4:   Questions to use in evaluating day-care centers

Table 31-5:   Nursing actions that encourage a sense of initiative in the disabled or chronically ill preschool child

Displays

Focus on National Health Goals

Focus on Family Teaching

Focus on Nursing Research

Focus on Cultural Awareness

Critical Thinking Questions:

1. Marty is a 3-year-old who is going to start day care because his mother is returning to work to help support the family. What suggestions could you make to his mother about choosing a safe setting? How should she prepare Marty for the experience?

2. Kathy is a preschool child. Her parents tell you that Kathy keeps the entire family awake at night because she is so afraid of the dark. What suggestions could you make to her family to help Kathy sleep?

3. Barry is a 4-year-old you see in a well child conference. His mother tells you she can not stand messy activities. What are activities you could suggest to Barry's mother that would stimulate a sense of initiative but not be messy?

Media Resources

The Preschool Years (17-minute video)

An overview of assessment and nursing care for children during preschool. Normal growth and development are highlighted, along with guidelines for planning care to enhance development in light of a childhood illness and emotional support for family members.

Source: Medcom/Trainex-Nasco Health Care Educational Materials

The Preschool Child (41-minute videocassette)

The rapid development of gross motor skills and beginning development of fine motor skills is shown through the medium of play activities. The emergence of the child as a social being and as functioning more fully as a member of the family unit is stressed.

Source: AJN Educational Services

Smart, Safe, and Sure: Preventing Child Abduction (28-minute videocassette)

Practical and essential advice on preventing abduction is presented. Suggestions on how children can protect themselves and the responsibility of health care professionals to teach the public to avoid high-risk situations are discussed.

Communications and education emphasizing open lines of communication with children are stressed.

Source: AJN Educational Services

Parenting Preschoolers (55-minute videocassette)

A visual presentation of the challenges and rewards of being a parent of a preschool child. Topics such as sibling rivalry, temper tantrums, meal time, toy management, and public behavior are discussed.

Source: Cambridge Educational

I'm a Little Jealous of that Baby (11-minute videocassette; film)

Puppets are used to follow a child's adjustment to the birth of a sibling. The child is able to work through feelings of jealousy and be reassured about her place in the family.

Source: Kid's Corner

Physical Examination of the Preschool Child (32-minute videocassette)

Physical assessment techniques for the examination of the preschool child are shown.

Source: Career Aids

Hug 'n' Kids: Parenting Your Preschooler (36-minute videocassette)

Thirteen dramatizations of problem situations involving parent—child conflicts are shown. The tape freezes at the point of conflict to allow time for discussion about the problem. The situation is then reenacted to show several possible approaches to resolve the conflict.

Source: Film Fair Communications

An Instant of Time (13-minute film)

Scenes are shown in which tragic accidents involving small children are about to occur; then measures to avoid them are shown.

Source: Perennial Education, Inc.

Human Development: 2 $\frac{1}{2}$ Years to 6 Years (filmstrip/videotransfer)

Preschool development including physical, cognitive, and motor development, language, intelligence, environment, sex differences and socialization, play, and expressions of feelings are discussed.

Source: Concept Media

Discussion Questions

1. The preschool period is a time for beginning moral development or learning to tell right from wrong. How might these concepts affect a child's notion of why he or she is ill?

2. Choosing a day-care center for a preschool child can be difficult for parents. How would you help parents decide whether or not child-care center experience would be acceptable for their child?

3. Preschool children fear mutilation and abandonment. How do these factors influence your nursing care of children in this age group?

Written Assignments

1. The toys that parents choose for preschool children have to be different from those they chose when the child was a toddler. What are ways that toys should differ? What are examples of good preschool toys?

2. Preschool children are such active children that keeping them safe is difficult. List specific ways that parents should "childproof" a house for a preschool child. What are measures to take on a hospital unit? An ambulatory clinic?

3. The mother of Becky, who is 4 years old, asks you to help her prepare Becky for the arrival of a new sibling. What advice would you give her?

Laboratory Experiences

1. Assign students to a setting such as a day-care center and ask them to assess a preschool child for growth and development parameters. Compare with the standard for the age.

2. Ask an acquaintance with a preschool child to bring his or her to postconference. Allow the class to interview both the parent and the child about growth and development and any problems encountered in care. See if the class can identify if a sense of initiative is being promoted.

3. Ask students who are caring for ill preschool children in hospital or ambulatory settings to include assessment of growth and development and a nursing diagnosis in relationship to this on all nursing care plans. Requiring this helps students look at the child and not the illness and improves their ability to give comprehensive care.

Care Study: A Preschool Child With a Rash

Darnell Tiffany is a 4-year-old seen in a hospital emergency room.

Health History

- Chief Concern: "She has a rash all over her."

- History of Present Concern: Family moved into an older (1845) but restored home yesterday. Darnell woke during the night crying with pain. On examination, his legs and arms were found covered with red oozing blisters. Mother is concerned that child has lead poisoning from moving into restored house. No allergies previously identified; no new foods eaten yesterday; no exposure to other children with rashes. Child has not had chickenpox.

- Family Profile: Family was previously living in a 10-year-old home in the suburbs; father has been restoring previous house for a year. Child was not allowed to visit in house until all old paint was removed. Mother works part-time as a nurse's aide; father has his own plumbing and furnace installation business. Finances are "tight because of new mortgage."

- History of Past Illnesses: No childhood illnesses; no hospitalizations. Health maintenance at City Well Child Conference. Seen once before in emergency room for a fall from an upper bunk bed. X-ray of shoulder taken; no fracture present.

- Pregnancy History: Planned pregnancy. Prenatal care from 3rd month. Had extensive hypertension of pregnancy requiring hospitalization and treatment with magnesium sulfate last 2 months. Birth was induced at 38 weeks after amniocentesis. Birth weight: 6 lb, 12 oz. Apgars: 8 and 9. Breathed spontaneously. Both infant and mother discharged in 3 days.

- Growth and Development: 2 months, social smile; 5 months, rolled over; 6 months, sat steady; 8 months, walked; 9 months, first word. Mother unsure when child first spoke in sentences. Child uses clear and long sentence structure now. Described large back yard and how she rolled with family dog in tall grass with no difficulty.

- Review of Systems: Symptoms as noted in Chief Concern. Occasional functional murmur has been heard at health maintenance visits. Has not ever had either vision or hearing screened. Needs preschool DPT and oral poliomyelitis boosters.

Physical Examination

- General Appearance: Crying and distressed, tall for age, 4-year-old with erythematous lesions present on all extremities. Height: 110 cms. Weight: 15.2 kg.

- Head: Normocephalic; fontanelles closed. One or two 0.5-cm vesicular lesions present on right cheek.

- Eyes: PERLA; red reflex. Follows to all fields. No erythema of conjunctivae.

- Nose: Nares patent; midline septum; no rhinitis.

- Neck: Full range of motion; no lymph nodes palpable. Midline trachea. Numerous 0.5-cm vesicular lesions with clear fluid oozing and several linear abrasions on back of neck.

- Chest: Lung sounds clear to auscultation. Respiratory rate: 22/min. No lesions present on chest.

- Heart: Rate 82/min. Grade I systolic murmur present; heard best at left intercostal margin.

- Abdomen: Bowel sounds present in all quadrants; no tenderness or masses. Liver palpable 1 cm under right lower costal margin. No lesions present on abdomen.

- Genitalia: Normal female; no discharge or erythema or lesions.

- Extremities: Wide areas of vesicular lesions on erythematous bases on posterior and anterior surfaces of arms and legs. Linear tracts are interspaced with lesions. Some lesions open and oozing clear fluid. Additional linear abrasions that appear to be scratch marks also present.

- Neurologic: Patellar reflex 2. Motor and sensory nerves grossly intact. Alert and oriented to place and name.

Care Study Questions

1. Darnell's mother had a number of complications during pregnancy. Based on the reported growth and development milestones, is Darnell presently developing normally?

2. Darnell's parents are concerned she might have lead poisoning. Is a rash a symptom of this? Did these parents take sensible precautions to prevent this from occurring?

3. Darnell was diagnosed as having poison ivy, probably contracted from the yard of the new home. Complete a nursing care plan that would identify and meet the needs of the Tiffany family.

The Family With a School-Age child

Chapter 32 discusses growth and development of the school-age child. Physical growth, language development, and emotional, cognitive, and moral growth are discussed. Ways to promote the developmental task of the school-age child, to develop a sense of industry, are stressed. The nursing role in health promotion with this age group includes safety, care, and interventions for parent's concerns. Problems associated with the age period and concerns of the family with a disabled or chronically ill child are included.

Most students have some understanding of childhood growth and development from previous course work. Their task, before caring for school-age children, is to apply this knowledge to a specific child. Concrete examples of ways that care needs to be modified because of the individual child's developmental level help students to appreciate the importance of learning growth and development as preparation for child care.

Chapter Objectives

After mastering the contents of this chapter, students should be able to:

1. Describe the normal growth and development pattern and common parental concerns of the school-age period.

2. Assess a school-age child for normal growth and development milestones.

3. Formulate nursing diagnoses for the family of a school-age child.

4. Plan anticipatory guidance to prevent problems of growth and development in the school-age child (eg, teaching about normal puberty).

5. Implement nursing care to help achieve normal growth and development of the school-age child, such as counseling parents about helping their child adjust to a new school.

6. Evaluate outcome criteria to be certain that goals of care have been achieved.

7. Identify national health goals related to the school-age child that nurses can be instrumental in in helping the nation achieve.

8. Identify areas related to care of school-age children that could benefit from additional nursing research.

9. Use critical thinking to analyze ways in which the care of the school-age child can be more family centered.

10. Synthesize knowledge of school-age growth and development with the nursing process to achieve quality maternal and child health nursing care.

Key Points

- School-age children mature slowly but steadily. Their annual average weight gain is 3 to 5 lb; their increase in height, 1 to 2 inches.

- At about 10 years of age, children begin to develop secondary sex characteristics. Preparation for this helps them to accept these changes positively.

- Deciduous teeth are lost and permanent teeth erupt during the school-age period.

- Erikson's developmental task for the school-age period is to gain a sense of industry or how to do things well.

- Common health problems during the school-age period are dental caries and malocclusion.

- Common parental concerns are language development, fears and anxieties, and behavior problems such as stealing and using recreational drugs.

- About 50 of families of school-age children are dual-earner families. This means many school-age children return home before their parents (latchkey children). Counseling families how to make this time of day a positive experience for the child is a nursing responsibility.

- Children in a concrete stage of operational thought are limited to understanding concepts they can actually see. When doing health teaching, use concrete examples (actually letting them hold a syringe, not just talking about it) to increase understanding.

- School-age children thrive on set rules. It is confusing for them when rules are changed (eg, giving medicine four rather than three times a day) unless they have a clear explanation why the change is occurring.

- School-age children are looking for good adult role models; it is hard for them to feel confidence in an adult who isn't honest with them or who fails to live up to their expectations by not following through on promises.

Definitions of Key Terms

accommodation: the ability to adapt thought processes to fit what is perceived

caries: destruction of the tooth enamel (dental cavities)

class inclusion: the concept that objects can belong to more than one classification

conservation: the ability to discern that although substances change their shape they do not change their basic composition

decenter: the ability to focus on others' views rather than your own

inclusion: the concept that children with disabilities should attend school classes with children without disabilities (formerly mainstreaming)

latchkey child: a child who is without adult supervision for a part of each weekday

malocclusion: abnormal alignment of the upper and lower jaw

nocturnal emissions: ejaculation during sleep

preconventional reasoning: the type of moral reasoning according to Kohlberg that occurs in the young child

Nursing Process Overview

The Nursing Process Overview in this chapter concentrates on helping the student adapt nursing care planning to the unique needs of the school-age child. Including the entire family in planning is stressed. Discussion notes the necessity to plan for ongoing evaluation as to whether goals or interventions remain appropriate in the light of the child's increasing need to be independent.

Study Aids

Boxes

Box 32-1:   Teaching points to help children avoid sexual abuse

Box 32-2:   Teaching points for the parents of latchkey children

Tables

Table 32-1: Chronologic development of secondary sex characteristics

Table 32-2: Summary of school-age development

Table 32-3: Health maintenance schedule, school-age period

Table 32-4: Parental difficulties evaluating illnesses in the school-age child

Table 32-5: Nursing actions that encourage a sense of industry in the disabled or chronically ill school-age child

Displays

Focus on National Health Goals

Focus on Family Teaching

Focus on Nursing Research

Focus on Cultural Awareness

Critical Thinking Questions

1. Martha is a 6-year-old who tells you she "hates school." What areas would you want to explore with her to document the extent of the problem? What are suggestions you might make to her parents to make school more appealing?

2. Debbie is a 9-year-old you see at a health maintenance visit. Her father tells you she is a "behavior problem" in school. What special physical assessments would you want to make of Debbie? What questions would you want to ask to discover the extent of the problem?

3. Russell is a 12-year-old who is confined to a wheelchair from muscular dystrophy. Why might developing a sense of industry be particularly difficult for him? What are specific suggestions you might make to encourage this?

Media Resources

The School Age Years (16-minute videocassette)

An overview of assessment and nursing care for children during school age years. Normal growth and development are highlighted along with guidelines for planning care to enhance development in light of a childhood illness and emotional support for family members.

> Source: Medcom/Trainex-Nasco Health Care Educational Materials

The Pre-adolescent Years (19-minute videocassette)

An overview of assessment and nursing care for the adolescent. Normal growth and development are highlighted along with guidelines for planning care to enhance development in light of a childhood illness and emotional support for family members.

> Source: Medcom/Trainex-Nasco Health Care Educational Materials

The School-Age Child (41-minute videocassette)

Refinement of motor skills and the seemingly continuous activity of the child in this age group. Continual socialization activities via play activities are demonstrated. The drive to learn and cognitive development are stressed. The effect of entering school and the importance of family are discussed.

> Source: AJN Educational Services{

Human Development: Six to Twelve Years (filmstrip/videotransfer)

School-age growth and development is described. Major topics include cognitive, social, physical, memory, and personality development.

> Source: Concept Media

Growing up: Body, Feelings, Behavior (18-minute film)

Preadolescent development of sexual characteristics, the changes in the way children feel about themselves and others, and expected changes in behavior during the school-age years are presented. Normal individual growth differences are demonstrated.

Source: Churchill Films

Better Safe Than Sorry (60-minute videocassette)

Four tapes of 15 minutes each addressing the issue of child sexual abuse. Designed to teach school-age children and adolescents about potentially dangerous situations involving strangers, friends, and family members. Children are challenged to problem solve how to avoid dangerous situations.

Source: Film Fair Communications

How to Develop Self-Confidence When You're not the Fastest, the Smartest, the Prettiest or the Funniest (videocassette)

Four scenarios that depict preadolescent children in situations that illustrate the importance and difficulties associated with developing independence and self-confidence. Suggestions for handling disappointment, making responsible decisions, and realizing personal goals are included.

Source: Guidance Associates

Discussion Questions

1. Moral development in children follows cognitive development. How would a 7-year-old answer the question, "Is it right to tell on a friend?" Would a 10-year-old's answer be different?

2. School-age children need orientation to adult sexual roles. How would you explain menstruation to a class of 10-year-old girls? Would you do it any differently if boys were also present? What if the entire class was boys?

3. School-age children enjoy projects that are short-term and offer a reward. How does this factor influence your nursing care of children in this age group?

Written Assignments

1. The toys that parents choose for school-age children have to be different from those they chose when the child was preschool age. What are ways that toys should differ? What are examples of good school-age toys?

2. School-age children are so adventurous that keeping them safe is difficult. List specific things that parents should teach this age child to keep him or her safe in the community. What are measures to take on a hospital unit? In an ambulatory clinic?

3. It is easy for parents to feel they are losing contact with school-age children because children are away from home so long each day. List suggestions you could make to parents to increase their contact time with children this age.

Laboratory Assignments

1. Assign students to a setting such as a grade school and ask them to assess a school-age child for growth and development parameters. Compare with the standards for the age.

2. Ask an acquaintance with a school-age child to bring him or her to a postconference. Allow the class to interview both the parent and child about growth and development and any problems encountered in care. See if the class can identify if a sense of industry is being promoted.

3. Ask students who are caring for ill school-age children in hospital or ambulatory settings to include assessment of growth and development and a nursing diagnosis in relation to this on all nursing care plans. Requiring this helps students look at the child and not the illness and improves their ability to give comprehensive care.

Care Study: A School-age Child With Obesity

Candy Ralston is a 9-year-old you care for in an ambulatory clinic.

Health History

- Chief Concern: "She's too fat to fit any clothes."

- History of Present Concern: Child was normal weight for height until about 2 years ago when according to mother she began gaining excessive weight (no previous health records to trace weight increase are available).

- Family Profile: Mother and daughter are homeless and have been living at City Mission shelter for last month; depend on donations for clothing. Mother concerned because child is so heavy at present that no donated clothes fit her. Mother states her age is 26 although she looks much older. She has an eighth grade education; ran away from home at age 13 because of sexually abusive father. Candy is the result of her being raped and impregnated at 17.

  Child currently attends school program at Mission; eats meals furnished by Mission. Describes finances as "better than before."

- History of Past Illnesses: No major illnesses; no hospitalizations. Mother unsure about immunizations (thinks she had "some" as a baby in Michigan). Child has many colds during the winter; has not had a documented otitis media. Pregnancy History: Mother received no prenatal care during pregnancy. Child was born vaginally in hospital emergency room. Birth weight: 6 lbs, 10 oz.

- Growth and Development: Developmental milestones not recalled. Child is described by mother as "smarter than me." Mother is pleased with child's ability to read and add and subtract. Child has attended no more than three months of school in any one year because of frequent moves.

- Nutrition: Child eats all meals at Mission. 24-hour recall: Breakfast: 1 bowl of Cheerios, 3 slices toast, 1 glass orange juice, 1 glass milk. Lunch: 1 bowl chicken soup, 1 serving beef stew, 1 peanut butter and jelly sandwich, 1 glass milk. Dinner: 1 green salad, 1 serving roast beef, 1 serving mashed potatoes, 1 serving corn, 2 slices bread and butter, 1 serving apple pie. Snacks: 1 bowl popcorn with butter, 2 candy bars, 1 dish gelatin with peaches, 3 cans cola.

- Review of systems: Head: lice infestation 2.

- Eyes and Ears: Had screening check at Mission last week; reported as normal.

- Gastrointestinal: Numerous episodes of diarrhea; dates unknown.

Physical Examination

- General Appearance: Very obese, alert-appearing 9-year-old.

  Height: 130 cms. Weight: 132 lbs.

- Head: Normocephalic; sand-colored grains present on hair shafts. Linear abrasions on scalp.

- Eyes: red reflex present. Follows to all fields of vision.

- Ears: Normal alignment. Unable to view tympanic membranes because of accumulated cerumen. Responded to whispered word.

- Nose: Nares patent; midline septum.

- Mouth and Throat: Palate intact; 24 teeth present; 6 caries present. One central upper incisor missing. Gag reflex intact. Geographic tongue noted.

- Neck: Full range of motion. Two ''shotty'' nodes palpable on right posterior cervical chain; one palpable in left submental chain.

- Chest: Lungs clear by auscultation. Respiratory rate: 20/min. No pubertal breast development as yet. Right

clavicle elevated as right shoulder is held higher than the left.

- Heart: Rate 88/min. No murmurs heard.

- Abdomen: Protuberant. Bowel sounds heard in all four quadrants. No masses present, although it is difficult to palpate because of obesity. Right hip is elevated in relation to left.

- Genitalia: Normal female. No discharge present.

- Extremities: Full range of motion. Fingernails are short and ragged as if bitten.

- Back: Lateral curve of spine present about 10 degrees on standing; accentuated on bending to about 30 degrees. Vertebrae not tender to palpation. Right scapula elevated.

- Neurologic: Patellar reflex 2. Motor and sensory nerves grossly intact. Alert and oriented to place and name.

Care Study Questions

1. Candy's mother is most concerned because Candy is overweight. Plot Candy's height and weight on a standard growth chart to see the extent of the problem.

2. Candy has two other health problems that are revealed on physical examination. What are these?

3. Complete a nursing care plan that would identify and meet Candy's needs.

The Family With an Adolescent

Chapter 33 discusses growth and development of the adolescent. The chapter begins with an overview of the nursing process specific to care of the adolescent. Physical growth, including puberty changes, and emotional, cognitive, and moral growth are discussed. Ways to promote the developmental task of the adolescent, to develop a sense of identity, are stressed. The nursing role in health promotion with the age group, including adolescent safety, care, and healthy family functioning, is discussed. Problems and concerns associated with the adolescent period such as fatigue, acne, sexuality, substance abuse, suicide, and runaways are discussed. Unique concerns of the family with a disabled or chronically ill adolescent are included.

Most students have some understanding of childhood growth and development from previous course work. Their task, before caring for adolescents, is to apply this knowledge to a specific child. Concrete examples of ways that care needs to be modified because of the individual child's developmental level helps students appreciate the importance of learning growth and development.

Chapter Objectives

After mastering the contents of this chapter, students should be able to:

1. Describe the normal growth and development pattern and common parental concerns of the adolescent period.
2. Assess adolescents for normal growth and development milestones.
3. Formulate nursing diagnoses for the family of an adolescent.
4. Plan nursing care related to growth and development concerns, such as planning health teaching necessary to accept puberty changes.
5. Implement nursing care related to growth and development or special needs of the adolescent, such as organizing a discussion group on ways to prevent drug abuse.
6. Evaluate outcome criteria to be certain that nursing goals were achieved.

7. Identify national health goals related to the adolescent that nurses could be instrumental in in helping the nation to achieve.
8. Identify areas related to care of adolescents that could benefit from additional nursing research.
9. Use critical thinking to analyze ways in which care of the adolescent could be more family centered.
10. Synthesize knowledge of adolescent growth and development with nursing process to achieve quality maternal and child health nursing care.

Key Points

- The major milestones of development in the adolescent period are onset of puberty and cessation of body growth. Between these milestones, physical growth is rapid and the development of adult coordination and thought processes is slow.

- The development task of the adolescent according to Erikson is to establish independence from parents through gaining a sense of identity. Adolescents, therefore, usually respond best to health care personnel who respect their attempts at independence and allow them as many choices as possible in care.

- The development of secondary sex characteristics is completed during adolescence. These are rated according to Tanner stages.

- Adolescents reach a point of cognitive development termed formal operation. At this stage, they are able to think in abstract terms and use the scientific method to arrive at conclusions.

- To appear older than they are, some adolescents present an assured, "I know that" attitude. To be effective, health teaching may have to be introduced with, "I know you know this, so I'll just review it" approach that allows the child to maintain a mature front, yet allows him or her to gain additional information.

- Being an adolescent is difficult in today's world. Be aware that to reduce stress, some adolescents begin to abuse drugs. Asking what an adolescent's experiences with this are during the health assessment is not intruding; it is conducting safe health assessment.

- Promoting adolescent safety is an important nursing role. Motor vehicle accidents are a leading cause of death in the age group.

- Common health problems in the adolescent are sometimes minor such as poor posture, fatigue, or acne; or they can be serious such as beginning hypertension, substance abuse, and suicide. Identifying these problems and referring the adolescent for help are important nursing actions.

Definitions of Key Terms

adolescence: the time period between 12 and 18 years

comedones: the lesion of acne arising from a plugged sebaceous gland

formal operational thought: a cognitive stage in which abstract thought is possible

identity: the developmental task of the adolescent: learning what kind of person he or she is

puberty: the period of life at which the ability to reproduce becomes possible

role confusion: the sense that develops if identity is not achieved

substance abuse: the use of chemicals to improve the mental state or induce euphoria

Nursing Process Overview

The Nursing Process Overview in this chapter concentrates on helping the student adapt nursing care planning to the unique needs of the adolescent. Including the entire family in planning is stressed. Planning must include ongoing evaluation as to whether goals or interventions remain appropriate in the light of the adolescent's increasing need to be independent.

Study Aids

Boxes

Box 33-1:   Health teaching guidelines for the prevention and treatment of acne

Box 33-2:   Health teaching guidelines for adolescents regarding sexuality

Box 33-3:   Measures to teach adolescents to prevent rape

Box 33-4:   Health teaching guidelines for the prevention of substance abuse in adolescents

Tables

Table 33-1:   Sexual maturation in adolescents

Table 33-2:   Health maintenance schedule, adolescent period

Table 33-3:   Stages of substance abuse

Table 33-4:   Symptoms to help identify drug abusers

Table 33-5:   Nursing actions that encourage a sense of identity in the disabled or chronically ill adolescent

Displays

Focus on National Health Goals

Focus on Family Teaching

Focus on Nursing Research

Focus on Cultural Awareness

Critical Thinking Questions

1.   Kenneth is a 16-year-old whom you meet in an ambulatory clinic. Although he tells you during history taking that he does not smoke, you notice his clothes smell like cigarette smoke. Although he says he doesn't use drugs, a number of blue and white capsules fall out of his shirt pocket when he unbuttons his shirt. What techniques could you use to see if Kenneth is smoking cigarettes or using drugs? What is your obligation to Kenneth's parents if Kenneth does admit he is not only heavily into drugs but does not intend to stop using them?

2.   Mary is a shy, quiet 14-year-old you care for in a hospital setting. She tells you she is concerned because she has not menstruated as yet. This is making her feel "left out" at school. How would you counsel Mary? What if she were 16 and had the same concern?

3.   Harry is a 15-year-old who enjoys rap music and has been collecting baseball cards since he was 8. He has recently started listening to classical music and he gave his collection of cards away to a neighbor boy because he "wouldn't need them where he's going." Would you be concerned about Harry? What if you learned Harry is about to leave to be an exchange student in England. Would you be more or less concerned?

Media Resources

Human Development: The Adolescent Years, 12 to 16 (filmstrip, videotransfer)

Adolescent physical development and its psychological effects, cognitive development, and the role of parents and peers are examined.

Source: Concept Media

Implication of Nursing Care--The Adolescent Years (18-minute videocassette)

An overview of assessment and nursing care for the adolescent. Normal growth and development are highlighted along with guidelines for planning care to enhance development in light of a childhood illness, and emotional support for family members is stressed.

Source: Medcom/Trainex-Nasco Health Care Educational Materials

All the kids do it (30-minute videocassette)

The danger of drinking alcohol and driving is dramatized. Statistical information relating to adolescents and alcohol-related vehicular accidents is presented. The adolescent's responsibility for safe drinking practices is emphasized.

Source: Pyramid Films

The Drug Tape (30-minute videocassette)

The effects of various drugs from alcohol to heroin are realistically portrayed. Presentation is designed to halt adolescents from experimenting with drugs.

Source: Cambridge Educational

Condoms: More Than Birth Control (11-minute videocassette)

The use of condoms, why it is important to use them, and how they should be used. Women are presented with a number of ways in which they can persuade a reluctant partner to use a condom for mutual protection.

Source: Polymorph Films

The Adolescent (44-minute videocassette)

Concepts of growth and development of adolescence are presented. Content includes rapid growth patterns that lead to sexual maturation, identity conflicts associated with wide mood swings, and problems important to the adolescent. Substance abuse, pregnancy, and sexually transmitted diseases are discussed with emphasis on health promotion and protection during adolescence.

Source: AJN Educational Services

Sex and the American Teenager (32-minute videocassette)

Adolescent and parental feelings about sexuality and life are presented. The film is intended to challenge adolescents to examine their values and to consider consequences of sexual activity. It also emphasizes the need for open communication between parents and adolescents.

Source: Pyramid Films

Youth Stress (24-minute videocassette)

Normal stressors for adolescents, including parental and peer pressure, lack of confidence, fear of failure, and unattainable expectations are presented. Suggestions are offered for counteracting the stress that adolescents are likely to experience in today's society.

Source: AJN Educational Services

Adolescent Physical and Psychosocial Changes: Basis for Nursing Approaches (30-minute videocassette)

Three phases of adolescence and the hormonal, musculoskeletal, integumentary, respiratory, and cardiovascular changes associated with each phase are discussed. The psychosocial and cognitive changes in the adolescent during each of the three phases of growth are discussed.

Source: Health Sciences Consortium

Suicide: A Teenage Dilemma

The necessity for young people to have adults listen to them is conveyed by conversations among groups of young people or parents who have attempted suicide or have a friend or family members who have. Clues and behavior changes to help identify adolescents who are potentially suicidal are given.

Source: Health Sciences Consortium

Discussion Questions

nts is that children change so much during this time. How is a 13-year-old different from a 14-year-old? A 15-year-old different from a 16-year-old?

2. Although age 18 is usually accepted as the beginning of adult life, many 18-year-olds are not emotionally ma-

ture. What are the ways in which you could help a hospitalized 18-year-old achieve more maturity?

3. Acne is a common adolescent health concern. What are ways you could help an adolescent increase his or her self-esteem until acne therapy is successful?

Written Assignments

1. Suicide counseling is a role for people experienced in crisis counseling. If you identified an adolescent contemplating suicide in your community, what are the resources you could use for referral?

2. It is generally accepted that programs to prevent drug abuse have a low rate of success. For what reasons are adolescents so prone to chemical dependency? Why are adolescent programs unsuccessful?

3. Steroids are a new type of drug abused by adolescents. Describe why this is a dangerous practice for adolescents.

Laboratory Experiences

1. Assign students to observe at a site where adolescents congregate, such as a shopping mall. What actions do they see that denote adolescents who are struggling to gain a sense of identity?

2. Ask an acquaintance with an adolescent to bring him or her to a postconference. Allow the class to interview the parent and the child about growth and development and any problems encountered in care. See if the class can identify if a sense of identity is being promoted.

3. Ask students who are caring for ill adolescents in hospital or ambulatory settings to include assessment of growth and development and a nursing diagnosis in relation to this on all nursing care plans. Requiring this helps students look at the adolescent and not the illness and improves their ability to give comprehensive care.

Care Study: An Adolescent With Depression

Wayne Pulvino is a 17-year-old brought to an ambulatory clinic by his father.

Health History

- Chief Concern: "He sleeps all the time. Has absolutely no energy."

- History of Present Concern: Father states that son's behavior has changed over the past year from an active sports-minded teenager to one who presently participates in no sports and misses school at least one day a week from "fatigue." Adolescent says he doesn't think there is anything wrong with him: "A person doesn't have to play football to be all right." Adolescent appeared self-conscious talking about self; very often spoke to hands instead of examiner. Sighs frequently and maintains sad facial expression.

- Family Profile: Father and son live in a rented apartment on west side of city. Parents were divorced one year ago. Wayne's sister and mother remain living in the family house. Wayne spoke of that bitterly, as his sister was able to remain in old school after divorce. He and mother had numerous arguments; when Wayne was suspended from school for smoking, his mother asked if he could live with his father. This required him to change schools. Described new school as ''a school; they're all the same'' when his father was in the examining room; as ''a high school from hell'' when he was alone.

Father works as a real estate salesman. Son described finances as ''okay'' but ''What good does working all your life do when all you end up with is a (adjective deleted) rented apartment while your wife takes everything?''

- History of Past Illnesses: Chickenpox about age 7 years. Stepped on a rusty nail at 12 years and had tetanus immunization booster; no sequelae. ''Bad acne'' since he was 14; used to take a prescribed medication for this: hasn't had the energy to go back to former doctor to have prescription renewed, so hasn't used anything for last 3 months.

- Growth and Development: Is a senior in high school (no failed grades); admits he was an A student in previous school; is ''closer to a D'' in new school. Attributes change in grades to ''things being taught differently at new school.'' Is sexually active; states he is aware of the symptoms of STDs and necessity to use condoms. Admitted to experimenting with cocaine on one occasion; smokes one pack of cigarettes daily (father is a chain smoker).

- Activity: 24-hour recall: Got up at 7:00 am ; rode ½ hour bus ride to school; rode back again at 3:30 pm. Participates in no after school activities. ''Hung out'' at city mall until 6:00 pm when he walked two blocks home for dinner. Father bought fast food dinner and they ate together. In the evening he visited at a girlfriend's house until 10:00 pm. Was asleep by 11:00 pm.

- Nutrition: 24-hour recall: Breakfast: 1 bowl cereal, 1 glass milk. Lunch: 1 cheese sandwich, two apples, 1 carton milk. Dinner: 1 cheeseburger, a serving French fries, 1 cup coffee. Snack: 1 bowl popcorn, 1 beer.

- Review of systems: Negative but for chief concern. No recent vision of hearing examination or immunizations.

Physical Examination

- General Appearance: Tall, rangy-appearing 17-year-old with bored expression on face.

- Head: Normocephalic. Numerous black comedones on erythematous bases present on forehead and cheeks.

- Eyes: Red reflex; pupils equal in size. React to light and accommodate. Tested by Snellen chart: 20/30 both eyes.

- Ears: Normal alignment. Tympanic membranes pink; landmarks present. Responds to whispered words.

- Nose: Midline septum; nares patent.

- Mouth and Throat: Palate intact. Lower third molars partially erupted. Areas tender to touch. Midline uvula. Gag reflex intact. Tonsilar issue not inflamed.

- Neck: Full range of motion. No nodes palpable. Midline trachea: thyroid not enlarged.

- Chest: Supernumerary nipple present, 3 cm below left nipple. Rhonchi heard in all four lobes of lungs; respiratory rate: 18/min.

- Heart: Rate 72/min. Marked sinus arrhythmia.

- Abdomen: Bowel sounds heard in all four quadrants. No masses. Neither spleen nor liver palpable.

- Genitalia: Normal circumcised male; Tanner 4. Testes descended.

- Extremities: Full range of motion. Walks with easy relaxed gait.

- Neurologic: Deep tendon reflexes 2. Nose to finger, Romberg accomplished without difficulty. Sensory and motor responses grossly intact.

Care Study Questions

1. Wayne's father is concerned that his son has a physical problem causing fatigue. Does Wayne's physical examination or history reveal any signs of illness?

2. Some adolescents are fatigued because of an excessive level of activity. Does Wayne's history reveal this? Poor nutrition can also lead to fatigue. Is Wayne's diet adequate? Could his diet be a factor? Is it more likely Wayne is demonstrating depression?

3. Complete a nursing care plan that would identify and meet the needs of Wayne and his father.

Nutritional Needs Through Childhood and Adolescence

Chapter 34 discusses nutritional concerns of children from the infant period through adolescence. The chapter begins with a Nursing Process Overview that summarizes ways to obtain an accurate nutrition history and develop nursing diagnoses that speak to the entire family's nutritional needs. The recommended daily dietary allowances for healthy children as well as nutrition problems of different age groups such as introducing solid food and weaning are stressed. Common childhood nutritional disorders such as lactose intolerance, iron-deficiency anemia, and obesity and ways to promote nutrition in the hospitalized child are included. Specific care of the child with total parenteral nutrition or gastrostomy and enteral feedings is included.

Chapter Objectives

After mastering the contents of this chapter, students should be able to:

1. Describe the differences in nutritional needs of children during the infancy, toddler, preschool, school-age, and adolescent periods.

2. Assess a child's eating patterns and determine nutritional needs.

3. Formulate nursing diagnoses regarding nutritional needs of the well child.

4. Plan nursing care for the specific nutritional needs of a hospitalized or well child.

5. Implement nursing care to meet the specific nutritional needs of the child, such as instituting total parenteral nutrition (TPN).

6. Evaluate outcomes established for care to ascertain whether goals have been achieved.

7. Identify national health goals related to nutrition and children that nurses could be instrumental in in helping the nation to achieve.

8. Identify areas related to nutrition and children that could benefit from additional nursing research.

9. Use critical thinking to analyze methods that will help parents improve nutrition throughout their child's life span.

10. Synthesize the elements of knowledge about childhood nutrition with nursing process to achieve quality maternal and child health nursing care.

Key Points

- Children need to follow basic guidelines for a healthy diet, such as eating a variety of foods; maintaining ideal weight; avoiding too much fat, saturated fat, and cholesterol; eating foods with adequate starch and fiber; avoiding too much sugar, and drinking alcohol in moderation, the same as adults.

- The best method for assessing nutritional intake is to take a 24-hour-recall history. Cultural and social considerations must be respected before assessing or planning nutrition for children.

- Solid food is generally introduced into the infant's diet at 5 to 6 months of age. Before infants can eat solid food effectively, they must lose their extrusion reflex.

- Infants are weaned from breast or bottle beginning at 6 to 9 months of age, depending on the parent's time preference. By 6 months, infants can begin to use a spoon to feed themselves.

- Toddlers are interested in finger foods because these can be eaten independently. The preschool child and school-age child enjoy helping to prepare food and plan menus. Encouraging them to plan their school lunch helps them maintain a healthy diet during the school year.

- Adolescents are interested in eating what their friends eat. Nutition planning must be creative to include basic food groups within this pattern.

- Vegetarian diets are adequate for children. Vitamn B_{12}, because it is found almost exclusively in animal sources, may need to be supplemented.

- Glycogen loading is inappropriate for children until the long-term consequences of carbohydrate deprivation are better studied.

- Children of African-American, Asian, and Mexican-American children may have lactase insufficiency and therefore lactose intolerance. They are unable to drink milk or eat milk products if this is present.

- Preventing obesity is an important concern in childhood nutrition. All children should be urged to engage in regular exercise and eat a sensible diet.

- Illnesses such as hypertension and hyperlipidemia occur during childhood. Measures such as reducing salt or saturated fat in the diet cann be implemented to reduce symptoms. Children under 2 years of age should not have fat restricted to ensure proper myelination of nerve cells.

- Actions that are necessary for promoting nutritional health in the hospitalized child include measuring fluid intake and output and providing enteral, gastrostomy, and total parenteral nutrition.

Definitions of Key Terms

adipocyte: a fat cell

calorie counting: calculation of calories ingested in 24 hours

gavage: To feed by means of a tube passed into the stomach

glycogen loading: excessively decreasing and then increasing carbohydrate intake to better sustain energy for a sporting event

lacto-ovovegetarian: a diet mainly of fruits and vegetables but also dairy and egg products

lactose intolerance: the inability to digest lactose due to lactase deficiency

lactovegetarian: a diet of mainly fruits and vegetables but with some added dairy products

macrobiotic: a diet in which protein is derived mainly from grains and seeds

macronutrient: a mineral needed by the body in an amount over 100 mg daily

micronutrient: a mineral needed by the body in an amount under 100 mg daily

ovovegetarian: a diet mainly of fruits and vegetables with some egg products allowed

total parenteral nutrition: a method whereby total body nutritional needs are supplied intravenously

Vegan: a strict vegetarian

Nursing Process Overview

The Nursing Process Overview in this chapter focuses on ways to assess nutrition using a 24-hour recall. Nursing diagnoses suggested are family centered, since children's nutrition is dependent on the entire family's nutrition.

Study Aids

Tables

Table 34-1:   Servings of the five pyramid food groups

Table 34-2:   Vitamins essential for health

Table 34-3:   Minerals essential for health

Table 34-4:   Recommended daily dietary allowances for children, birth through adolescence

Table 34-5:   Physical signs of adequate nutrition

Table 34-6:   Suggested schedule for introduction of solid foods

Table 34-7:   Areas to consider when planning nutrition for hospitalized children

Table 34-8:   Methods to determine proper gavage tube placement

Displays

Focus on National Health Goals

Focus on Family Teaching

Focus on Nursing Research

Focus on Cultural Awareness

Critical Thinking Exercises:

1. Renie is a 2-year-old whose mother tells you that she "eats nothing." What would be the best way to assess what she eats? What suggestions could you make to her mother to increase the amount of food she eats daily?

2. Sam is a 12-year-old whose mother wants him to take a meat sandwich for lunch at school daily. He refuses to take anything but a peanut butter and pickle sandwich. They argue about this daily. How could you help them resolve this conflict?

3. Karen is a preschool child. Her parents want her to follow a vegetarian diet but she doesn't seem to like any vegetables. What suggestions could you make to them to help Karen improve her nutrition?

Media Resources

Insertion of an Infant Gavage Feeding Tube (11-minute videocassette)

The insertion of an orogastric-nasogastric feeding tube in an infant is demonstrated. Tube placement verification measures and interventions for insertion problems are discussed.

Source: Ross Laboratories

Development of Infant Feeding Skills (24-minute videocassette)

Normal infant and young child feeding patterns including stages of development, transition to solid foods, and self-feeding skills.

Source: Churchill Films

Unfinished Child (30-minute videocassette)

The impact of maternal, fetal, and infant nutrition on physical and mental development is presented by Patricia Neal. Poor nutrition is identified as a factor in the perpetuation of the poverty cycle.

Source: March of Dimes Birth Defects Foundation

Warmth, Involvement, Caring: The WIC Success Story (14-minute videocassette)

The purposes of the WIC program, the eligibility requirements, and the role of WIC in overall health care are presented. The immediate and long-term benefits and cost of the program are discussed.

Source: Ross Laboratories

Nutrition: Foods, Fads, Frauds, Facts (Filmstrip/videocassette)

The physiology of hunger and appetite are presented. Cultural and psychosocial influences on eating habits and food selection and the effects of advertising and packaging on food choices are discussed. The way that taste and eating habits develop early in life and how eating relates to stress are discussed, as well as the nutritional role of vitamins, minerals, proteins, fats, and carbohydrates.

Source: Guidance Associates

Discussion Questions

1. Most parents enjoy preparing finger foods. Plan an entire day's menu using only finger foods.

2. Introducing solid food as early as 1 week of life is still common practice in some communities. What would you teach about infant growth and development to try to discourage this practice?

3. Adolescent obesity is a concern because it interferes with self-esteem. What are some ways to improve self-esteem in an obese adolescent?

Written Assignments

1. Feeding problems often begin in the toddler years. What are common reasons for this and how can you help a parent prevent it from happening?

2. School-age children may not be interested in learning good nutrition because they do not see it as important. What methods could you use to interest this age group in better nutrition?

3. School-age children and adolescents typically eat at least one meal away from home each day. What are five different lunches a child could bring to school that would be nutritionally adequate yet not be boring?

Laboratory Experiences

1. Assign students to care for children who are hospitalized or on home care with specific nutrition concerns, such as children who require enteral feedings or who are receiving total parenteral nutrition.

2. Assign students to a day's experience in an ambulatory nutrition clinic where children with problems such as obesity or failure to thrive are seen; assign them to obtain a nutrition history.

3. Assign students to a well child conference or other setting where infants are seen for health maintenance care. Assign students to obtain a nutrition history to allow them to discover the wide range of methods of introducing solid food that parents use.

Care Study: An Infant With Gastrostomy Feedings

Michelle Endria is a 4-month-old infant born with a tracheoesophageal fistula. She receives feedings by a gastrostomy tube.

Health History

- Chief Concern: "She's thrown up twice this morning."
- History of Present Concern: Child has been cared for at home by parents since first stage of surgery for tracheoesophageal fistula 1 month ago. Either mother or father or grandmother gives feedings. Child has been fretful and crying since early morning; threw up by tube immediately after 8 am feeding and again after noon feeding. Vomitus was sour milk; slight fresh bleeding with second vomiting episode. Bowel movement this morning was moderate in amount; yellow and semiformed.
- Family Profile: Family intact; both parents attend college and support selves by teaching assistantships. Live in 1-bedroom apartment in student housing project. Admit that finances are "bad." Maternal grandmother who lives nearby babysits at times both parents have classes.
- Pregnancy History: Pregnancy unplanned and at first undesired. Mother decided against abortion after "deep thought." Hydramnios diagnosed at 8th month of pregnancy. Infant born at 36 weeks' gestation after premature labor could not be effectively halted. Respirations were spontaneous; inability to pass orogastric tube into stomach in delivery room revealed esophageal stenosis.
- Growth and Development: Infant lifts head and trunk off bed when prone; turns front to back. Demonstrates social smile; laughs out loud.
- Past Medical History: Infant was maintained on total parenteral nutrition for 2 months; has been maintained on gastrostomy feedings for 1 month after first stage of surgery.

  Infant hospitalized for 1 month after birth for pneumonia; received intravenous antibiotics and was on ventilator. Infant has been gaining weight since on home care.
- Family Medical History: Mother had cleft lip as infant; repair left almost no scar.

  Paternal grandfather: epilepsy since childhood; takes phenobarbital and dilantin daily.

Physical Examination

- General Appearance: Crying, distressed appearing, small-for-age infant.
- Head: Normocephalic; anterior fontanelle 2 cm 3 cm; posterior closed.
- Eyes: TMs pink; landmarks visible.
- Nose: Midline septum; no discharge.
- Neck: Full range of motion; no palpable nodes; midline trachea.
- Chest: Lungs clear to auscultation and percussion. Respiratory rate: 20/min. Well healed surgery scar on sternal midline.
- Heart: Rate 100/min; no murmurs.
- Abdomen: Distended. Gastrostomy tube inserted in left upper quadrant; skin slightly erythematous around opening. No bowel sounds heard in any quadrant. Infant cries as if abdomen is tender to touch on palpation.
- Genitalia: Normal female; no erythema or discharge.

- Extremities: Full range of motion; hips abduct to 180 degrees.
- Neurologic: Moro, tonic neck, step-in-place, trunk innervation intact. Patellar reflex: 2 bilaterally.

Care Study Questions

1. Michelle was diagnosed as having a pyloric obstruction from migration of the gastrostomy tube. What signs and symptoms was she showing that would have alerted you this was happening?

2. Michelle has been ill since birth. She was hospitalized for a long time immediately after birth. Has this interfered with growth and development?

3. Complete a nursing care plan that would both identify and meet the needs of Michelle and her family.

The Effects of Hospitalization on Children and Their Families

Chapter 35 discusses the meaning of illness to children and the damaging effect of separation that can occur with hospitalization. The chapter begins with an overview of nursing process specific to the care of children in the hospital. Ways to prepare a child for hospitalization are reviewed, such as providing necessary preliminary information, sound orientation to the hospital, encouraging parent and sibling participation in care, providing substitute parents for children during hospitalization, and providing play space to encourage normal development. The value of play to the hospitalized child is discussed along with the value and techniques of therapeutic play in helping children master and grow from a hospital experience.

Few students in nursing have been hospitalized, so they may have little concept of how damaging a hospital experience can be without proper preparation. The concept of therapeutic play is new to students and is one they need to be introduced to in order for them to incorporate it into nursing care planning.

Chapter Objectives

After mastering the contents of this chapter, students should be able to:

1. Describe the meaning of ambulatory and in-hospital experiences to children.

2. Describe the meaning of play and preferred types of play for children of different ages.

3. Assess the impact of a health care visit or hospital stay on a child.

4. Formulate a nursing diagnosis related to the stress of a health care visit or hospital stay.

5. Plan nursing care to reduce the stress of a health care visit or hospital stay, such as helping parents plan for the experience.

6. Implement measures such as orientation, education, and therapeutic play to reduce the stress of health care visits.

7. Evaluate outcome criteria to be certain nursing goals were achieved.

8. Identify national health goals related to hospitalization or health care that nurses can be instrumental in in helping the nation to achieve.

9. Identify areas related to hospitalization or health care of children that could benefit from additional nursing research.

10. Use critical thinking to analyze ways in which a hospital experience can be made more family centered and less traumatic for children.

11. Synthesize knowledge about the child's response to illness and hospitalization with the nursing process to achieve quality maternal and child health nursing care.

Key Points

- Hospitalization may be more traumatic for children than adults because of their inability to communicate and monitor their own care, and because they have different nutritional, fluid, and electrolyte needs.

- Separation from parents can have permanent psychologic effects on children. Methods to reduce this are keeping hospital stays as brief as possible, promoting open parent and sibling visiting, and providing primary nursing.

- Preschool children may have the most difficult time during a hospital experience because they have so many fears. Preparation and promotion of therapeutic play are essential to reduce the trauma to a tolerable level.

- Currently, many medical procedures can be done on an ambulatory basis. Advocating for care to be done in such settings is a nursing responsibility.

- The presence of parents can help reduce trauma to children. Making parents welcome makes it possible for them to room-in. Include the parents in both the planning and implementation of care. Parents reinfect children with fear if their own fear is not reduced.

- Because hospitalizations currently are so brief, parents need good discharge instructions to continue to care for children safely at home. Providing clear instructions and danger signs for parents to watch for is important.

Definition of Key Terms

accommodation: the ability to adapt thought processes to fit what is perceived

assimilation: the ability to change how a situation is perceived to coincide with beliefs

case management nursing: a method of nursing which features total care and planning for an individual client

play therapy: a form of psychotherapy in which children are helped to confront and gain insight into their fears

primary nursing: a method of nursing in which the nurse assumes primary responsibility for planning care for an individual client

therapeutic play: a technique useful to help children express fears or concerns

triage: the classification of injured persons as to degree of injury and priority for treatment

Nursing Process Overview

The Nursing Process Overview in this chapter concentrates on helping the student adapt nursing care to meet the unique needs of the hospitalized child. The importance of assessment to learn what the child expects from hospitalization, the importance of individualizing nursing diagnoses, and planning care that promotes a family-centered experience are stressed.

Study Aids

Boxes

Box 35-1:   Books on hospitalization for children

Box 35-2:   Guidelines for conducting hospital tours with early school-age children

Box 35-3:   Nursing interventions to meet children's spiritual needs

Box 35-4:   Guidelines for therapeutic play

Tables

Table 35-1:   Stages of separation anxiety

Table 35-2:   Information necessary for nursing care plan on admission

Table 35-3:   Ways to incorporate play into ambulatory nursing care

Table 35-4:   Ways to incorporate play into inpatient children's nursing care

Table 35-5:   Games and activities using materials available on a nursing unit

Table 35-6:   Therapeutic play techniques for children after procedures

Displays

Focus on National Health Goals

Focus on Family Teaching

Focus on Nursing Research

Focus on Cultural Awareness

Critical Thinking Questions

1. Devon is a 3-year-old who had emergency surgery while on vacation with her single mother. Her mother has returned home because of work responsibilities so Devon will have no family with her for a week. What measures could you take to help hospitalization and separation less traumatic for her?

2. The administration of a hospital has asked you to help them plan a playroom on a hospital unit for toddlers and preschoolers. What toys would you suggest?

3. Many people suggest that children be allowed to play with syringes with actual needles attached. How do you feel about his? What would be advantages and disadvantages of this?

Media Resources

Initial Nursing Assessment of a Hospitalized Child: Basis for Developing a Nursing Care Plan (36-minute videocassette)

A method of developing a nursing care plan for a hospitalized child is demonstrated through Robyn, a $3\frac{1}{2}$-year-old admitted to the hospital for chemotherapy. The nursing team assesses Robyn's physical, psychologic, cognitive, and language development and develops a plan of care based on these findings.

Source: Health Sciences Consortium

Nursing Care of the Hospitalized Child With a Chronic Health Problem (28-minute videocassette)

Explanations of how long-term illness affects developmentally on infants and children and how the admission of a chronically ill child to the hospital is different from the admission of a child who anticipates complete recovery. Parenting patterns which prevent opti mal growth of the chronically ill child are also described.

Source: Health Sciences Consortium

Utilizing the Nursing Process in Pediatric Care (31-minute videocassette)

An overview of the nursing process, stressing its importance in optimizing the nursing care of the hospitalized child.

Source: Health Sciences Consortium

Preparing Children for the Hospital Experience (28-minute videocassette)

A review of child cognitive development levels is given to help nurses key their explanations of hospitalization to the level of understanding of each child. The use of books, diagrams, dolls, and actual hospital equipment in patient teaching is demonstrated.

Source: AJN Educational Services

Promoting Normal Growth in the Hospitalized Child (12-minute videocassette)

Details of the stages of development from infancy to adolescence, emphasizing the particular care that can be given to acknowledge these stages in a hospitalized child. Such concepts as the need to encourage infant stimulation, toddler autonomy, preschool imagination, school-age industry, and adolescent peer interaction are stressed.

Source: AJN Educational Services

Caring for the Parents of Critically Ill Children (28-minute videocassette)

Ways to help parents maintain an active, vital role during hospitalization are shown. Methods to promote a caring attitude toward the parent, how to ascertain parental goals and expectations, how to assess a parent's perception of a child's illness, and suggestions for care are included.

Source: AJN Educational Services

A Hospital Adventure: Starring Boris the Bear (11-minute videocassette)

Boris the Bear guides the viewer through a first hospital experience, recounting being scared and the nurses who comforted him and helped him recover. Intended to help children learn more about hospitalization.

Source: AJN Educational Services

Young Children's Reactions to Hospitalization (14-minute videocassette)

Candid interviews with parents and children portray how a child can undergo behavior changes during hospitalization. Parents are urged to be open with children about the problems of separation.

Source: AJN Educational Services

Coping with Cancer: the Early School Years (36-minute videocassette)

An 8-year-old boy and a 9-year-old girl in play therapy explore their fears, anxieties, understanding, and ways of coping with their cancer experiences. The use of puppets and modified hospital equipment with play techniques is shown.

Source: AJN Educational Services

Discharge Planning in Pediatric Catastrophic Illness (56-minute videocassette in 2 parts)

A two-part video that (1) focuses on the planning process while the child is still in the hospital, illustrating steps in the process of discharge planning and (2) examines planning when the child is at home. The role of the pediatric home care nurse and the necessity of coordinating health care are stressed.

Source: AJN Educational Service

A Safe Place for Children (7-minute film)

Play techniques in a pediatric clinic waiting room and activities to help children understand procedures and to reduce fear are shown.

Source: The Little Red Filmhouse

Peace Has Not Been Made: A Case History of a Hmong Family's Encounter with a Hospital (25-minute videocassette)

The events surrounding a southeast Asian family's misunderstanding about their son's diagnosis is shown. Discussion about the situation takes place between the hospital staff and Hmong community leaders.

Source: Rhode Island Office of Refugee Resettlement

Play in the Hospital (50-minute film)

Supervised play activities for the hospitalized child. Fears and anxieties that confront children in the hospital are discussed. Examples of children acting out their reactions during play are shown.

Source: Campus Films

Discussion Questions

1. A child's first impression of a hospital is gained on admission. What are steps to take to make admission atraumatic?

2. The way that children think of illness affects how you prepare them for procedures. How would you prepare a preschool child for a lumbar puncture? How would you prepare a school-age child?

3. Sibling visitation helps a hospitalized child continue to feel a part of his or her family. What considerations for safety do you have to think about when siblings are visiting a child?

Written Assignments

1. Providing toys can be costly for a hospital unit. What resources are there in your community which you could depend on to provide toys for the use of ill children?

2. Reserving time for play is not regarded as a priority by all nurses. How would you introduce the idea of providing a set time for play every day to a nursing staff?

3. Observe the behavior of a toddler when his parents visit him or her in the hospital. Did the child show any signs of parental separation? How did the parents react to this?

Laboratory Experiences

1. Assign students to a hospital playroom. Ask them to observe one child as to the child's level of development as revealed through play.

2. Assign students to design an inexpensive toy that would be age-appropriate for a child they care for. Donate the toys to the hospital unit after grading is completed.

3. Assign students to observe with a child life specialist for a day and participate or observe therapeutic play being conducted to relieve anxiety in hospitalized children.

Health Teaching With Children

Chapter 36 discusses of techniques of health teaching that are pertinent for use with children. The chapter begins with an overview of the nursing process specific to health teaching with children. Types of learning, the influence of age on learning, and techniques for developing and implementing a teaching plan are included. Health teaching for a surgical experience is used as an example.

Although students have had an orientation to health teaching in previous course work, teaching with children is often new content. As students begin to incorporate health teaching into nursing plans and care, the chapter should serve as an often-consulted resource.

Chapter Objectives

After mastering the contents of this chapter, students should be able to:

1. Describe principles of teaching and learning and their specific application to health teaching with children.
2. Assess children for their readiness to learn.
3. State nursing diagnoses related to the need for health teaching.
4. Establish health teaching priorities for a specific child based on the child's age, developmental maturity, emotional needs, and learning style.
5. Implement health teaching (eg, devising a puppet show) using principles of teaching-learning.
6. Evaluate outcome criteria to be certain that nursing goals established for care have been achieved.
7. Identify national health goals related to teaching and children that nurses could be instrumental in in helping the nation achieve.
8. Identify areas of care related to health teaching of children that could benefit from additional nursing research.
9. Use critical thinking to analyze ways that health teaching can be further incorporated into the nursing care of children and families.
10. Synthesize knowledge of teaching-learning with nursing process to achieve quality maternal and child health nursing care.

Key Points

- Children's cognitive development must be evaluated to ensure that material being presented can be easily comprehended. Preschool children, for example, are egotistic and are able only to see situations from their standpoint, not others. They ''center'' and are only able to grasp one idea from a visual aid. School-age children are concrete thinkers. They learn best what they can see and touch and handle. Abstract concepts cannot be grasped until adolescence.

- The type of teaching used with children varies depending on the child's age. Various types to consider are formal vs informal, single or group teaching, lecture, discussion, and role playing.

- Behavior modification is a special technique aimed at erasing some form of behavior that interferes with health functioning.

- There are three types of learning: cognitive, psychomotor, and affective. In order for something to be learned well, all these areas must be involved.

- To individualize a teaching program for a child, assess the child's attention span, cognitive intellectual capability, lifestyle, learning style, and your own teaching strengths and limitations.

- In many instances there is a great deal of material that a child must learn about an illness. If taught all at once, however, it would be overwhelming. Divide material into lessons to be taught immediately and lessons that can be taught at spaced, return health visits.

- Remember that children are present-oriented. They learn information that they can see will immediately benefit them more easily than information that has future benefits.

- Children are learning a great deal of other things besides health information every day. This may make the retention of information not as great as you would like. Frequent reviews and updates may need to be scheduled to keep them current.

Definitions of Key Terms

<u>affective learning:</u> the acquisition of behaviors involved in expressing feelings or attitudes

<u>behavior modification:</u> a form of therapy in which acceptable patterns of behavior are substituted for unacceptable patterns

cognitive learning: the acquisition of behaviors concerned with problem-solving ability

demonstration: performing an action to demonstrate the correct way for it to be done

positive reinforcement: offering praise to motivate a child to learn

psychomotor learning: the acquisition of motor skills

redemonstration: imitating an action which has just been demonstrated

teaching plan: a prescription of goals and actions to ensure learning success

Nursing Process Overview

The Nursing Process Overview in this chapter concentrates on helping the student identify his or her role as a health educator with children. The importance of constructing a teaching plan that lists goals and includes measures for evaluation are stressed. Teaching interventions that are especially effective with children such as puppet play or drawing are included.

Study Aids

Tables

Table 36-1: Principles of teaching

Table 36-2: Ways to incorporate teaching into care

Table 36-3: Principles of learning

Displays

Focus on National Health Goals

Focus on Nursing Research

Focus on Cultural Awareness

Critical Thinking Questions

1. Bobby is a ten-year-old with asthma who has to learn how to monitor his medication needs by using a peak flow meter at least once daily. How would you teach this to him? Suppose he states he has no intention of learning how to read the meter because his mother can do this for him. Would your teaching plan be different?

2. Chuck is an adolescent who has familial hypercholesteremia. His physician has prescribed a low cholesterol diet for him. What are teaching techniques that would be especially effective teaching a new diet to Chuck? His mother has to learn this too. Would you teach her any differently?

3. Mary is a preschooler who will be having surgery in a week for bilateral syndactyly. Her mother asks you how to prepare her for this. What suggestions would you make? Mary will be left with a noticeable scar and some lack of function following surgery so she can not be reassured that everything will be all right. Will this affect your teaching?

Media Resources

Pediatrics: Psychosocial Implications: The Nursing Challenge (18-minute filmstrip or videotransfer)

The developmental knowledge and observational skills necessary for communication with children are demonstrated. The nurse's relationship with the family is stressed as a means of involving parents in children's care.

Source: Concept Media

Knowing, Feeling, Growing (videocassette)

Puppetry is used to demonstrate coping techniques to solve problems and to decrease anxiety.

Source: University of Minnesota

Parents and Children Series: How to Play With a Child (36-minute videocassette)

Ways to interact with children in play through the use of vignette demonstrations. Parents are shown ways to identify children's capabilities and needs, provide positive support for play, and help children develop imaginative and creative play.

Source: Health Sciences Consortium

Parents and Children Series: Helping Children Learn (35-minute videocassette)

Ways that learning can be fostered in play situations without adult direction are shown. Vignettes show how to talk to children, foster their language development, build confidence in their learning ability, and help them learn to problem-solve and deal with frustration.

Source: Health Sciences Consortium

Discussion Questions

1. Most preschool children watch television programs such as ''Sesame Street.'' How does this type of creative program affect the way you teach children?

2. Kate, a 4-year-old, and Tom, a 10-year-old, both need to learn more about preventing accidents. What techniques would you use to teach them? How would your technique differ because of their ages?

3. Teaching psychomotor skills differs a great deal from teaching affective skills. What teaching techniques work best for these two different types of learning?

Written Assignments

1. Select some knowledge or task a child you care for needs to learn. Construct a teaching plan that speaks to cognitive, psychomotor, and affective learning.

2. Some people are naturally better teachers than others. Survey students in your class as to who was their favorite teacher and what were the special qualities that made that teacher so effective.

3. Watch a children's program on television and analyze for what age child the program's commercials are targeted, based on the information supplied and techniques of presentation.

Laboratory Experiences

1. Assign students to observe for a day with a nurse clinician skilled in teaching children, such as a diabetic teaching nurse. Ask them to note how the teaching level is adapted to the child's cognitive level.

2. Assign students to observe in a day-care or school setting. Ask them to prepare a health promotion teaching method to meet the age of the children in that setting.

3. Ask the parents of a hospitalized child to come to a postconference and discuss their satisfaction with the health teaching they themselves or their child have received. What are ways health teaching could have been improved to better meet their needs?

Nursing Care of the Hospitalized Child and Family: Diagnostic and Therapeutic Techniques

Chapter 37 discusses the ways that diagnostic and therapeutic techniques must be modified in order to be effective with children. The chapter begins with an overview of the nursing process specific to modifying care with children. Common diagnostic techniques are presented and how these may be perceived by children. These include vital sign assessment, specimen collection, medication administration, intravenous therapy, hot and cold therapy, preparation of the child for a surgical experience, providing a safe environment, promotion of sleep, spiritual health, assessing and relieving pain, providing stimulation, encouraging self-care, and establishing elimination.

Although students have had an orientation to these topics in previous course work, they may not have had a chance to apply them in a clinical setting and so have little practical knowledge of them. The chapter should serve as a resource as students begin to include these techniques into nursing care planning with specific children.

Chapter Objectives

After mastering the contents of this chapter, students should be able to:

1. Describe common nursing interventions used in the health care of children to aid diagnosis and therapy.

2. Assess children as to developmental stage and knowledge level before beginning any diagnostic technique, therapeutic procedure, or other nursing intervention.

3. Formulate nursing diagnoses related to common diagnostic therapeutic techniques used with children.

4. Plan nursing interventions to aid in diagnosis or therapy for children, such as obtaining specimens or administering medicine.

5. Implement nursing procedures such as beginning intravenous therapy, while respecting the individuality and special needs of each child.

6. Evaluate outcome criteria to be certain that nursing goals related to diagnostic and therapeutic techniques were achieved.

7. Identify national health goals related to care of children that nurses could be instrumental in in helping the nation achieve.

8. Identify areas related to nursing procedures with children that could benefit from additional nursing research.

9. Use critical thinking to analyze ways that procedures can be modified to meet the needs of children of all ages.

10. Synthesize knowledge of common procedures with nursing process to achieve quality maternal and child health nursing.

Key Points

- Preparing children for procedures reduces anxiety. Prepare a child by trying to relate a procedure to something he or she is already familiar with, such as comparing an x-ray machine to a camera.

- Include parents in both the planning and implementation of care. Parents reinfect children with fear if their own fear is uncontrolled. Give explanations on two levels: ''I'm going to change the dressing on her suture line'' for a parent, but ''I'm going to put a clean bandage on your tummy'' for the child.

- Reduce painful procedures to the minimum possible (combine blood sampling procedures, if possible).

- Perform any procedures that will cause pain in a treatment room or away from the child's bedside so the bed remains a ''safe place.''

- Perform treatments without chilling or exposure. Be aware that even small children expect modesty to be respected.

- Allow the child to voice anger or fear of a procedure. Provide therapeutic play following the procedure to help reduce anger or fear.

- Identify a child well before a procedure; children do not monitor their own care as do adults.

- Children enjoy adults who are secure in their actions. Practice as necessary the steps of a procedure before you begin, in order to radiate confidence in your manner.

- Once you have announced that a procedure needs to be done, proceed to do it; waiting for something to happen is often as stressful as actually having it done.

- Respect time for play for children. This is not ''free'' time to be filled with procedures, but a time for learning.

- Involve children in procedures, because this gives them a sense of control. Allow a child to examine electrodes or apply lubricant for electrode contact. Give the child a portion of an ECG strip as a badge of courage following the procedure, or let the child apply his or her own adhesive bandage.

- Praise children for cooperation, even if none was visibly obvious. For painful procedures, any behavior short of hysterical screaming counts as cooperation.

Definitions of Key Terms

aspiration studies: diagnostic studies involving the withdrawal of a body fluid by suction

barium contrast studies: diagnostic procedures carried out by instillation of a radiopaque substance and x-ray.

battered child syndrome: a child who has been physically, sexually, or emotionally abused

bronchoscopy: the visual examination of the respiratory tree by means of an endoscope

central venous access devices: entrance to the superior vena cava

clean-catch urine specimen: a urine that is as free of bacterial contamination as possible without the use of catheterization

computed tomography: an x-ray technique that displays the appearance of a cross-section of tissue

distraction: a process that prevents or lessens the perception of pain by focusing attention on an object other than the pain

electrical impulse studies: diagnostic studies that analyze the electrical activity of body cells

endoscopy: inspection of a body cavity by means of an endoscope

gating theory: a theory of pain relief that acts to prevent pain stimulation from being received or interpreted as pain in the brain cortex

intermittent infusion devices: a device inserted in an intravenous line that allows for intermittent infusion of fluid or insertion of medicine (heparin trap)

magnetic resonance imaging: a diagnostic technique that uses magnetic and sound waves to reveal body composition and appearance

nocturnal enuresis: involuntary release of urine at night (bed-wetting)

non-rapid-eye movement sleep: A type of sleep during which physiologic growth occurs

positron emission tomograph (PET): a diagnostic technique involving a radioisotope and computed tomography

radiopharmaceutical: a radioactive substance injected or swallowed for diagnostic procedures

rapid-eye movement (REM) sleep: a pattern of sleep during which dreams and movement of the eyes under closed eyelids occurs

sensory overload: the overbombardment of stimuli to the senses

single photon emission computerized tomography (SPECT): a diagnostic procedure combining tomography and a radioisotope

sleep deprivation: a state of confusion or depression caused by inadequate sleep

ultrasound: a diagnostic study made by high frequency sound waves to reveal body organs

venipuncture: the entrance into a vein to withdraw blood or instill medication or fluid

Nursing Process Overview

The Nursing Process Overview in this chapter concentrates on helping the student modify nursing interventions to meet the needs of young clients. Topics include careful assessment to determine the developmental level of the child; planning for short-term goals that will be consistent with children's shorter attention spans, and evaluation techniques that speak to the psychologic effect of a therapy on a child as well as the physical effects.

Study Aids

Boxes

Box 37-1:   Guidelines for hot and cold applications with children

Tables

Table 37-1:   A method to calculate caloric expenditure

Table 37-2:   Stages of sleep in children

Table 37-3:   Myths and facts about pain in children

Table 37-4:   Calculating acetaminophen (Tylenol) doses

Procedures

Procedure 37-1:   Technique for fingertip or heel capillary puncture

Procedure 37-2:   Obtaining a clean-catch urine specimen on a young child

Displays

Focus on National Health Goals

Focus on Family Teaching

Focus on Nursing Research

Focus on Cultural Awareness

Critical Thinking Exercises

1. John is a 2-ear-old who is very frightened of dark places. He is scheduled to have an MRI of his head done, which means he will be wheeled into a huge, dark, hollow tube. How could you prepare him for this?

2. Megan is a 6-year-old who has to have debridement for burns done daily, a very painful procedure. She screams from fright when you bring in an analgesic injection to give her, however. Which would be better: to give the injection and risk frightening her, or not give it and allow her to experience more pain?

3. Jeff is an adolescent who is scheduled for a series of diagnostic tests for chronic abdominal pain. He always says, "I'm not a kid, you know," and refuses to listen when you start to explain any procedure. Later, he acts angry because he feels he has been "tricked" into having a procedure. How could you give explanations to Jeff without offending him? Why do you think he acts this way?

Media Resources

Restraints: Restraining Infants and Children (16-minute filmstrip/videocassette)

Commonly used restraining procedures and devices for children are shown.

> Source: J.B. Lippincott Company

Physical Care: Administering Oral and IM Medications (filmstrip/videotransfer)

The preparation of oral medications and the selection of sites for injections of various age groups of children. Techniques of medication administration are discussed and illustrated.

> Source: Concept Media

Your Child has a Fever (20-minute videocassette)

Basic information for parents describing normal temperature and fever that is potentially dangerous. How to recognize a fever, the use of a thermometer, and when to seek professional advice are discussed.

> Source: Churchill Films

Fever in Children: Fears and Facts (videocassette)

Common myths about fever and techniques for taking temperatures of children are explained. Guidelines are given for when to ask for professional help and ways to make the child with fever more comfortable.

> Source: Concept Media

Special Issues in Pain Control: Pediatric Pain (19-minute videocassette)

The physiology of the pain response is outlined, as are techniques for response assessment. Pain intervention options are discussed. Ethical and legal parameters are presented. The common misconceptions surrounding pain and management for children are included.

> Source: Health Sciences Consortium

Special Pain Problems: Pediatric and Elderly Patients (28-minute videocassette)

Discussion of why pain is underestimated or undertreated in the infant, child, adolescent and elderly patient. Effective communication techniques to assist the nurse in assessment and management of pain in pediatric and elderly patients are identified.

> Source: AJN Educational Services

Instrument Preparation and Care for Pediatric Endoscopic Procedures (20-minute videocassette)

How to assemble, maintain, and handle the instruments used in pediatric endoscopic procedures. Commonly used instruments such as the bronchoscope, bronchoscopic bridge, telescope, laryngoscope, and nasal endoscope are shown and described.

> Source: Health Sciences Consortium

Jeannie (6-minute videocassette)

The thoughts and emotions of an 11-year-old who is about to have heart surgery are captured. As the tape shows the removal of a tumor from her heart, a voice reenacts in a stream-of-consciousness technique what she is thinking and feeling. Fright and confusion as well as optimism are conveyed.

> Source: Health Sciences Consortium

With Care and Caring... Pediatric Medication Administration (30-minute videocassette)

How to administer medication to children of various ages is demonstrated. Specific physical techniques and practical considerations in how to approach a child based on the child's stage of development are demonstrated with real-life situations.

> Source: Health Sciences Consortium

Medicating Children (23-minute videocassette)

Important information about administering medications to children of various ages is presented. General considerations and details related to routes of medication administration, safety factors in calculation and administration, and comfort measures are discussed. The child's developmental, psychosocial, and communication skills are considered.

> Source: AJN Educational Services

Pediatric IV Therapy (40-minute videocassette)

The assembly of IV flow devices and electronic infusion monitors is shown. An exploration of children's needs, physiologic aspects, cognitive factors, psychosocial needs, and teaching needs for IV therapy is discussed. Providing opportunities for play and maintaining observation of each child are stressed.

> Source: AJN Educational Services

Why Do I Have to Cry? Assessment of Pain in Children (25-minute videocassette)

Common myths and misconceptions about pain in children are presented. Research-based strategies for assessing pain in children and developmental stage differences in pain response are discussed. Three pain assessment "tools" including poker chips, the "oucher," and the adolescent pediatric pain tool are shown.

Source: AJN Educational Services

Pediatric procedures: Module I (videocassette with CAI instruction)

Pediatric nursing procedures such as lumbar puncture, bone marrow aspiration, and central line placements are described and shown. Indications, location, techniques, and complications are stressed. A quiz and feedback complete the program.

Source: Health Sciences Consortium

Discussion Questions

1. The introduction of universal health goals has changed nursing practice. What are ways that newborn care has changed owing to these precautions?

2. Interview a child or adolescent who has pain as to how the child would rate the pain and the child's satisfaction with health care personnel in relieving the pain. What was the best pain rating technique for this child?

3. Caring for a child with a parent always present has both good and bad points. Discuss the pros and cons.

Written Assignments

1. Choose a procedure you have done recently with a child and list the specific ways you needed to modify the procedure because of the child's age or understanding.

2. Medication administration poses particular risks with children because they are unable to identify themselves adequately. Suppose you are about to give a medication to Jamie Tyson, an infant and realize he wears no arm band. No parent is present. How would you identify the infant as Jamie Tyson?

3. Using restraints with children requires concern for the child's safety. What are the situations in which you might consider using a restraint? What special precautions would you take to ensure child safety with the restraint in place?

Clinical Experiences

1. Assign students to a clinical area where they can experience procedures with children. Discuss at a postconference the different procedures carried out, so that all students can benefit from the learning experience.

2. Giving injections to children is a procedure not readily available clinically, since children tend to receive either intravenous or oral medication. Assigning students to ambulatory settings where immunizations are given can provide opportunity for this experience.

3. Adapting procedures to children is difficult for students who have not had prior experience with children. Role-playing adaptation of procedures in a laboratory setting can be helpful to students in developing this technique.

Nursing Care of Children and Their Families in the Home

*C*hapter 38 discusses ways that nursing care can be adapted to make home care successful. The chapter begins with an overview of the nursing process specific to care of the child at home. The nursing responsibility for home care is outlined, as well as related techniques such as intravenous therapy, oxygenation, nutrition, medication administration, phototherapy, promoting healthy family functioning, and providing a therapeutic environment.

Students are aware that a great deal of nursing care is presently conducted in homes. They may not be aware how advantageous home care is for children until they are exposed to it.

Chapter Objectives

After mastering the contents of this chapter, students should be able to:

1. Outline the advantages and disadvantages of home care.
2. Assess the appropriateness of home care for a particular child and family.
3. Formulate nursing diagnoses related to care of a child at home.
4. Plan modifications of nursing care, such as administration of intravenous therapy for the home setting.
5. Implement care (eg, supervising safe oxygen administration) for a child in the home.
6. Evaluate goal criteria to be certain that nursing goals were achieved.
7. Identify national health goals related to home care that nurses can be instrumental in in helping the nation to achieve.
8. Identify areas related to home care that could benefit from additional nursing research.

9. Use critical thinking to analyze ways that nursing interventions can promote healthy family functioning when care is delivered in the home as well as ways that the link between hospital and home care can be strengthened.
10. Synthesize principles of home care with nursing process to achieve quality maternal and child health care.

Key Points

- Home care is increasing as a way to provide care for chronically ill children. It has advantages of being cost effective and providing meaningful comfort and ready support to the child. Disadvantages are that parents can become fatigued, cost can cause financial hardship, and families can experience social isolation and the disruption of normal home life.

- Important in planning is to consider ways to provide a therapeutic environment, adequate nutrition, adequate mobility, respiratory function, elimination, administer medication, and encourage self-care.

- Be certain parents truly are comfortable and skilled at performing procedures by asking them to demonstrate how to perform a procedure such as a gastrostomy tube feeding they will need to do at home. This is a rewarding time for them if they are comfortable and skilled; if they are not, it is a time to review the skill.

- Home care is exhausting for parents. Be certain they devise a schedule of care that allows them enough rest.

- Advocate for medicine schedules that will allow parents to get adequate sleep, such as administering a medication once a day rather than around the clock.

- Parents need respite care to continue to be effective care providers, just as professionals need time off. Help parents to relieve each other so each has some free time each week. Urge them to do something they truly enjoy during this time (read a good book, try a new recipe, and so forth).

- Home health care can continue for years. Help parents to discover ways to meet the child's growth and development needs during this time. Adult caregivers also have growth needs. Both child and parents taking a continuing education course, reading library books, or learning a new hobby together might fulfill both of their needs.

- Not all homes are ideal for home care. Assess if a primary care provider is present, if the family is knowledgeable about the care necessary, if necessary resources are available, and if safety features such as a smoke detector, a safe area for oxygen storage, and a safe refrigerator for food or medicine are present.

Definitions of Key Terms

direct care: nursing care provided by the primary care nurse

home care: nursing care conducted in a client's place of residence

hospice care: care of a terminally ill individual in a facility designed to maintain a satisfactory lifestyle until death

indirect care: nursing care which is completed by an auxiliary person under the supervision of a nurse

phototherapy blanket: a commercial pad which emits ultraviolet rays; used in treatment of hyperbilirubinemia

skilled home care: nursing care which includes physician-prescribed procedures such as a dressing change

Nursing Process Overview

The Nursing Process Overview in this chapter concentrates on helping the student adapt nursing care to the child being cared for at home. The importance of including the entire family in assessment and planning is stressed. Nursing diagnoses are suggested that speak not only to the physical condition of the child but the psychologic strain that is placed on a family by home care.

Study Aids

Tables

Table 38-1:   Assessment criteria for home care by age group

Displays

Focus on National Health Goals

Focus on Family Teaching

Focus on Nursing Research

Focus on Cultural Awareness

Critical Thinking Exercises:

1. Terry is a 4-year-old on home care for chronic respiratory disease. His parents state that they are exhausted because of the necessity of round-the-clock care. What suggestions could you make to them to make care easier?

2. Celeste is a 14-year-old who will be cared for at home following orthopedic surgery. She is concerned that because her home stay will be lengthy, she will be cut off from her friends for a long time. What suggestions could you make to Celeste to help her maintain contact with friends?

3. Mario is a newborn who will be cared for at home because of hyperbilirubinemia. His parents tell you that they are inexperienced and are worried they are not up to providing care to an ill newborn. How would you support them until they grow more confident?

Media Resources

Discharge Planning in Pediatric Catastrophic Illness (56-minute videocassette in two parts)

A two-part video that (1) focuses on the planning process while the child is still in the hospital, with steps in the process of discharge planning, and (2) examines planning when the child is at home. The role of the pediatric home care nurse and the necessity of coordinating health care is stressed.

Source: AJN Educational Services

Caring for the Parents of Critically Ill Children (28-minute videocassette)

Nurse—parent interactions that establish a caring attitude toward the parent, help ascertain parental goals and expectations, and assess the parent's perception of a child's illness and attitudes. Designed to espouse family-centered care.

Source: AJN Educational Services

Only a Breath (30-minute videocassette)

The lives of five families with ventilator-assisted children on home care are shown. The problems of learning to live with technology problems and the importance of support systems are stressed. Concerns of health care providers are discussed.

Source: Medical Electronic Educational Services, Inc.

Discussion Questions

1. Children on home care miss interaction with peers. What are suggestions to help a child maintain this kind of contact?

2. Providing nutrition for a child on home care can be a challenge because the child grows bored with mealtime. What are suggestions for making mealtime more interesting?

3. Preparing a child for home care involves careful assessment of the home and family. What are specific questions you would want to ask to help ensure safe home care?

Written Assignments

1. Parents often need "respite" time in order to continue to care for a child at home. What organizations in your community provide this type of care you could use for referral sources?

2. Families often need help in remembering to give medicine to a child on home care. List five suggestions to help parents accomplish this successfully.

3. Caring for a child with oxygen administration at home requires parents to enforce precautions to prevent fire. List specific measures for parents to take.

Laboratory Experiences

1. Assign students to observe with a home care nurse or a community health nurse for a day so they have a chance to see children being cared for at home.

2. Ask a parent who is caring for a child at home to come to a postconference and describe specific problems she or he has encountered in home care. How could health care personnel have been more help? Would the parent do anything different another time?

3. Ask students to make a follow-up home visit on a child they have cared for so they have a chance to evaluate their discharge instructions. Ask them to describe what they would have done differently now that they fully understand the child's home circumstances.

Care Study: An Early Adolescent With Crohn's Disease

Beth is a 14-year-old with Crohn's disease on home care.

Health History

- Chief Concern: "Beth is bored and we're tired."

- History of Present Concern: For the last 6 months, Beth has had a history of frequent loose bowel movements, 4—5 times a day plus anorexia. Had frequent flatulence and sometimes noticed blood in stool. Lost 8 pounds over past 6 months. Was diagnosed 1 month ago as having Crohn's disease and hospitalized for 2 weeks. Was discharged home on total parenteral nutrition plus Azulfidine and prednisone to reduce bowel inflammation. At first she was cooperative about helping out with household chores; she has spent the last week crying about having to stay home and being so ill. Insists that one parent stay awake during night to watch TPN infusion. Is refusing to take prednisone because of publicity that steroid use is bad for athletes.

- Family Profile: Beth is a high school freshman. She was an A student before becoming ill. Her marks have begun to fall over the last 6 months and she has missed considerable school (20 days) this semester. She also was active in sports as a member and captain of the high school varsity soccer and basketball teams and a coach for a city soccer team of 6-year-olds.

  Father works as the high school football coach in Beth's school. Mother is primary caregiver (works part-time selling cosmetics). Family lives in a neatly kept ranch home on a quiet, tree-lined street. Siblings are a brother 10-years-old and twin sisters 8-years-old. Finances are described as "not a problem."

- Past Medical History: Roseola at 8 months; no other childhood diseases. No hospitalizations prior to diagnosis of Crohn's disease. Immunizations up to date.

- Family Medical History: Hypertension in maternal grandfather; diabetes mellitus in paternal aunt. A brother of child's father "always complains of stomach trouble."

- Review of Systems: Neuropsychiatric: Child is "high-strung"; works very hard to be the best at what she does. No history of seizures.

- HEENT: Wears glasses for reading; vision 20/30 and 20/40. Hearing was assessed in school and rated adequate. No otitis media.

- Gastrointestinal: Had an allergy to milk when first born. Formula was changed four times, finally to soybean base, which was tolerated. When milk was reintroduced again at 1 year, Beth had no difficulty digesting it. Has had numerous "canker sores" during last year.

Physical Examination

- General Appearance: White, thin-appearing, adolescent female with uncombed hair and still wearing nightgown at 2:00 pm. Height: 164 cms. Weight: 81 lbs.

- Head: Normocephalic; hair oily; unbrushed.

- Eyes: Red reflex. Follows through fields of vision. No erythema of conjunctiva.

- Ears: TMs pink and subtle; landmarks and light cone visible.

- Nose: Nares patent; midline septum.

- Mouth and Throat: Midline uvula; intact palate. Thirty teeth present; no caries. Mucous membrane moist; no ulcerations.

- Neck: Subtle; no palpable lymph nodes. No thyroid hypertrophy; midline trachea.

- Chest: Lungs clear to percussion and auscultation. Respiratory rate 20/min.

- Heart: PMI at left 5th intercostal space. Rate 84/min. No murmurs.

- Abdomen: Tenderness elicited in all four quadrants on palpation. Bowel sounds hyperactive in upper quadrants.

- Genitourinary: Tanner stage 2. Perineal and rectal area is erythematous with a pinpoint rash.

- Back: No curvature of spine; no tenderness of vertebrae.

- Extremities: Full range of motion; normal gait.

- Neurologic: Patellar reflex: 3; sensation and gross motor grossly intact. Fully oriented to place and person.

Care Study Questions

1. One of the reasons that home care is so difficult for many parents is because they grow so exhausted with 24-hour care. What suggestions could you make to Beth's parents to help them with this problem?

2. Beth is refusing to take her medication because of wrong information about the drug. What are measures you could take to help Beth with medicine compliance?

3. Complete a nursing care plan that would identify and meet the needs of Beth's family.

Nursing Care of the Child Born With a Physical Developmental Disorder

Chapter 39 discusses care of infants born with physical concerns. The chapter begins with a Nursing Process Overview to assist the student with assessment of such infants and to suggest nursing diagnoses that are pertinent to their care. Care is described for children with gastrointestinal disorders such as cleft lip and palate, tracheoesophageal fistula, and omphalocele, neural tube disorders such as meningocele, and orthopedic disorders such as the talipes deformities and subluxated hips. The role of the nurse as advocate and the necessity to incorporate the entire family in care of these infants are stressed.

Key Points

- The earlier parents learn about a child's health problem, the easier it is for them to adjust to it. Advocate for parents to help them obtain as much information as they need.

- Cleft lip and palate result from failure of the maxillary process to fuse in intrauterine life. The chief nursing diagnoses for these conditions are high risk for altered nutrition and ineffective airway clearance, impaired tissue integrity, infection, altered parenting, self-esteem disturbance, and altered pattern of communication. Surgical repair is possible early in life with good prognosis for both these conditions.

- Tracheoesophageal atresia and fistula occur from failure of the trachea and esophagus to divide appropriately in intrauterine life. The nursing diagnoses most frequently identified for these conditions are high risk for altered nutrition and infection. Surgical intervention often requires several procedures to complete.

- Omphalocele is the protrusion of abdominal contents through the abdominal wall at birth, protected only by a peritoneal membrane. When the membrane is not present, this is gastroschisis. Nursing diagnoses most frequently identified are high risk for infection and altered nutrition. Although several stages of repair are often necessary, surgical correction has a good outcome.

- Intestinal obstruction can result from atresia (complete closure) or stenosis (narrowing) of a part of the bowel. It is associated with hydramnios in pregnancy. The nursing diagnosis most frequently identified is high risk for fluid volume deficit related to vomiting.

- A meconium plug occurs when an extremely hard portion of meconium blocks the lumen of the intestine. Infants with this need to be observed for continued bowel function and may have a sweat test done for cystic fibrosis (CF), because children with CF often have this symptom.

- Diaphragmatic hernia occurs when the abdominal organ protrudes through a defect in the diaphragm into the chest cavity. This prevents the lungs from fully expanding at birth. The nursing diagnoses for this are ineffective airway clearance and altered nutrition related to the misplaced bowel. These infants are critically ill at birth and need extensive surgical correction.

- Imperforate anus is stricture of the anus resulting in inability to pass stool. Nursing diagnoses identified for this are altered nutrition, impaired tissue integrity following surgery, and altered parenting related to a lengthy hospitalization. The infant may have a temporary colostomy done before a final surgical correction.

- Physical anomalies of the nervous system that may occur are hydrocephalus (excess of cerebrospinal fluid in the ventricles) and spina bifida (incomplete closure of the spinal cord). Nursing diagnoses identified for the infant with hydrocephalus are high risk for altered nutrition, altered skin integrity, altered cerebral tissue perfusion, knowledge deficit, and altered growth and development. Those for the infant with spina bifida are high risk for infection, altered nutrition, altered cerebral tissue perfusion, altered skin integrity, impaired physical mobility, and altered elimination. Infants with hydrocephalus have a shunt implanted from their ventricles to the perineum to remove excess CSF. Children with myelomeningocele, the most severe form of spinal cord defect, will have a permanent loss of lower neuron function that requires continued habilitation.

- Absent or malformed extremities may occur ranging from absence of a finger to absence of an entire limb. Children may need physical therapy and to learn to use a prosthesis to have full function.

- Hip dysplasia is the improper formation and function of the hip socket; talipes deformities are foot and ankle deformities. Children may need extensive bracing and casting to correct these disorders.

- Any child who is hospitalized at birth is at high risk for child abuse. Assess family relationships at health maintenance visits to see that bonding has occurred.

Definitions of Key Terms

ankyloglossia: tongue-tie

atresia: absence or closure of a normal body passage

cleft lip: incomplete fusion of the lip during intrauterine life

cleft palate: incomplete fusion of the palate during intrauterine life

dislocated hip: a congenital orthopedic condition in which a shallow acetabulum allows the femur head to slip from the socket

fistula: an abnormal passage or communication between two organs

frenulum: the attachment of the inferior surface of the tongue to the oral mucous membrane

hip dysplasia: a subluxated or dislocated hip

hydrocephalus: an abnormally enlarged head size due to accumulated cerebrospinal fluid distending the cerebral ventricles

meconium plug: an unusually thickened portion of intestinal contents formed during fetal life which obstructs the intestine at birth. Associated with cystic fibrosis

omphalocele: a congenital protrusion of intestine through a defect in the abdominal wall at the umbilicus

polydactyly: an extra digit on the hand or foot

spina bifida: a congenital vertebra defect

stenosis: a narrowing in a passageway

subluxated hip: a congenital orthopedic condition in which a shallow acetabulum allows the femur head excess freedom of movement

syndactyly: webbing or joining of fingers or toes

transillumination: a diagnostic technique utilizing the phenomenon that a bright light shown on a body part will reveal if the contents of the part are fluid

Nursing Process Overview

The Nursing Process Overview in this chapter stresses the importance of careful assessment of all newborns in order that congenital disorders can be identified as early as possible. Nursing diagnoses that stress the long-term aspects of these disorders as well as the difficulty new parents may have accepting the conditions are discussed.

Study Aids

Boxes

Box 39-1:   Instructions for self-catheterization

Tables

Table 39-1:   Motor function disability in myelomeningocele

Displays

Focus on National Health Goals

Focus on Family Teaching

Focus on Nursing Research

Focus on Cultural Awareness

Critical Thinking Exercises:

1. Joshua is a newborn who has been diagnosed with a tracheoesophageal fistula and is waiting transport to an intensive care nursery. What would be important assessments to make of him? How would you explain this disorder to his parents? They ask you how this could have happened. What would be your answer?

2. Children with subluxated hip may be in casts for a full year or more. What suggestions could you make to a parent to help her instill a strong sense of trust in her child? A sense of autonomy?

3. You notice that the 16-year-old mother of a child born with a cleft lip is obviously upset at the child's appearance. She doesn't want to feed the baby and voices the thought of placing her for adoption. The child's father, a 22-year-old, in contrast, handles the baby warmly and asks questions about surgery. No grandparents visit. What interventions would you want to begin with this family?

Media Resources

Caring for the Child in a Hip Spica Cast (19-minute slide/audiocassette)

A parent education program describing the application of a hip spica cast and related care necessary. Included are techniques for keeping the cast clean and dry, checking circulation, protecting the skin, planning play activities, and ensuring safety.

Source: University of Michigan

Mobility Problems in Children (28-minute videocassette)

The physical manifestations and nursing care of children with congenital orthopedic anomalies including talipes disorders, hip dislocation, and spina bifida are presented. Muscular dystrophy, cerebral palsy, and scoliosis are also discussed.

Source: Medical Electronic Educational Services, Inc.

How to Feed Your Baby Who Has a Cleft Lip or Palate (11-minute slide/audiocassette)

Safe and effective feeding techniques for the baby with a cleft lip or palate is shown. Equipment, positioning, and mouth care are illustrated. Guidelines for food selection and introduction are discussed.

Source: Health Sciences Consortium

Neonatal Problems: Jaundice (14-minute slide/audiocassette)

The methods of diagnosing neonatal jaundice, history, examination, and laboratory tests are presented. The causes of jaundice are discussed. Clinical manifestations and appropriate treatment are included.

Source: Health Sciences Consortium

Crisis for the Unborn (8-minute film)

Fetal alcohol syndrome and its effects on fetal growth are discussed.

Source: March of Dimes Birth Defects Foundation

Dental Care for the Cleft Lip/Cleft Palate Child (11-minute slide/audiocassette)

The procedures for the maintenance of children's teeth, normal dental development, proper nutrition, and the value of fluoride is presented. Information specific to children with cleft lip or palate is stressed.

Source: Health Sciences Consortium

Neurologic Insults in the Neonate (24-minute slide-audiocassette)

The more common congenital and acquired neurologic defects in the neonate are discussed. Signs of neurologic damage and the importance of prevention are included.

Source: Master Concepts

Hospital Infection Control Series: Common Neonatal Viral Infections (28-minute videocassette)

A moderator conducts a discussion with two physicians on the causes, incidence, transfer, diagnosis, and therapy for herpes simplex, congenital rubella, and cytomegalovirus infections. Emphasis is placed on the education of both the mother and the hospital staff to prevent spread of these diseases.

Source: Health Sciences Consortium

Children at risk: Alcohol and Pregnancy (17-minute videocassette)

The argument that an expectant mother should take no risks with her child and so avoid consumption of any alcohol during pregnancy is presented. The specific effects of fetal alcohol syndrome are discussed.

Source: Health Sciences Consortium

Phenylketonuria (27-minute slide-audiocassette)

The definition, pathophysiology, and characteristic signs of phenylketonuria are described. Methods of screening are discussed. Early detection is stressed to prevent brain involvement.

Source: Mead Johnson and Company

Discussion Questions

1. Anomalies such as tracheoesophageal fistula and omphalocele create secondary problems of nutrition, because infants with these disorders are unable to breast- or bottle-feed. This can limit a mother's ability to feel like a parent because she can not feed the child. How can nurses help mothers overcome this feeling?

2. A parent may have more difficulty discussing a congenital anomaly when it involves a part of the body such as the rectum. What are the implications for this for the parents of the child born with imperforate anus?

3. In the past, the parents of infants with myelomeningocele were told that the child had no chance for any quality of life. Discuss whether this is still true. How has this influenced care?

Written Assignments

1. Caring for the child with hydrocephalus requires long-term care. List the specific precautions you would want to discuss with the parents of such a child. How do these precautions change as the child grows older?

2. Infants with diaphragmatic hernia are treated today with extracorporeal membrane oxygenation. As this is specialized therapy, it is only available in regional centers. Suppose a parent objects to his baby being transferred for this high technology care? What would be your role?

3. Infants born with anencephaly will predictably have a limited life span. Often parents of these infants sign permission for organ transplants when these infants die. List the pros and cons of using organ transplants from such infants.

Laboratory Experiences

1. Assign students to observe for a day in an intensive care nursery. Ask them to assess the impact on the family when a child is born with a congenital anomaly.

2. Ask a parent of a child born with a congenital anomaly who has required extensive follow-up care to attend a postconference and describe the experience. Were there things the parent would have preferred be done differently another time? How could nurses have been more of a help to her?

3. Assign students to a follow-up clinic for infants who were cared for in an intensive care nursery because of an anomaly at birth. Ask them to assess the quality of life of a particular infant they see.

Care Study: An Infant With Hydrocephalus

Sheldon Suderman is a 2-month-old brought to a private pediatrician for a well child visit.

Health History

- Chief Concern: "His eyes seem funny to me."

- History of Present Concern: Child was born with a meningocele that was repaired at birth. Child discharged from hospital at 7 days; infant has apparently full use of legs. Mother reports that child's eyes "roll down" as if he's "blinking at a light" for past week.

- Family Profile: Family intact. Father is a full-time student studying to be a rabbi; mother sells real estate. Family lives in a two-bedroom condominium. Finances are "adequate."

- Pregnancy History: At 15 weeks of pregnancy alphafetoprotein level revealed that child might have an open spinal disorder; sonogram confirmed the open lesion and it seemed to be a meningocele. Defect was diagnosed definitely at birth as meningocele; repaired by 6 hours post birth.

- Past Medical History: No illnesses other than meningocele. Indirect bilirubin rose to 12 mg/dL at second day of life.

  No immunizations as yet.

- Growth and Development: Infant lifts head when prone; demonstrates social smile. Nutrition: takes SMA with iron 4 ounces q4h.

- Family Medical History: Maternal grandmother: diabetes, adult onset; has received hemodialysis four times a week for kidney failure for past year.

  Mother: Severe PMS manifested as migraine headache for 2 days prior to menses.

- Review of Systems: Mother feels anterior fontanelle is growing in size.

- Extremities; Diagnosed as having talipes equinovarus at birth; casted before discharge from hospital; has had cast changed twice since then. Infant kicks symmetrically.

- Urinary: voids about every 3 hours with dry periods in between.

- Neurologic: No seizures. Child has seemed irritable for past week.

Physical Examination

- General Appearance: Alert appearing 2-month-old male; prominent anterior bossing of forehead; cry high and shrill.

- Head: Anterior fontanelle 4 cm 4 cm; posterior fontanelle 3 cm. Anterior fontanelle transilluminates 3 cms. Sagittal suture line separated 1/4 inch. Forehead bossed forward; scalp veins prominent.

- Eyes: Normal alignment; sclera visible over pupils bilaterally. PERL but response is not immediate; consensual constriction present.

- Ears: Normal alignment. TMs pink; landmarks visible. Slight brown cerumen in both canals. Infant attunes to sound of examiner's voice.

- Nose: Midline septum; no discharge.

- Mouth and Throat: No teeth; midline uvula; mucous membrane moist.

- Neck: Full range of motion; child holds head upright but only momentarily. No palpable lymph nodes.

- Lungs: Clear to auscultation and percussion; no adventitious sounds. Respiratory rate 18/min.

- Heart: Rate 90/min; no murmurs

- Abdomen: Soft; no masses; liver palpable 1 cm below right costal margin.

- Back: Well healed surgery scar at level of sacral vertebrae; vertebrae in good alignment.

- Extremities: Full range of motion; hips abduct to 180 degrees. Talipes equinovarus cast in place on left leg from midfoot to over knee.

- Genitalia: Circumcised male; testes descended.

- Neurologic: Unable to elicit moro or patellar reflexes; tonic neck intact. Babinski flares.

Care Study Questions

1. Sheldon does not demonstrate either a moro or patellar reflex. Should these still be present at 4 months of age?

2. Compare Sheldon's head circumference to a standard for a 2-month-old. Is the circumference increased?

3. Sheldon was diagnosed as having increased intracranial pressure from developing hydrocephalus. Complete a nursing care plan that would identify and meet the needs of Sheldon and his family.

Care of the Child With a Respiratory Disorder

Chapter 40 discusses care of the child with a disorder of the respiratory tract. The chapter begins with a nursing process overview stressing the nurse's role in assessing children for respiratory illness and establishing nursing diagnoses that speak to the effect of such disorders. Both upper respiratory tract disorders (eg, the common cold, streptococcal pharyngitis, tonsillitis, laryngotracheobronchitis, and epiglottitis) and lower respiratory tract disorders (eg, bronchitis, bronchiolitis, respiratory syncytial virus infection, pneumonia, atelectasis, tuberculosis, cystic fibrosis, and pneumothorax) are discussed. Sudden infant death syndrome is also included.

Students need to review respiratory physiology before studying care of the child with a respiratory disorder in order that they can fully appreciate the effect of poor respiratory exchange on body functions. Respiratory disease occurs frequently in children, and learning care of these children is essential to maternal child health nursing.

Chapter Objectives

After mastering the contents of this chapter, students should be able to:

1. Describe common respiratory illnesses in children.
2. Assess the child with a respiratory illness.
3. Formulate nursing diagnoses related to respiratory illness in children.
4. Plan the nursing care of the child with a respiratory illness, such as planning times for postural therapy.
5. Implement nursing care (eg, providing oxygen therapy) for the child with a respiratory illness.
6. Evaluate outcome criteria to be certain that nursing goals established for care have been achieved.

7. Identify national health goals related to children with respiratory disorders that nurses could be instrumental in in helping the nation achieve.
8. Identify areas related to care of children with respiratory disorders that could benefit from additional nursing research.
9. Use critical thinking to analyze ways that nursing care for a child with a respiratory illness could be more family centered.
10. Synthesize knowledge of respiratory illness in children with nursing process to achieve quality maternal and child health nursing care.

Key Points

- Respiratory tract disorders tend to occur more frequently in children than adults because the lumen of bronchi are narrow and obstruction can occur more easily.

- Acute nasopharyngitis (common cold) is the most frequently seen infectious disease in children. There is no specific therapy for a cold. The nursing diagnosis—health seeking behaviors—is usually most fitting because it describes the parents' response to illness in their child.

- Tonsillitis is infection and inflammation of the palatine tonsils. Adenitis is infection and inflammation of the adenoid tonsils. The nursing diagnoses identified for this are usually "High risk for fluid volume deficit" and "Pain" because of the surgery required to remove the infected tonsils.

- Laryngotracheobronchitis (croup) is inflammation of the larynx, trachea, and major bronchi. Epiglottitis is inflammation of the epiglottis. Both of these conditions can cause severe impairment of the airway. The nursing diagnosis associated with the disorders is "High risk for ineffective airway clearance." Children with epiglottis should never be gagged with a tongue blade, or the elevated epiglottis may completely occlude the airway.

- Bronchitis is inflammation of the major bronchi and trachea. Bronchiolitis is inflammation of the fine bronchioles. Children are administered antibiotics and usually oxygen therapy. The nursing diagnosis "Parental anxiety related to sudden onset of symptoms" is generally appropriate.

- Respiratory syncytial virus (RSV) infection is an infection that accounts for the majority of lower respiratory infection in young children. Infants with RSV infections must be observed closely since they are prone to apnea.

- Pneumonia may occur from a variety of organisms (viral, pneumococcal, chlamydial, mycoplasmal, lipid, and hydrocarbon). Children need specific antibiotics depending on the organism present.

- Sudden infant death syndrome (SIDS) is the most frequent cause of death from a respiratory illness in infants under 6 months of age. Parents need concerned support when SIDS occurs, since it is so unexpected and not preventable.

- Tuberculosis is an illness growing in incidence. One strain is very resistant to the usual therapy and presents a risk to health care providers. Nurses are well advised to maintain a current PPD status so they can be aware if exposure occurs.

- Cystic fibrosis is a disease in which there is generalized dysfunction of the exocrine glands. Nursing diagnoses chosen are often "Altered nutrition," "High risk for ineffective airway clearance," "Altered skin integrity," and "Ineffective family coping."

- Infants need extremely close observation with respiratory illness, because they cannot describe oxygen hunger. Young children do not appreciate the fact that oxygen supports combustion. They need more observation than adults do to be certain that no flames, such as birthday candles, are brought within 10 ft of an oxygen source.

Definitions of Key Terms

adventitious sounds: abnormal sounds heard on auscultation of the lungs

aspiration: inhalation of a foreign object

atelectasis: collapse of a lung

bronchial breathing: the sound heard over the trachea and main stem bronchus; the expiratory sound is longer than inspiratory

clubbing: abnormal enlargement of the distal fingers

cupping: a technique of postural drainage in which the chest is struck with the curved palm

cyanosis: a bluish discoloration of the skin

expiration: exhalation

hypoxemia: deficient oxygenation of the blood

hypoxia: deficient oxygenation of body cells

inspiration: inhalation

paroxysmal coughing: a series of loud exhalations usually followed by a deep inspiration

percussion: striking the fingers on a body surface to produce sound

pneumothorax: collapse of the lung due to air in the pleural space

postural drainage: positioning of a client in order to drain secretions from the pulmonary tree

rales: the sound of air moving through fluid in alveoli; a crackling sound

retraction: inward movement of the chest wall on inspiration

stridor: a high-pitched inspiratory sound

tachypnea: rapid respirations

vesicular breathing: the type of breath sounds heard over lung periphery; inspiration is longer than expiration

wheezing: a whistling expiratory sound

Nursing Process Overview

The Nursing Process Overview for this chapter concentrates on the importance of recognizing signs and symptoms of respiratory illness and nursing diagnoses that speak to the effect of such illnesses, such as "Activity intolerance related to insufficient oxygenation."

Study Aids

Boxes

Box 40-1:   Interpreting ABGs

Box 40-2:   Allen test

Tables

Table 40-1:   Commonly used respiratory assessment terms

Table 40-2:   Adventitious findings revealed by auscultation and palpation in respiratory disease

Table 40-3:   Blood gas values

Table 40-4:   Comparison of respiratory alkalosis and respiratory acidosis

Table 40-5:   Pulmonary function tests

Table 40-6:   Drugs commonly used with respiratory disorders

Table 40-7:   Terms commonly used with ventilator therapy

Table 40-8:   Common problems with assisted ventilation

Table 40-9:   Comparison of laryngotracheobronchitis (croup) and epiglottitis

Table 40-10: Comparison of bronchiolitis and pneumonia

Procedures

Procedure 40-1: Postural drainage

Procedure 40-2: Tracheotomy suction

Displays

Focus on National Health Goals

Focus on Family Teaching

Focus on Nursing Research

Focus on Cultural Awareness

Critical Thinking Questions:

1. Mary is a 3-year-old who has a permanent tracheotomy tube in place. Her parents are going to enroll her in a preschool center. What precautions would you want to review with the parents to keep this experience safe for Mary?

2. Bryan is a 10-year-old who has just returned from tonsillectomy surgery. What observations would be important to make with Bryan? Why is the 7th day following tonsillectomy surgery a particularly important day?

3. Karen is a 16-year-old with cystic fibrosis. Her parents want to take her on an extended vacation in the Caribbean next summer. What anticipatory guidance would give Karen and her parents?

Media Resources

Suctioning Techniques for the Pediatric Patient (16-minute videocassette)

}The procedure for tracheal suctioning of the pediatric patient is illustrated. Types of tracheostomy tubes, humidification, frequency of suctioning, complications that can occur, and the emotional needs of the child needing suctioning are included.

Source: Health Sciences Consortium

Pediatric Physiotherapy (20-minute videocassette)

The procedure for postural drainage and percussion, examination of the chest, and breathing exercises for children are presented. Knowledge of the basics of chest physiotherapy is necessary before viewing the video. The program is self-instructional and includes a workbook.

Source: Medical Electronic Educational Services, Inc.

The Story of Susan McKellar (20-minute videocassette, film)

A young woman with cystic fibrosis who has learned to cope with her disease describes how a positive attitude has enabled her to marry, lead a full life, and pursue her career as a nurse. She is shown performing respiratory therapy on herself and discussing how she is able to manage her physical limitations.

Source: Filmmakers Library

Bronchiolitis (26-minute slide/audiocassette)

A detailed discussion of the pathology, incidence, clinical manifestations, and chronic effects of bronchiolitis. The reasons for the severity of symptoms in infants and young children are discussed. A workbook accompanies the program.

Source: American Lung Association

Children with Croup (9-minute slide/audiocassette)

The major forms of croup and the appropriate therapeutic management of each type are described.

Source: University of Michigan

An Orientation to Asthma (slide/audiocassette)

An overview of asthma including pathology, clinical manifestations, and precipitating stimuli. The mechanisms that produce air flow obstruction such as bronchoconstriction, inflammation, and edema are illustrated and the drug management to reverse these conditions is explained. Asthma is a chronic childhood condition, and the ways it influences children's lifestyles are examined.

Source: American Lung Association

Suctioning Techniques for the Pediatric Patient (16-minute videocassette)

The procedure for tracheal suctioning is demonstrated. The use of cuffed tubes and humidifiers, frequency of suctioning, complications, and the emotional needs of the child during suctioning are discussed.

Source: Health Sciences Consortium

The Story of Sixty-five Roses (10-minute film)

}The ability of girl to adapt to a diagnosis of cystic fibrosis as she grows from preschool-age to young adult. Family concerns and support are identified. The title is derived from the name she gave her disease before she was able to pronounce it clearly.

Source: Cystic Fibrosis Foundation

Discussion Questions

1. Observing a child with croup for respiratory obstruction is an important nursing responsibility. Which signs or symptoms would alert you that the child is developing increased obstruction?

2. Tracheotomies may lead to the development of pneumonia. What kind of care would you plan for a child with a tracheotomy to help keep pneumonia from developing?

3. Infants with acute nasopharyngitis (a common cold) have difficulty sucking. What measures would you suggest to a parent to help maintain hydration in the child?

Written Assignments

1. Various adventitious sounds can be heard on auscultation of the lungs. Write a paragraph describing the sound of rhonchi, rales, wheezing, and stridor and the importance of these sounds.

2. Children who are being cared for at home on apnea monitors create a care problem for parents. What are suggestions you could make to parents to help keep the child safe while on this form of monitoring?

3. Many children with respiratory illness are prescribed postural drainage daily. Describe the positions you would place a child in to perform this in order to drain each lung lobe.

Laboratory Experiences

1. Assign students to clinical areas that are caring for children with respiratory disorders such as cystic fibrosis and pneumonia. Stress with students that parents are very frightened when their children have these illnesses and will need a great deal of support.

2. Assign students to spend a day with a respiratory therapist to increase student understanding of oxygen therapy and postural drainage.

3. Assign students to a home care service so they can have an experience with a child on an apnea monitor or with ventilator assistance at home.

Care Study: An Adolescent With Cystic Fibrosis

Billy Denman is a 16-year-old with cystic fibrosis admitted to your hospital unit.

Health History

- Chief Concern: "The usual. Pneumonia for sure."

- History of Present Concern: Billy was diagnosed as having cystic fibrosis at 8 months of age. Has been hospitalized 68 previous times for pneumonia. The present complication began 3 days ago with elevated temperature (102gF), loss of energy, and persistent green-colored sputum on postural drainage. Delayed reporting symptoms to mother because he wanted to attend a school dance this evening; by mid-morning this day he realized he was too sick to delay reporting symptoms any longer. Temperature is now 104gF; respiratory rate: 28/min; pulse: 132/min. Adolescent is coughing frequently but nonproductively.

- Family Profile: Billy lives with mother. Parents were divorced when he was 4 years old because "father couldn't stand knowing he had a kid with CF." Father has never contributed to Billy's care despite the fact he lives in the city and knows of Billy's large medical bills. Mother is a nurse; history was obtained from Billy since she had not arrived at hospital yet. Billy rated their finances as "hanging in there." Family lives in a 3-bedroom house; "one bedroom for mom, one for me, and one for a slant board." Billy does own postural drainage on anterior lobes with automatic vibrator; mother does posterior surface; a home care aide visits two times a week to supplement therapy.

- History of Past Illnesses: Chickenpox at 4 years (contracted while in hospital).

  Hospital admissions for CF average 4 times a year since diagnosis; "severe" congestion with heart failure 2 times in last 2 years.

  One ER admission for swallowing "too many aspirin" last May. Treated with stomach lavage, 24-hour observation, and discharged. Adolescent states episode occurred from "trying to stop a headache, nothing else."

- Immunizations: Up to date. Received pneumococcal and meningococcal vaccines.

- Pregnancy History: Planned pregnancy; first pregnancy for mother; no complications. Spontaneous respirations at birth. No bowel movement for 30 hours post birth; then meconium plug was expelled. Billy was kept in hospital 3 extra days for failure to regain birthweight and excessive jaundice.

- Growth and Development: Was breast-fed as an infant; weight gain continued to be slow; bowel movements large and foul-smelling. Was changed to formula at 3 months in an attempt to increase weight. Weight and height both continued to follow 10th percentile. Infant and preschool motor milestones achieved late; didn't walk until 24 months. Language: normal; spoke in sentences by 2 years.

Currently attends high school in sophomore year (1 year behind); has had extra hours of tutoring to maintain school placement.

Participates in the school science and computer clubs; participates in no school sports. Maintains an active walking program; uses treadmill in home on rainy or cold days. States he is normally able to do "things he wants to do." Admits to using illness to not do things he does not want to do on occasion. Has regular household chores: cleaning own room and doing own laundry; mowing lawn with power mower.

- Family Medical History: No other person with illness in family, although maternal grandmother who lives in Switzerland had 2 infants die at birth for "unknown reasons." Mother: hysterectomy 3 years ago for dermoid cysts of ovaries. Father's family history: not known.

- Review of Systems: Head; occasional headaches when using computer too long.

- Eyes: vision 20/50 L, 20/70 R; wears corrective glasses.

- Ears: No otitis media; hearing tested in school in 8th grade and found to be adequate.

- Gastrointestinal: Takes pancreatin with meals; no rectal prolapse.

- Integumentary: Had heat prostration in 6th grade from running in a foot race in hot sun. Treated with intravenous fluid in emergency room. Now more careful to reduce activities in hot weather.

- Neurosych: "Resigned" to having chronic illness, although does experience occasional episodes of depression thinking about future. Mother concerned that poisoning episode last year was not a pure accident.

Physical Examination

- General Appearance: Underweight pale-appearing adolescent male; sad facial expression. Height: 5'4"; Weight: 92 lbs. Blood pressure: 90/50.

- Head: Normocephalic; 2 blackened comedones present on forehead.

- Eyes: Red reflex present; follows to all fields of vision; no erythema or discharge present.

- Ears: TMs reddened bilaterally; landmarks not distinct; hearing equal to examiners.

- Nose: Midline septum; mucous membrane reddened; yellow pustular discharge present.

- Mouth and Throat: Prominent anterior overbite; no cavities; geographic tongue. Yellow drainage present on posterior throat; tonsils and posterior palate slightly erythematous; no pus in tonsillar crypts.

- Neck: Subtle, no pain on forward flexion; midline trachea; no nodes palpable in thyroid; 3 palpable lymph nodes on left; 2 on right in posterior cervical chains.

- Chest: Scattered rhonchi in all lobes; decreased breath sounds in right lower lobes; moist crackling in both lower lobes.

- Heart: Rate 80/min; third heart sound audible. Marked sinus arrhythmia.
- Abdomen: Liver palpable 2 cms below right costal margin; no masses. Bowel sounds at 2—3 per minute in all quadrants.
- Genitalia: Adolescent male; Tanner 5; testes descended; midline meatus.
- Extremities: Full ROM, poor muscle tone in upper extremities.
- Neurologic: Patellar and brachial reflexes 2; sensory and motor nerves grossly intact.

Care Study Questions

1. Billy is an adolescent who is very knowledgeable about his disease. Is it easier or more difficult to take care of a child who is an "expert" on a disease?

2. Billy had an episode last year during which he swallowed too many aspirin. He said this was because he had a severe headache. Is this a realistic explanation for a child as knowledgeable as Billy?

3. Billy has the problem of dealing with a long-term illness. Billy was diagnosed as having pneumonia. Complete a nursing care plan that would identify and meet his needs.

The Child With a Cardiovascular Disorder

Chapter 41 discusses care of the child with a cardiovascular disorder. The chapter begins with a Nursing Process Overview suggesting nursing diagnoses pertinent to the area and ways that nursing care can be modified to meet the special needs of the child with a cardiovascular disorder. Care of the child with both congenital disorders and acquired disorders such as rheumatic fever, Kawasaki disease, congestive heart disease, and hypertension are discussed. Care of the child undergoing cardiac catheterization, heart transplant, and cardiac surgery is described, as well as the technique of cardiopulmonary resuscitation. The importance of recognizing the stress engendered by a diagnosis of heart disease and initiating measures to reduce parents' and children's fears is stressed.

Nursing care of children with cardiac disorders calls for responsible assessment and evaluation by students, since the signs and symptoms of a heart failing to compensate are subtle. Students should be certain to review cardiopulmonary resuscitation skills before beginning care of children with these disorders.

Chapter Objectives

After mastering the contents of this chapter students should be able to:

1. Describe the common cardiovascular disorders of childhood.
2. Assess a child with cardiovascular dysfunction.
3. Formulate nursing diagnoses for the child with a cardiovascular disorder such as congenital heart disease, rheumatic fever, and hypertension.
4. Plan nursing care for the child with a cardiovascular disorder such as preparing a child for cardiac catheterization.
5. Implement nursing care such as teaching parents how to administer a cardiac medication for the child with a cardiovascular disorder.

6. Evaluate outcome criteria to be certain that nursing care goals were accomplished.
7. Identify national health goals related to cardiovascular disorders and children that nurses could be instrumental in in helping the nation achieve.
8. Identify areas related to the care of children with cardiovascular problems that could benefit from additional nursing research.
9. Use critical thinking to analyze ways that nursing care of children with cardiovascular disorders could be more family centered.
10. Synthesize knowledge of cardiovascular disorders with nursing process to achieve quality maternal and child health nursing care.

Key Points

- Cardiac anomalies are the most frequently occurring type of congenital anomaly. Observing for cyanosis in newborns to help detect this is a major nursing responsibility. Assessing the femoral pulses in newborns helps rule out coarctation of the aorta.

- Cardiovascular disorders in children may be either structural such as congenital heart disease or acquired such as Kawasaki disease and rheumatic fever.

- Assessment of children with heart disease includes history and physical examination. Many children have cardiac catheterizations done for diagnosis. Nursing diagnoses associated with this are Anxiety, and High risk for altered tissue perfusion, and infection.

- Preoperative care is an important concern in cardiovascular surgery. Nursing diagnoses commonly identified in connection with this are "Fear,""High risk for altered cardiopulmonary tissue perfusion,""Ineffective airway clearance,""Hypothermia,"and "Parental anxiety."

- Post—cardiac surgery syndrome and postperfusion syndrome are two complications that may occur after cardiac surgery because of the extracorporal circulation used during the procedure.

- Children such as those born with hypoplastic left heart syndrome may undergo cardiac transplant. Children born with ineffective SA node function may have pacemakers implanted to improve heart function.

- Common types of acyanotic heart defects are ventricular or atrial septal defect, coarctation of the aorta, patent ductus arteriosus, pulmonary or aortic stenosis, duplication of the aortic arch, and an endocardial cushion defect.

- Cyanotic heart defects commonly seen are tetralogy of Fallot, transportation of the great arteries, total anomalous pulmonary venous return, truncus arteriosus, tricuspid atresia, and hypoplastic left heart syndrome. Children with cyanotic heart disease are prone to "tet" or cyanotic episodes. The emergency intervention when this occurs is to place the child in a knee—chest position.

- The families of children undergoing cardiac surgery need a great deal of support to help them cope well enough with this major event to be a support for the child.

- Common signs of congestive heart failure seen in children are tachycardia, tachypnea, enlarged liver, dyspnea, and cyanosis. Signs tend to be subtle in infants and may be manifested chiefly by difficulty in feeding from exhaustion and dyspnea. Nursing diagnoses identified for congestive heart failure include "High risk for altered nutrition," "Altered cardiopulmonary tissue perfusion," and "Fear."

- Rheumatic fever is an autoimmune disease that occurs following a group A, beta-hemolytic streptococcal infection. Common signs and symptoms are fever, chorea, arthralgia, polyarthritis, erythema marginatum, subcutaneous nodules, and an elevated sedimentation rate. Helping parents (and the child) remember to administer prophylactic penicillin following the illness until age 18 helps prevent further recurrence and cardiac involvement. Children with congenital heart disease may also need to maintain this same protection routine.

- Kawasaki disease results from altered immune function. The inflammation of blood vessels occurs, leading to platelet accumulation and the formation of thrombi.

- Infectious endocarditis is infection of the endocardium of the valves of the heart. It may be a complication of congenital heart disease.

- Children with cardiac disease may fall behind in developmental progress because they do not have the energy to play the usual childhood games. Help parents to think of games that are intellectually or developmentally stimulating without being physically exhausting.

- Hypertension usually occurs as a secondary manifestation, not a primary one, in children. Cardiac disease in adults can be reduced if, as children, they eat a moderate-cholesterol diet, exercise regularly, and maintain a weight proportional to height. Counseling children to follow these "heart healthy" guidelines calls for tact and persistence.

- Children with heart disease are at high risk for cardiopulmonary arrest. Cardiac resuscitation in a newborn is done by a light touch: pressing a thumb or two fingers on the mid-sternum. Drugs commonly used in resuscitation procedures are epinephrine, atropine, and calcium chloride.

Definitions of Key Terms

acyanotic heart disease: heart disease involving a left to right shunt or a stricture in blood flow

afterload: the systemic resistance against which the heart ventricles must pump

balloon stenotomy: the technique of inserting a catheter with a deflated balloon attached through a narrow passageway, inflating the balloon, and withdrawing the catheter to widen the constricted portion

cardiac catheterization: a diagnostic procedure in which a catheter is introduced into a vein or artery and threaded into the heart

congestive heart failure: a condition characterized by inability of the heart to move blood received forward

contractility: ability of a muscle to tighten and produce tension

cyanosis: bluish discoloration of the skin and mucous membrane

cyanotic heart disease: heart disease marked by a right to left shunt or unoxygenated blood entering the oxygenated circulation

diastole: contraction of the heart atria

echocardiography: ultrasonic examination of the heart

electrocardiography: a study of the electrical activity of the heart

extracorporeal membrane oxygenation: oxygenation of the blood by a heart—lung machine

fluoroscopy: a radiology study that offers serial images

hypertension: elevated blood pressure

innocent heart murmur: an accessory heart sound that represents a benign origin

left-to-right shunt: a passageway in the heart allowing oxygenated blood to pass into unoxygenated blood

organic heart murmur: an accessory heart sound that signifies a structural heart defect

phonocardiogram: a record of heart sounds recorded by microphone

polycythemia: an excess of red blood cells

post—cardiac surgery syndrome: a febrile episode occurring following extracorporal perfusion

postperfusion syndrome: a febrile illness following extracorporal perfusion possibly caused by a cytomegalovirus

preload: the volume of blood in the heart ventricles at the end of diastole

right-to-left shunt: a passageway in the heart allowing unoxygenated blood to pass into oxygenated blood

systole: contraction of the ventricles

Nursing Process Overview

The Nursing Process Overview in this chapter concentrates on formulating nursing diagnoses that speak not only to physical problems such as "Altered tissue perfusion" but also to psychological ones that arise from the stress of having a child with a cardiac disorder such as "High risk for altered parenting.'' The role of the nurse as the health care provider who is responsible for assessing vital signs —important indications of cardiac illness—is stressed.

Study Aids

Tables

Table 41-1:   Abnormal pulse patterns

Table 41-2:   Comparison of innocent and organic murmurs

Table 41-3:   Criteria for diagnosis of Kawasaki disease

Displays

Focus on National Health Goals

Focus on Family Teaching

Focus on Nursing Research

Focus on Cultural Awareness

Critical Thinking Exercises:

1. Joey is a newborn who has been diagnosed as having congenital heart disease. He will be living at home with his parents for a month before he returns for surgery. His doctor told his parents to "watch him carefully" during this time. They ask you what this means. How would you answer them?

2. Heather, 10 years old, is a child who is recovering from rheumatic fever. She lives during the week with her mother and visits her father on the weekends. She will need to continue to take penicillin daily for the next 8 years. What steps would you take to ensure compliance over this long a period of time?

3. You have been asked to prepare a class for a group of parents on cardiopulmonary resuscitation for newborns. How would you teach this?

Media Resources

It's Time for Your Cardiac Catheterization (10-minute slide/audiocassette)

The preparation of a school-age child for cardiac catheterization is presented. The procedure and equipment used are described and illustrated using simple language. This program could be used to prepare children for the procedure.

Source: University of Indiana

Infant Cardiopulmonary Resuscitation for Parents (15-minute videocassette)

The American Heart Association standards are demonstrated on how to perform cardiopulmonary resuscitation (CPR) on an infant and what to do if choking occurs. Available in both English and Spanish.

Source: AJN Educational Services

Your Baby with a Congenital Heart Defect (29-minute videocassette)

Interviews with three families as they describe their feelings and experiences with caring for infants with congenital heart defects. Such problems as crying, cyanosis, feeding, and meeting developmental and health needs are discussed.

Source: University of Michigan

Cardiac Failure in Infancy (30-minute film)

The physical signs found on examination of infants with cardiac failure are presented. The diagnostic workup and principles of immediate medical treatment of infants with cardiac failure, of either gradual or sudden onset, are outlined.

Source: American Heart Association

Congenital Malformations of the Heart: Cyanotic Congenital Heart Disease (30-minute film)

The contrasts between normal oxygenation and conditions that cause cyanosis are presented. Included defects are tricuspid atresia, tetralogy of Fallot, Eisenmenger complex, truncus arteriosus, and transposition of the great vessels.

Source: Universal Education and Visual Arts

Congenital Malformations of the Heart: Acyanotic Congenital Heart Disease (14-minute film)

The most common acyanotic heart defects are presented: patent ductus arteriosus, atrial septal defect, and ventricular septal defect. Anatomic structure, clinical manifestations, and principles upon which a differential diagnosis can be made are included.

Source: Universal Education and Visual Arts

Leonard Z Lion Presents: Learning About Your Heart (Catheterization; Learning about Your Heart Operation; Taking Care of Your Teeth to Protect Your Heart) (15-minute videocassette)

These three programs are designed to explain to school-age children with heart disease the importance of dental care and what to expect during cardiac catheterization and heart surgery. The tape would be useful for orienting school-age children to these procedures.

Source: University of Michigan

Jeannie (6-minute videocassette)

An 11-year-old is prepared for cardiac surgery. The child's thoughts and feelings during surgery and afterward are illustrated. The impact of cardiac disease and surgery on a child is stressed.

Source: Health Sciences Consortium

Discussion Questions

1. An important nursing care measure for the child with congestive heart failure is to protect the child from tiring easily. How would you do this with an infant? A school-age child?

2. Cardiac surgery is a strain for both parents and children because of its seriousness. What special measures would you take before surgery to prepare parents and children for this?

3. Kawasaki disease is an illness that most parents do not know exists. How would you explain this illness to parents? To a six-year-old child?

Written Assignments

1. All nurses should know cardiopulmonary resuscitation technique. List the steps you would take if you found a child with congestive heart failure not breathing.

2. Children with rheumatic fever, hypertension, and some congenital heart disorders need to take medication for years. What are methods to help parents remember to give medication? What are methods to help the children themselves remember?

3. Most parents are not aware of the existence of a ductus arteriosis. How would you explain the purpose and flow of blood in this structure during intrauterine life? How does this change after birth?

Laboratory Experiences

1. Assign students to observe in a cardiac catheterization laboratory for a day so they can better appreciate exactly what the procedure entails and so can better prepare children and parents for the experience.

2. Require that students complete a course in CPR before beginning clinical skills and to update these skills yearly. Assign them to teach the technique to parents of children with high risk status.

3. Assign students to observe in an intensive care unit so they can see the clinical appearance of children with heart disorders so they can develop an appreciation for the parents' concern about having a child with so serious a disorder.

Care Study

Heather is an 8-year-old brought to a pediatrician's office by her mother because of a sore knee.

Health History

- Chief Concern: "Her right knee is swollen; yesterday her left one was that way."

- History of Present Concern: Child has been listless and complaining of many small aches in her arms, stomach, and legs for the past week. Today her right knee is warm to touch, obviously swollen, and too sore for the child to walk on comfortably. Child cannot remember falling or bumping the knee. Her temperature yesterday was 100.2gF; today is 100.5gF. Child had sore throat 10 days ago; this resolved by itself with only warm salt gargles; child not seen by pediatrician; no antibiotic therapy prescribed.

- Family Profile: Parents are married; mother works as flight attendant part-time; is overnight in distant cities at least once a week. Father is a roofer; is receiving unemployment at present because weather is still too cold for seasonal construction work. Father is primary caregiver when mother is out of town. Finances described as "fair this time of year. Good as soon as construction season begins."

- Pregnancy History: Planned pregnancy. Mother developed urinary tract infection during pregnancy; was treated with penicillin for 10 days. Child was born by cesarean due to a breech presentation; spinal anesthesia used. Infant cried spontaneously; Apgars 8 and 9.

- Growth and Development: Child followed regularly by pediatrician; developmental milestones of infant and preschool periods all met. Child is in 3rd grade at present (age appropriate). Active in swimming club; has won medals for breast stroke and diving. Appetite: "no problem; eats everything."

- History of Past Illnesses: No major illnesses; no hospitalizations. Seen in emergency room once for falling from bicycle at age 6. Knocked out right upper deciduous central incisor. As tooth was not a permanent one, it was not replaced. Permanent tooth erupted at $6\frac{1}{2}$ years with no discoloration or malalignment.

- Family Medical History: Father and paternal grandfather both have hypertension. A 2-year-old cousin of Heather's (living in St. Louis) was identified as having lead poisoning.

- Review of Systems: HEENT: Received eye and ear exams in school during last year. Both reported as within normal limits. Has had about 2 colds a year since first year.

  Heart: No murmurs previously documented.

  Immunizations: Up to date.

Physical Examination

- General Appearance; Distressed-appearing thin 8-year-old, Caucasian female with reddened, swollen right knee. Temperature 100.6gF oral; pulse: 94/min; respirations: 20/min; blood pressure: 90/50.

- Head: Normocephalic; fontanelles closed.

- Eyes: Red reflex; follows to 6 positions of gaze. Lower conjunctivae appear pale.

- Ears: Normal alignment; TMs pink; landmarks discernible. Right canal slightly reddened; pain present on movement of pinna; no lateralization on Weber test.

- Nose: Midline septum; no discharge; mucus membrane pink.

- Mouth and Throat: Teeth in good alignment; mucous membrane pink and moist; no caries. No erythema in throat; gag reflex intact; midline uvula.

- Neck: Midline trachea; full range of motion; no pain on flexion; one "shotty" node in right posterior cervical chain.

- Lungs: Respiratory rate: 20/min; no adventitious sounds.

- Heart: PMI observed at 4th left intercostal interspace. Grade I blowing systolic murmur present; marked sinus arrhythmia.

- Abdomen: Macular rash with ill defined border present; bowel sounds heard in all 4 quadrants; no masses; both lower quadrants tender to palpation; liver palpated 1 cm below right subcostal margin.

- Genitalia: Normal female.

- Extremities: Two subcutaneous nodules, 1 cm in diameter, present by right elbow; nontender; non erythematous. One by right knee; tenderness of right elbow and left knee elicited on movement. Right knee is markedly swollen; warm to touch; very tender on flexion. Child walks with limp, favoring right leg.

- Neurologic: Patellar reflex: 2; **sensory and motor nerves grossly intact.**

Laboratory Results

- Erythrocyte sedimentation rate: 25/mm/hr.
- C-reactive protein: **3**
- ASO titer: 500 Todd u/mL{/UL}

Care Study Questions

1. Heather's parents vary their roles as primary caregiver. If Heather has a long-term illness, will this make enforcing medicine compliance difficult? What could you suggest to this family to help them with this?

2. Heather has been ill for a week but her mother didn't bring her for care because the signs were so subtle. If the illness turns out to be serious, this can make parents feel guilty that they weren't concerned earlier. How can you help parents when they feel this way?

3. Heather was diagnosed as having rheumatic fever. Complete a nursing care plan that would identify and meet Heather's needs.

Nursing Care of the Child With an Immune Disorder

Chapter 42 begins with a Nursing Process Overview describing nursing diagnoses and care pertinent to the care of the child with an immune disorder. Discussion also pertains to care of the child with an atopic disorder such as infantile dermatitis, eczema, and asthma, and of the child with a contact dermatitis and anaphylactic shock. The importance of parents and children taking active steps to reduce environmental exposure is stressed.

Students may not appreciate the seriousness of immune disorders if they have thought of these as "only allergies" in the past. They may need exposure to children with these disorders before they can appreciate how these disorders affect and can limit almost all aspects of children's lives.

Chapter Objectives

After mastering the contents of this chapter, students should be able to:

1. Describe the immune process as it relates to childhood illness.
2. Assess the child with a disorder of the immune system.
3. Formulate nursing diagnoses for the child with a disorder of the immune system.
4. Plan nursing care pertinent to the child with an immune system disorder such as teaching a parent ways to make a house environmentally safe for the child.
5. Implement nursing care related to the child with an immune disorder, for example, teaching breathing exercises to a child with asthma.
6. Evaluate outcome criteria to be certain that goals established for care of the child with an immune disorder have been achieved.
7. Identify national health goals related to immune disorders and children that nurses could be instrumental in in helping the nation achieve.

8. Identify areas related to care of the child with an immune disorder that could benefit from additional nursing research.
9. Use critical thinking to analyze ways that nursing care for the child with an immune disorder can be more family centered.
10. Synthesize knowledge of immune disorders and nursing process to achieve quality maternal child health nursing care.

Key Points

- An antigen is a foreign substance capable of stimulating an immune response. The immune system protects the body from invasion of foreign substances by leukocyte activity.

- Humoral immunity refers to immunity created by antibody production. B cells are involved in this type of reaction.

- Autoimmunity results from an inability to distinguish self from nonself, causing the immune system to carry out immune responses against normal cells.

- Immunodeficiency disorders can be primary, such as B-cell and T-cell deficiencies, or secondary, such as acquired immunodeficiency syndrome (AIDS). AIDS is spread by the retrovirus HIV through blood and body secretions. By following universal precautions, health care personnel can prevent the spread of this illness in the hospital setting.

- Allergic disorders occur as a result of an abnormal antigen—antibody response. About one in every five children suffer from some form of allergy.

- Immune disorders, as a category, are long-term disorders, and children must participate in their own care in order to remain well (avoiding allergens or avoiding a child at school with an infection, for example). Involving children from the start helps them achieve an active role in their own care.

- Anaphylactic shock is an acute reaction characterized by extreme vasodilation and circulatory shock. Know the procedure for care at your care site so you can act quickly to alleviate symptoms if it occurs.

- Environmental control refers to ways to reduce the number of allergens to which children are exposed. Hyposensitization is increasing the plasma concentration of IgG antibodies to prevent or block IgE antibody formation and allergic symptoms.

- Atopic disorders include hay fever (allergic rhinitis), atopic dermatitis, and asthma.
- Asthma is a diffuse obstructive disease of the airway. Parents of children with asthma need to be well informed about emergency measures to take during an acute attack. Review these measures with them at health assessments, particularly if they will be administering an injection, so they remain well prepared to act in an emergency. Nursing diagnoses commonly identified for children with asthma include ''Fear,'' ''Health-seeking behaviors,'' and ''High risk for ineffective airway clearance.''
- Promoting breast-feeding may be a prime intervention to help prevent allergies in allergy-prone families.

Definitions of Key Terms

allergen: a substance that can produce a hypersensitivity reaction

anaphylaxis: an unusual or exaggerated reaction of the body to foreign protein that could result in death

angioedema: temporary swelling of areas of the skin

antigen: a foreign body protein capable of evoking an antibody response

atopy: a hypersensitivity state

autoimmunity: an immune response to one's own tissues

B lymphocyte: the form of white blood cell responsible for producing antibodies

cell-mediated immunity: a delayed type IV hypersensitivity reaction initiated by T lymphocytes

chemotaxis: movement of an organism from a region of high to low (or low to high) concentration

complement: enzymatic serum proteins arising from an antigen—antibody reaction

contact dermatitis: skin inflammation related to irritation by an object touching the skin

cytotoxic response: a substance such as an antibody which has a specific harmful reaction against body cells

delayed hypersensitivity: cell-mediated immunity

hapten: a nonprotein substance that acts as an antigen by combining with particular bonding sites on an antibody

helper T cell: a type of white blood cell that stimulates B lymphocyte production

humoral immunity: immunity created by antibody production

hypersensitivity response: an immune response in which histamine is released

hypersensitization: the state of being sensitive to allergens

immune response: the body's ability to combat outside invading organisms by leukocyte activity

immunity: the state of being nonsusceptible to an organism

immunocompetent: capable of producing an effective immune response

immunogen: an antigen that produces an immune response

killer T cell: a specialized lymphocyte that is able to bind to the surface of an antigen and destroy it

lymphokines: a substance secreted by killer cells to prevent migration of antigens

lysis: dissolution

macrophage: a phagocytic cell

memory cell: a form of B lymphocyte that maintains the formula for producing antibodies

phagocytosis: killing of cells

plasma cell: a form of B lymphocyte that produces antibodies

specificity: the concept that antibodies destroy only like antigens

suppressor T cell: specialized T lymphocytes that reduce the production of immunoglobulins

T lymphocyte: a form of white blood cell involved in the immune response

tolerance: progressive diminution of response to the effects of a substance introduced into the body

urticaria: swelling and itching

vaccine: a substance composed of microorganisms administered to create immunity

Nursing Process Overview

The Nursing Process Overview in this chapter focuses on ways to improve assessment techniques in order to better detect the subtle ways that immune disorders can present and on formulating nursing diagnoses specific to care of the child with an immune disorder. The importance of including the entire family in care, especially in steps to reduce environmental exposure to allergies, is stressed.

Study Aids

Boxes

Box 42-1:   Emergency measures for anaphylactic shock

Focus on Nursing Care: Nursing actions for drugs used to treat allergy

Tables

Table 42-1: Location and function of immunoglobulins

Table 42-2: CDC classification system for HIV in children

Table 42-3: Classification of hypersensitivity reactions

Table 42-4: Common measures for environmental control of allergens

Table 42-5: Comparison of seborrheic dermatitis and infantile eczema

Displays

Focus on National Health Goals

Focus on Family Teaching

Focus on Nursing Research

Critical Thinking Exercises:

1. Jose is a 4-year-old who has a primary B-cell immune deficiency. His teacher calls you; she is afraid to have him in her classroom because he will spread the HIV

virus to classmates. What would you want to explain to Jose's teacher about immune deficiency disorders?

2. Ellen is a 10-year-old who has allergic rhinitis (hay fever). She notices symptoms most strongly in the late spring while in school. What environmental control measures would you suggest to her parents to improve her symptoms?

3. Samuel is a 12-year-old with asthma you care for in the emergency room. His mother states the first thing she did when Samuel became ill was to bring him to the hospital even though she had been taught to inject epinephrine possibly to prevent a hospital admission. Why do you think the mother reacted this way? What steps could you take to help the mother follow a specified emergency protocol next time?

Media Resources

Allergies: The Twentieth Century Disease (42-minute videocassette)

The types, causes, and treatment of allergies are presented through interviews with patients and physicians. Physical and psychologic responses that alter lifestyle are discussed. The controversy between medicinal therapy and environmental exposure is presented.

Source: Filmmakers Library

Allergy (22-minute filmstrip)

Antigen—antibody reactions in immunity and allergy are discussed. Typical allergic reactions and desensitization are explained, with an overview given of diagnostic tests, environmental allergy elimination, and prevention measures.

Source: Medical Electronic Educational Systems

The Terror of Anaphylaxis (14-minute slide/tape or videotransfer)

The clinical manifestations of an anaphylactic reaction and differences between laryngospasm and bronchospasm are presented. Treatment modalities and precautions that decrease the risk of a serious anaphylactic reaction are identified.

Source: University of Michigan

AIDS (28-minute videocassette)

The epidemiology and pathophysiology of AIDS including responsibilities for infection control and recommendations from the Centers for Disease Control are presented. The physical and emotional needs of patients with AIDS are described, and a comprehensive nursing diagnosis listing is included. Two adult patients with AIDS are interviewed.

Source: AJN Educational Services

AIDS (45-minute videocassette)

A dramatization of the fears and uncertainty that surround the diagnosis of a 16-year-old who has contracted the HIV virus through a blood transfusion. An immunologist explains the disease to the teenager's family, peers, and the community.

Source: Churchill Films

A Regular Kid (20-minute film)

Children who have asthma and their families are interviewed. Children discuss their coping methods and concerns related to having a chronic respiratory disease. A positive approach toward psychosocial adaptation to asthma is emphasized.

Source: American Lung Association

Superstuff (Self-help information package)

The package contains a record, poster, news magazine, book, and games designed to educate school-age children with asthma about their illness. Topics include learning to recognize physical and environmental "triggers" of an asthma attack, steps to take to prevent attacks, and ways to develop healthy lifestyles.

Source: American Lung Association

Discussion Questions

1. Children with asthma often respond well to environmental control. What specific steps should parents take to reduce environmental contaminants in their home?

2. Caring for a child with atopic dermatitis can be frustrating for parents because the child can be extremely irritable. What suggestions could you make to parents to help them find more satisfaction in caring for their child?

3. Caring for a child who is HIV positive requires strict adherence to universal precautions. What are these precautions?

Written Assignments

1. A reaction from a stinging insect bite calls for immediate action. List specific actions to take.

2. Contact dermatitis is seen less frequently in children than adults. What are some objects or plants that can cause this?

3. Therapy for a food allergy requires that a parent eliminate the offending food from a child's diet. How would you describe an elimination diet to a child's parent?

Laboratory Experiences

1. Assign students to a hospital unit where children with asthma are cared for so they can appreciate the stress such an illness creates for a family.

2. Assign students to an allergy clinic so they have an opportunity to view allergy testing and can better appreciate the role of this in therapy.

3. Ask a parent of a child with extensive allergies to come to a postconference and explain how the illness affects the entire family. How could health care providers have been more helpful to the family?

Care Study: An Adolescent With Atopic Dermatitis

Sarah Tustin is a 13-year-old brought to a dermatology clinic by her grandmother for scaling lesions on her elbows and knees.

Health History

- Chief Concern: "My skin looks like a snake's."
- History of Present Illness: Skin condition began with irritation on flexor surfaces at elbows and knees 4 months ago. At first it was only reddened; then it became scaly and extremely pruritic. Mother tried applying calamine lotion to areas without improvement. Child is not aware of any new foods eaten in the last 4 months or any other irritating factor. No such involvement has occurred in other family members.
- Family Profile: Child is oldest of three children (brothers are 10 and 7) of a single parent. Mother lives with grandmother in two-bedroom apartment. Family is supported by public assistance. Mother is currently attending school to become a bartender. Grandmother states that money has "always been a problem;" is hopeful that mother's new job will improve situation.
- History of Past Illnesses: Has had "hay fever" since first grade. Sneezes and develops stuffy nose around Christmas trees and goldenrod. Had rubella at 6 years; head injury at 8 years from fall from swing; seen in ER; no sequelae.
- Growth and Development: Child met infant and preschool developmental milestones. Is presently in 8th grade (age appropriate) but is not doing well with school work. Has been told that she will not be promoted to high school unless there is a definite improvement in her work. Child states that "itchiness" interferes with concentration.

  Has not menstruated as yet.
- Nutrition: Grandmother states child "eats junk food" in preference to table food.
- Family Medical History: Mother has sickle cell trait. Maternal grandmother has adult onset diabetes mellitus. Both mother and maternal grandmother are obese. Health of child's father is unknown.
- Review of Systems: Essentially negative but for chief concern.

  Eyes: Tested in school in January and rated adequate.

  Ears: Tested in school last fall and rated normal.
- Extremities: Lesions as described in Chief Concern.

Physical Examination

- General Appearance: Obese 13-year-old with obvious lesions on flexor surfaces of both arms. Height: 5'4". Weight: 170 lbs. Blood pressure: 120/60.
- Head: Normocephalic; scattered reddened papules on chin.
- Eyes: Red reflex present. Follows to all fields of gaze. Able to read small print without difficulty.
- Ears: TMs pink; landmarks present. Good alignment.
- Nose: Midline septum; mucous membrane swollen; clear nasal discharge.
- Mouth and Throat: Thirty teeth present; one cavity in left lower molar. Geographic tongue observed.
- Neck: Midline trachea; full range of motion present.
- Lungs: Occasional rhonchi in upper lobes; respiratory rate: 20/min.
- Heart: Rate 80/min. No murmurs.
- Abdomen: Soft; no masses. No tenderness on palpation.
- Genitalia: Normal preadolescent female. Tanner 2.
- Extremities: Area 35 on flexor surfaces of both arms and legs at elbows and knees covered by white scales on erythematous base. Linear abrasions apparently from scratching also present. Full range of motion in joints present.
- Neurologic: Patellar reflex 2. **Sensory and motor nerves grossly intact.**

Care Study Questions

1. Many children are referred to health care providers because of school behavior problems when they actually have a physical illness. Could this be happening to Sarah? Is this the first physical illness she has had that would interfere with school performance?
2. Skin conditions such as atopic dermatitis are often ignored by parents because their chief symptoms are pruritus, not anything life threatening. Are there psychologic consequences of having such a condition? Should these be considered as well?
3. Sarah was diagnosed as having atopic dermatitis. Complete a nursing care plan that would identify and meet her needs.

Nursing Care of the Child With an Infectious Disorder

*C*hapter 43 discusses nursing care of children with the common infectious disorders of childhood. The chapter begins with an overview of the nursing process specific to care of children with infectious disorders. Common microorganisms that cause disease in children, the principles of immunization, and guidelines for isolation are discussed. Common therapies such as comfort measures for a rash are included. Viral, bacterial, rickettsial, parasitic, helminthic, protozoal, and fungal infections are discussed. Since most childhood infectious disorders can be prevented, emphasis is placed on the nursing role in prevention of these illnesses. With many parents caring for these children at home, the nursing role is to educate parents to give safe care to the child with an infectious disorder.

Some parents take the importance of having their child immunized lightly, having never seen a child with a serious infectious disorder before. Some students may also. Students need to learn about the severe consequences that can result from these disorders to help them give better well-child care and become better health educators.

Chapter Objectives

After mastering the contents of this chapter, students should be able to:

1. Describe the causes and course of common infectious disorders of childhood.
2. Assess the child with an infection, such as the common exanthems.
3. Formulate nursing diagnoses related to infection in children.
4. Plan nursing care, such as how to relieve the discomfort of a rash, for the child with an infection.
5. Implement nursing care specific to the child with an infection (eg, administer an antibiotic intravenously).

6. Evaluate outcome criteria to be certain that nursing goals for care of the child with an infection have been achieved.
7. Identify national health goals related to infectious disorders and children that nurses could be instrumental in in helping the nation achieve.
8. Identify areas of nursing care related to children with infectious disease that could benefit from additional nursing research.
9. Use critical thinking to analyze ways that care of the child with an infection can be more family centered.
10. Synthesize knowledge of infectious diseases and nursing process to achieve quality maternal child health nursing care.

Key Points

- The incubation period of infectious disease is the time between the invasion of an organism and the onset of symptoms. A prodromal period is the time between the beginning of nonspecific symptoms and specific symptoms. Children are infectious during the prodromal period. Illness is the stage during which specific symptoms are evident. The convalescent period is the interval between the time symptoms begin to fade and return to full wellness.

- The chain of infection depends on the presence of a reservoir, a portal of exit, a means of transmission, a portal of entry, and a susceptible host.

- Immunization depends on the activation of the immune system. Both B-cell (humoral immunity) and T-cell (cellular immunity) are involved. Immunity may be **active** (the child has developed the disease or had antigens of the disease administered, or **passive** (antibodies against the disease are administered to the child by vaccines or placental transfer).

- Common viral infections of childhood are exanthem subitum (Roseola), rubella (German measles), measles (Rubeola), chickenpox (Varicella), herpes Zoster, erythema infectiosum (Fifth disease), pityriasis rosea, mumps (epidemic parotitis), infectious mononucleosis, and cat scratch disease. Other important viral infections are poliomyelitis (now almost extinct), herpesvirus infections, and verrucae (warts). Rabies continues to be a problem because of children's love of animals.

- Streptococcal diseases seen in children are scarlet fever and impetigo. Staphylococcal infections seen are furunculosis (boils), cellulitis, and scalded skin disease. Outbreaks of diphtheria, whooping cough (pertussis), and tetanus (lockjaw) still occur.

- Important rickettsial diseases seen are Rocky Mountain spotted fever and Lyme disease. Parasitic infections are pediculosis capitis (head lice), pediculosis pubis, and scabies. Helminthic infections are roundworm, hookworm, and pinworm. Fungal infections are tinea capitis and tinea corporis (ringworm).

- Teach parents and children that keeping immunizations up to date is the best protection against childhood communicable diseases.

- Teach children that careful handwashing and limiting the number of items shared in school can limit the spread of many childhood infections.

- Before a horse-based serum is administered, sensitivity testing must be done to rule out the possibility of antiphylactic shock.{/BL}

Definitions of Key Terms

anaerobic: able to grow and function without oxygen

antitoxin: the antibody to the toxin of an antigen

chain of infection: the interrelated steps that allow infection to result

communicability: the ability to be transmitted from one person to another

complement: a protein released from an antigen—antibody reaction

convalescent period: time span until recovery from an illness is complete

enanthem: a rash on the mucous membrane

exanthem: a rash present on the skin

fomites: nonliving materials (eg, combs) that spread infection

gamma globulin: antibodies

immune serum: a solution of plasma that contains those antibodies normally present in adult human blood

incubation period: time span from invasion of an organism until symptoms occur

interferon: a protein formed when cells are exposed to a virus that prohibits the growth of viruses

Koplik's spots: peculiar blue-and-white-centered red spots that occur on the mucous membrane in children with measles

means of transmission: the ways that communicable diseases can be spread

pathogen: any microorganism capable of producing disease

portal of entry: site at which an infectious organism enters a body

portal of exit: site at which an infectious organism leaves a body

prodromal period: expectant period, or the period during which a disease is infectious before clinical symptoms appear

reservoir: a container in which organisms grow

septicemia: infection of the blood

susceptible host: a person vulnerable to contracting a disease

toxoid: a solution of toxins that still stimulates the formation of antitoxins

Nursing Process Overview

The Nursing Process Overview in this chapter concentrates on helping the student plan care for situations in which he or she will serve as a health educator to teach parents more than the actual health care provider. The importance of promoting immunization to help eliminate childhood infectious diseases is stressed. The importance of evaluation following an infection to be certain that a long-term health problem such as hearing loss has not occurred is included.

Study Aids

Boxes

Box 43-1:   Misconceptions concerning contraindications to vaccination

Box 43-2:   Tips for avoiding exposure to Lyme disease

Tables

Table 43-1: Methods by which infections spread

Table 43-2: Types and functions of white blood cells (leukocytes)

Table 43-3: Schedule for the routine immunization of healthy infants and children (based on the recommendations of the American Academy of Pediatrics and the CDCP)

Table 43-4: Universal precautions to prevent infection

Displays

Focus on National Health Goals

Focus on Family Teaching

Focus on Nursing Research

Focus on Cultural Awareness

Critical Thinking Exercises:

1. Norman is a 2 year old who is found to have pediculosis on a routine health exam. His mother tells you she can't believe the diagnosis because she thought only poor children developed head lice. She is also very concerned that her son will have to have his head shaved to cure him. How would you advise her?

2. Mrs. Torrance tells you that she does not intend to have her newborn immunized because she feels the risk of developing a complication from vaccine administration is higher than letting her child contract simple childhood diseases. How would you counsel her?

3. Mrs. Bernicki's daughter developed chickenpox after attending a birthday party. She asks you why parents don't have common sense enough to keep an ill child at home so infectious diseases aren't spread this way? Is controlling infectious disease this simple? Can Mrs. Bernicki be certain her daughter didn't spread the disease to another before her disease became obvious?

Media Resources

Skin Rashes in Infants and Children (Programmed Instruction with Color Prints)

This series of photographs of various rashes is designed to assist the nurse in recognizing the most common and more serious conditions involving skin rashes in infants and children. Evaluation and nursing care strategies are given for each condition identified.

> Source: American Journal of Nursing Company

Recognizing Common Communicable Diseases (slides)

Illustrations of common communicable diseases of children such as measles, rubella, chickenpox, and scarlet fever. A program guide provides objectives, a glossary, and learning activities.

> Source: University of Minnesota

Common Neonatal Viral Infections (28-minute videocassette)

The causes, characteristics, transmission, sequelae, and management of herpes simplex, rubella, and cytomegalovirus infections in neonates are discussed.

> Source: Health Sciences Consortium

Controlling Transmission of Infection (28-minute videocassette)

The chain of infection transmission and an overview of nosocomial infection are presented. Category-specific and disease-specific Centers for Disease Control isolation precautions are identified.

> Source: AJN Educational Services

Lice are Not Nice. (11-minute film)

A program designed to teach the symptoms of head lice. Both home and school environments are used to acquaint children with the problem.

> Source: AIMS Media

Communicable Diseases (35-minute videocassette)

The physical findings of the common communicable diseases of childhood are explained and illustrated.

> Source: Wayne State University, College of Medicine

Discussion Questions

1. Pediculosis capitis is a common infection among school-age children. What measures should children take to prevent the spread of this in classrooms?

2. Children can easily become lonesome in isolation rooms. Think of two games to play with each age group of children that require no special materials and thus could be used in isolation?

3. Measles is most common in the college-age population. What symptoms would you assess for if a roommate of yours developed a rash?

Written Assignments

1. Rashes cause extreme distress in children because of pruritus. What are measures to reduce the discomfort of a rash?

2. Lyme disease is a newly identified disorder. List the common manifestations of this and prevention measures parents and children should take to prevent the spread of the disease.

3. Impetigo is a misunderstood disorder in children. Describe the cause, appearance, and therapy.

Laboratory Experiences

1. Assign students to attend a well-child conference to foster awareness of the importance of immunization.

2. Assign students to observe at a day-care center for the precautions taken to prevent the spread of infections, such as washing toys after use and cleaning a diaper changing area.

3. Assign students to spend a day with a hospital infection control officer to increase their awareness of the importance of nosocomial infections and the measures nurses can take to reduce the risk of this.

Care Study: An Adolescent With Infectious Mononucleosis

Lee Sukioto is a 14-year-old who comes to the school health office complaining of a sore throat.

Health History

- Chief Concern: "I feel like I'm swallowing broken glass my throat is so sore."

- History of Present Concern: Child began feeling "listless" a week ago and noticed a pink macular rash on arms and trunk. Developed a sore throat 4 days ago. Didn't take temperature but thinks it has been elevated. Temperature is 101.8gF orally now.

- Family Profile: Child is youngest of three children (a brother, 24; a sister, 18). Child lives with parents in a lakeside condominium. Parents own a doughnut franchise; Lee works at the counter most evenings after school; attends dance class every Monday evening.

- Growth and Development: Lee is a sophomore in high school (class is age appropriate); taking a college entrance curriculum. Currently dating a high school senior. Admits to being sexually active; takes prescribed birth control pill daily. Has taken dance lessons since age 4; active in drama club; starred in spring musical at school.

- Nutrition: Eats a vegetarian diet along with parents.

- Family Medical History: Aunt with breast cancer; cousin who is HIV positive from receiving a transfusion.

- Review of Systems: Essentially negative but for chief concern.

- Genitourinary: menarche at 11 years; menstrual cycle 28 days; menses for 5 days. Does self-breast examination following menses.

Physical Examination

- General Appearance: Well proportioned, listless-appearing 14-year-old female holding hand over anterior throat. Weight: 112 lbs. Height: 5'5". Blood pressure: 120/72.

- Head: Normocephalic; hair is full and well bodied; no tenderness over sinuses.

- Eyes: Red reflex present; follows to all fields of vision; slightly reddened conjunctivae.

- Nose: Midline septum; no discharge.

- Ears: TMs pink; landmarks present; moderate amount of cerumen in both canals. Hearing is equal to examiners.

- Mouth: Teeth in good alignment; 2 repaired cavities; none at present.

- Throat: Bright red, tonsillar tissue swollen; white pus present in crypts. Mucous membrane dry. Filmy exudate covering posterior throat.

- Neck: Midline trachea; thyroid not enlarged; two palpable submaxillary lymph nodes on right side. No pain on forward flexion.

- Chest: Lungs: coarse rhonchi in both upper lobes. Respiratory rate 20/min.

- Heart: Rate 80/min; no murmurs.

- Abdomen: Spleen palpable 3 cms under left costal margin; bowel sounds present in all quadrants; no masses. Scattered pink macular rash evident on abdomen.

- Back: Spine is in good alignment; no tenderness over vertebrae.

- Genitalia: Deferred.

- Extremities: No inflammation of joints; full ROM. A fading ecchymotic area (yellow/brown) 21 cm present over left tibia.

- Neurologic: DTRs 2; Kernig's sign negative. Babinski negative. Sensory and motor function grossly intact.

Care Study Questions

1. Lee was diagnosed as having infectious mononucleosis. Her family depends on her to watch her younger sibling after school. She is also active in school affairs and maintains good school marks. In light of this, what would a long period of bed rest mean to Lee?

2. Lee asks you how soon she can return to dance class. What factors would you weigh to make this judgment?

3. Complete a nursing care plan that would identify and meet Lee's needs.

Nursing Care of the Child With a Blood Disorder

Chapter 44 discusses care of the child with a disorder of the bone marrow or blood cells. The chapter begins with a Nursing Process Overview stressing assessment techniques for these disorders and suggestions for nursing diagnoses that speak to the long-term care involved with these processes. Disorders of the red blood cells such as iron-deficiency anemia, megaloblastic anemia, and hemolytic anemias such as thalassemia and sickle-cell disease are included. Disorders of the white cells such as neutrophilia and disorders of blood coagulation such as the purpuras, and hemophilia are also discussed.

Students may need to review the formation and function of blood cells, particularly the schema of blood coagulation, before they can grasp the importance of these disorders to life functions and the potential impact they have on growth and development.

Key Points

- Bone marrow transplant is therapy for a number of blood dyscrasias. Nursing diagnoses commonly identified in relation to this are ''Anxiety'' and ''High risk for altered growth and development and infection.''

- Disorders of the red blood cells that commonly occur in children are acute blood-loss anemia and anemia of acute infection. Aplastic and hypoplastic anemias occur from depression of hematopoietic activity in bone marrow. This can be congenital or acquired. Nursing diagnoses related to this are ''High risk for infection,''''Altered self-esteem,'' and ''Fluid volume deficit.''

- A major hypochromic anemia that develops in children is iron-deficiency anemia. The major nursing diagnosis associated with this is altered nutrition.

- Macrocytic anemias are from folic acid deficiency and pernicious anemia (vitamin B_{12} deficiency).

- Hemolytic anemias consist of congenital spherocytosis, glucose-6-dehydrogenase deficiency, sickle-cell ane-

mia, thalassemia, and autoimmune acquired hemolytic anemia. Sickle-cell anemia occurs most prominently in black children. Nursing diagnoses related to this are ''High risk for ineffective tissue perfusion'' and ''Altered health maintenance.''

- Disorders of white blood cells that occur are neutropenia and neutrophilia (reduced number of white blood cells). Both of these conditions make children susceptible to infection. Reverse isolation may be instituted to guard against infection. Health care personnel and family members with infections should be restricted access.

- Disorders of blood coagulation include the purpuras (idiopathic thrombocytopenic purpura, Henoch-Schönlein syndrome, disseminated intravascular coagulation, and the hemophilias. Nursing diagnoses identified with the hemophilias are ''Pain related to joint infiltration'' and ''Altered family processes related to the long-term nature of the illness.''

- Children with blood coagulation disorders must be guarded carefully against injury. This includes monitoring types of toys and activities. It may include padding crib or siderails.

- Children with anemia invariably fatigue easily because they are unable to oxygenate body cells well. Their care must include measures to keep them from tiring; oxygen administration may be necessary.

- Disorders of the blood tend to be long-term illnesses. Education of the parents and of the child is important so they can learn to adapt to the condition; long-term administration of medication needs planning so it is consistently maintained.

Definitions of Key Terms

agranulocyte: a white blood cell that does not contain cytoplasmic granules such as a monocyte

allogeneic transplantation: the grafting of tissue taken from the body of one person to another

aplastic anemia: a deficiency of blood components related to ineffective bone marrow production.

autologous transplantation: grafting of tissue from one part of the body to the other

bilirubin: a breakdown product from the destruction of red blood cells. It is unconjugated or insoluble and toxic to body cells until it is conjugated and made soluble to water by the liver

blood dyscrasias: abnormal or pathologic conditions of the blood

blood plasma: the liquid portion of the blood

erythroblast: an immature red blood cell

erythrocyte: a red blood cell

granulocyte: a white blood cell that contains cytoplasmic granules such as a neutrophil

hemochromatosis: excess iron deposits in the body that have caused tissue destruction

hemoglobin: the iron-containing portion of red blood cells responsible for the transportation of oxygen to body cells. Expressed in mg/100 mL.

hemosiderosis: excess deposits of iron in the body without tissue damage

leukocyte: a white blood cell

leukopenia: a decrease in the number of white blood cells

megakaryocyte: an immature platelet

normoblast: an immature red blood cell

pancytopenia: deficiency of all cell elements of the blood

petechiae: pinpoint nonraised, purplish spots on the skin caused by intradermal or submucosal hemorrhage

polycythemia: an excess of red blood cells

purpura: confluent small blood spots under the skin

reticulocyte: immature red blood cells

sickle cell crisis: an acute, episodic condition occurring with children with sickle cell anemia in which red blood cells cluster and cause circulatory obstruction and anoxia to tissue

sickle cell trait: the heterozygous form of sickle cell anemia; both hemoglobin S and hemoglobin A are present in red blood cells

synergeneic transplantation: the grafting of tissue from a genetically identical individual to another genetically identical individual

thrombocyte: a platelet

thrombocytopenia: deficiency of platelets{/GL}

Nursing Process Overview

The Nursing Process Overview in this chapter focuses on identifying ways to detect the illnesses which interfere with cell oxygenation or blood coagulation. Nursing diagnoses selected as examples speak to long-term care and family-centered concern, since these diseases concern the child for a lifetime and effect the entire family functioning. The role of the nurse as a member of a genetic counseling team is included.

Study Aids

Boxes

Box 44-1:   Blood coagulation factors

Focus on Nursing Care: Meathods to Reduce Bleeding with a Diminished Platelet Count

Tables

Table 44-1:   Tests for blood coagulation

Table 44-2:   Common blood transfusion reaction symptoms

Table 44-3   Effects of thalassemia

Displays

Focus on National Health Goals

Focus on Family Teaching

Focus on Nursing Research

Focus on Cultural Awareness

Critical Thinking Exercises:

1. Maria is a 12-year-old with sickle-cell anemia. You have noticed that every summer for the past five years while Maria has been home from school on summer vacation, she has had an acute episode of her illness. What assessments would you want to make of Maria's family before this summer? What precautions would you want to discuss with them?

2. Hillary is a 6-year-old who has developed neutrophilia from chemotherapy. What precautions to prevent infection would you want to encourage her family to take while Hillary attends a family reunion?

3. Kevin is a 3-year-old with hemophilia. He wants to join a preschool soccer program. How would you counsel his family regarding this?

Media Resources

Matter of Chance (28-minute videocassette)

The work of a hospital-based counseling program for people at risk for sickle cell anemia is shown. Genetic transmission of the disease and differentiation of sickle cell trait from sickle cell anemia are explained.

Source: National Audiovisual Center

Joey (18-minute film)

The etiology, mode of genetic transmission, types, diagnosis, and therapy for hemophilia are discussed. The film describes home care of the child with hemophilia including costs, criteria for participation in a home care program, and training needed.

Source: National Hemophilia Foundation

Heredity and Hemophilia (12-minute slide/audiocassette)

Harold, a boy with hemophilia, is presented in cartoon form discussing how he inherited hemophilia. Genetic principles involved, the implications of having hemophilia, and a positive view of living with a long-term disorder are presented. This program could be used as a teaching aid with preschool and school-age children.

Source: Cutter Biological Laboratories

Inside a Bleeding Joint (12-minute slide/audiocassette)

The underlying mechanisms of hemophilia are presented in cartoon form. A detailed look is given to joint changes and the need for immediate factor replacement infusion.

Source: Cutter Biological Laboratories

Home Infusion Techniques for Hemophiliacs (20-minute slide/audiocassette)

A step-by-step guide to administering antihemophilic agents in the home. It outlines necessary equipment, venipuncture technique, storage and transporting of the factor, disposing of syringes and needles, and record keeping.

Source: Abbott Scientific Products Division

Discussion Questions

1. Iron deficiency anemia is the major nutritional illness in the United States. What is its most common cause? How can it be prevented?

2. Many people confuse the terms sickle cell trait and sickle cell disease. How would you define them to a 12-year-old?

3. Having an illness of the blood-forming process often requires a child to undergo many painful procedures. What are ways you can minimize the number of these or help a child to accept them?

Written Assignments

1. Children with hemophilia need extra precautions taken in order to remain safe from hemorrhage into joints during childhood. What special precautions would you advise a parent to take to "childproof" a home for a child with hemophilia?

2. Children grow bored easily while receiving blood transfusions. List activities that would be appropriate to reserve for these times so the time becomes one that fosters development?

3. Children with sickle cell anemia need to avoid situations in which they will experience anoxia. What are common situations that parents should work to avoid happening to their child?

Laboratory Assignments

1. Assign students to hospital units where children with anemias are admitted for care so students can have experience with the interventions commonly used for the child with sickle cell crisis or iron-deficiency anemia.

2. Assign students to an ambulatory clinic where children with anemias are seen for follow-up care to help students better appreciate how these illnesses affect family as well as individual functioning.

3. Ask a parent of a child with sickle cell anemia or thalassemia to come to a postconference and discuss the family changes that have been necessary because of a long-term illness. How could health care personnel be more helpful to them?

Care Study: A Child With Hemophilia

Brian Winston is an 18-month-old with hemophilia. He is seen in the emergency room following a fall from a 2-foot-high wall at a shopping mall.

Health History

- Chief Concern: "He fell and his nose is bleeding and his knee is swelling."

- History of Present Concern: Brian was diagnosed as having hemophilia at birth because of history of disease in family. Mother has VIII factor replacement at home and is knowledgeable in how to administer it. Today, she only applied a cold compress to nose and knee and brought child directly to emergency room as this was closer than going home. Child's nose is still bleeding after 20 minutes; knee has discolored to a purplish blue and is swollen to twice the size of opposite knee. No loss of consciousness after injury.

- Family Profile: Family intact. Father, age 24, works as a parole officer. Mother, age 23, is homemaker while she is attending evening classes to become an accountant. Family lives in upstairs apartment over father's parents. Finances are rated as "doing all right."

- Pregnancy History: Pregnancy planned following loss of first pregnancy because of incompetent cervix. Sirodkar sutures placed at 14 weeks; removed at pregnancy term. Child born by vertex vaginal birth; no excessive bruising noticed at birth. Apgars: "good."

- Growth and Development: Child met infant developmental milestones: sat at 8 months; walked at 14 months. Speaks many words; mother not certain he actually forms noun—verb combinations yet.

- Family Medical History: Mother's brother has hemophilia; age is 24; attending college; has had little difficulty with illness. An uncle of mother's died of disease of cerebral hemorrhage at age 12.

  Paternal grandfather: left leg amputated for injury in World War II; ambulatory with prosthesis. Maternal grandmother: alcoholism and liver and esophageal varices.

- Past Medical History: Infant not circumcised at birth because of history of disease in family. Hospitalized at 6 months for bleeding on hand that would not stop after mother clipped fingernail too short. Child fell at 9, 12, and 14 months while learning to walk; factor replacement administered each time at home with no apparent long-term effect. No hospitalizations; no other major illnesses or childhood communicable diseases

- Review of Systems: Eyes: Eyes crossed frequently at birth; were straight without therapy by 3 months; no eye infections.

  Ears: Hearing never formally tested but mother feels it is adequate. No ear infections.

- Overall Health: Good. Child eats at table with parents; no special foods prepared for him.

Physical Examination

- General Appearance: Crying 18-month-old male with a bleeding nose and swollen, discolored left knee. Weight: 23.5 lbs. Height: 32 inches. Blood pressure: 80/50.

- Head: Normocephalic; posterior fontanelle closed; anterior fontanelle still palpable; Head circumference: 47 cms.

- Eyes: Red reflexes present bilaterally; child refused to follow light to test extraocular muscles; eyes in straight alignment by Hirschberg test.

- Ears: TMs: pink, landmarks prominent. Child responds to whispered word.

- Nose: Midline septum; point in left nares actively bleeding; bleeding does not halt in response to normal pressure.

- Mouth and Throat: 18 teeth; no caries. Midline uvula; no erythema.

- Neck: Full range of motion; no palpable lymph nodes; midline trachea.

- Chest: Lungs clear to auscultation and percussion; no adventitious sounds. Respiratory rate: 24/min (crying).

- Heart: Rate 110/min; no murmurs.

- Abdomen: Bowel sounds heard in all 4 quadrants; no masses; not tender to touch.

- Genitalia: Normal male; testes descended bilaterally; uncircumcised.

- Extremities: Full range of motion in all but left knee; child has limited motion in knee from pain and swelling; knee increased in size to twice that of opposite knee; has discolored to purple and is warm to touch.

- Neurologic: Child is aware of surroundings; answers to name. Reflexes not tested to avoid pressure near joints.

Care Study Questions

1. Mark had three separate incidences of bleeding while he was learning to walk. Does this seem excessive or normal? Are there steps you think his parents could have taken to reduce these accidents?

2. Mark has one relative who died young because of his illness and another who has little apparent involvement. How do you anticipate this history could influence his feelings about himself or his future plans?

3. Complete a nursing care plan that would identify and meet the needs of Mark and his family.

Nursing Care of the Child With a Disorder of the Gastrointestinal System

Chapter 45 discusses care of the child with a gastrointestinal disorder. The chapter begins with a Nursing Process Overview that provides suggestions on ways to modify care for the child when a disorder results in an interference with nutrition. Congenital disorders such as pyloric stenosis and Hirschsprung's disease as well as acquired disorders such as celiac disease, Crohn's disease, and vitamin deficiencies are discussed. Liver diseases such as hepatitis and cirrhosis and the nursing responsibility for care of the child following liver transplant are included.

The necessity of including the entire family in care when a nutritional problem is present is stressed. Before caring for a child with gastrointestinal disorders, students need to review basic nutrition information as well as anatomy and physiology of the gastrointestinal tract. This is an opportunity for students to learn the role of the nutritionist in health care and the need for nurses to collaborate with other health care providers in order for health planning to be optimum.

Chapter Objectives

After mastering the content of this chapter, students should be able to:

1. Describe common gastrointestinal disorders in children, such as appendicitis and pyloric stenosis and symptoms of disorders, such as vomiting and diarrhea.

2. Assess the child with a gastrointestinal disorder.

3. Formulate nursing diagnoses for the child with a gastrointestinal disorder.

4. Plan nursing care with specific goals for the child with a gastrointestinal disorder (eg, a plan that teaches parents about a special diet).

5. Implement nursing care for the child with a gastrointestinal disorder, such as administering a gastrostomy feeding.

6. Evaluate outcome criteria to ensure that goals of nursing care were achieved.

7. Identify national health goals related to gastrointestinal disorders and children that nurses could be instrumental in in helping the nation to achieve.

8. Identify areas of care related to gastrointestinal disorders and children that could benefit from additional nursing research.

9. Analyze ways that nursing care of the child with a gastrointestinal disorder can be more family centered.

10. Synthesize knowledge of gastrointestinal disorders with nursing process to achieve quality maternal child health nursing care.

Key Points

- Remember that children lose proportionately more fluid with vomiting and diarrhea than adults. For this reason, they need rapid assessment and interventions to avoid dehydration.

- Both fluid and electrolyte imbalances tend to occur rapidly with vomiting and diarrhea. Vomiting leads to alkalosis. Diarrhea leads to acidosis. Nursing diagnoses associated with diarrhea are ''High risk for fluid volume deficit,''''Altered skin integrity,'' and ''Anxiety.''

- Gastrointestinal disorders almost always interfere with nutrition at least to some degree. This is a greater problem in children than adults, since children need to take in enough nutrients and fluid daily for growth as well as body maintenance.

- Chalasia (gastroesophageal reflux) is a neuromuscular disturbance in which the cardiac sphincter is lax, which allows for easy regurgitation of gastric contents into the esophagus. It is treated by feeding a thickened formula and positioning the infant prone with head elevated.

- Pyloric stenosis is hypertrophy of the valve between the stomach and duodenum. It impedes the passage of feedings and leads to vomiting. Nursing diagnoses associated with this are ''High risk for fluid volume deficit'' and ''Infection.''

- Peptic ulcer may occur in even young children. This is a shallow excavation formed in the mucosal wall of the stomach. It is treated like adult ulcers, with medications to suppress gastric acidity.

- Hepatic disorders seen in children are hepatitis A (caused usually by eating contaminated shellfish) and hepatitis B (caused by contaminated blood or placental spread). Nursing diagnoses associated with these disorders are "High risk for infection transmission" and "Altered comfort."

- Congenital obstruction of the bile ducts occurs from failure of the bile duct to recanalize in utero. Cirrhosis is fibrotic scarring of the liver that occurs as a result of congenital biliary atresia. Most of these children need a liver transplant to restore liver function.

- Intussusception is the invagination of one portion of the intestine into another. Nursing diagnoses identified for this are "High risk for pain," "Fluid volume deficit," and "Altered parenting."

- Necrotizing enterocolitis is the development of necrotic patches on the intestine. It occurs almost exclusively in immature infants.

- Appendicitis is inflammation of the appendix. It is always an emergency situation and is the most common cause of abdominal surgery in children. Therapy is surgery to remove the appendix before it ruptures. Nursing diagnoses identified for this are "Pain," "Fear," and "High risk for fluid volume deficit."

- Celiac disease (gluten-induced enteropathy) is a change in the ability of the intestinal villi to absorb. It is apparently a dominantly inherited illness. Nursing diagnoses identified are "Altered family processes" and "Altered nutrition."

- A number of hernias can occur in children such as inguinal and hiatal hernia. These are surgically corrected when recognized.

- Hirschsprung's disease (aganglionic megacolon) is absence of ganglionic innervation in a section of the lower bowel. The therapy is possibly a temporary colostomy followed by surgery. Nursing diagnoses identified for this are "Altered bowel elimination," "Altered nutrition," and "High risk for ineffective family coping."

- Inflammatory bowel disease can occur as either ulcerative colitis or Crohn's disease. Children may have portions of their bowel removed to relieve these conditions.

- Kwashiorkor (protein deficiency), nutritional marasmus (starvation), and vitamin A, D (rickets), B₁ (beriberi), and C (scurvy) deficiencies occur in children when they are not provided with or cannot absorb adequate nutrients. Although associated with developing countries, these disorders can occur in a child in any community.

- Encourage children with nutrient disorders to join the family for mealtime if possible. Even if they cannot eat the same foods as other family members they benefit from the social interaction.

- Some gastrointestinal disorders lead to long-term therapies such as colostomy or gastrostomy feedings. Because these disorders interfere with common body functions, such as eating and elimination, they are difficult for children to accept without the support of concerned health care providers.{/BL}

Definitions of Key Terms

aganglionic megacolon: the congenital absence of nerve innervation of a portion of the large bowel

appendicitis: inflammation of the appendix

beriberi: polyneuritis caused by the deficiency of vitamin B₁ (thiamine)

celiac disease: a condition marked by malabsorption of the small bowel related to the intake of gluten

chalasia: relaxation of the cardiac sphincter leading to regurgitation

dehydration: Excessive loss of fluid from body tissues

hepatitis: inflammation of the liver

hiatal hernia: projection of the stomach into the chest through the diaphragm

hypertonic dehydration: excessive loss of fluid from body tissues in which a greater proportion of fluid than electrolytes are lost

hypotonic dehydration: excessive loss of fluid from body tissues in which a greater proportion of electrolytes than fluid is lost

inguinal hernia: projection of intestine into the inguinal canal

intussusception: prolapse of a portion of intestine into an adjacent portion

irritable bowel syndrome: inflammation of the bowel marked by diarrhea and pain

isotonic dehydration: an excessive loss of fluid from body tissues in which fluid and electrolytes are lost in proportion

keratomalacia: ulceration of the cornea resulting from vitamin A deficiency

kwashiorkor: a malnutrition syndrome caused by protein deficiency

liver transplantation: grafting of the liver from one individual to another

Meckel's diverticulum: outpouching of the ilium related to yolk sack retention

metabolic acidosis: excessive acid in the body resulting from a digestive or metabolic concern

metabolic alkalosis: decreased acid or increased bicarbonate in the body resulting from a digestive or metabolic concern

necrotizing enterocolitis: death of intestinal tissue related to ischemia of the bowel

nutritional marasmus: progressive wasting and emaciation from inadequate dietary intake

overhydration: excessive fluid in body tissue

pellagra: inflammation, weakness, and disability related to deficiency of niacin

peptic ulcer: an ulceration of the stomach or duodenum

pyloric stenosis: stricture of the valve between the stomach and duodenum

rickets: deficiency of vitamin D which leads to distortion of bones

steatorrhea: fat in stools

ulcerative colitis: inflammation of the bowel with shallow necrotic lesions

volvulus: a twisting of the intestine

xerophthalmia: a deficiency of vitamin A resulting in reduction of eye fluid and diminished sight

Nursing Process Overview

The Nursing Process Overview in this chapter focuses on helping the student identify signs and symptoms of gastrointestinal illnesses and formulating nursing diagnoses that include the entire family in order to reduce stress on the family. Making plans that can be sensibly maintained long-term is encouraged. Continuing evaluation is important to be certain that nutrition guidelines are being followed.

Study Aids

Tables

Table 45-1: Maintenance requirements of fluid based on caloric expenditure

Table 45-2: Signs of dehydration in children

Table 45-3: Maintenance requirements of sodium, chloride, and potassium for intravenous therapy in children

Table 45-4: Comparison of metabolic alkalosis and metabolic acidosis

Table 45-5: Differentiation between regurgitation and vomiting

Table 45-6: Liver function tests

Table 45-7: Gluten-restricted diet

Table 45-8: Minimum-residue diet

Displays

Focus on National Health Goals

Focus on Family Teaching

Focus on Nursing Research

Focus on Cultural Awareness

Critical Thinking Questions:

1. Anne is an 8-month-old girl admitted to the hospital with severe diarrhea. What emergency interventions does Anne need to prevent an electrolyte or fluid imbalance? What measures could you take to reduce her fear of the strange hospital environment?

2. John is a 12-year-old with Crohn's disease. He is being cared for at home with parenteral alimentation. How can you help John keep pace with his friends at school? How can yo help him maintain a sense of high self-esteem in the light of many hospitalizations and home care?

3. Pamula is a 4-year-old who is being transferred to a distant city to have a liver transplant because of congenital biliary atresia. Her parents ask you what they can expect at the distant hospital. How would you prepare them for this?

Media Resources

Care of the Patient with an "Ostomy" (30-minute slide-tape program)

The major types of ostomies such as ileal conduit, ileostomy, and colostomy are discussed and illustrated. The physiologic reasons for the creation of each type of diversion and the type of care required are explained.

Source: Communications in Learning, Inc.

Pediatric Enema Administration (35-minute filmstrip and audiocassette)

The techniques and precautions to follow when administering an enema to an infant or child are presented. A study guide is included.

Source: J.B. Lippincott

Living With Inflammatory Bowel Disease (15-minute videocassette)

Crohn's disease and ulcerative colitis are described, along with available treatments and ways to cope with problems. Interviews with adolescents describing their experiences and coping strategies are included. The tape is designed to assist adolescents with the disorders to understand and manage their disease in a healthy way.

Source: National Foundation for Ileitis and Colitis, Inc.

Scott Duchess, a Twelve-Year-Old Boy with Appendicitis (CAI)

A case study of a child with appendicitis is presented. The computer program discusses all aspects of nursing care for a child who requires abdominal surgery and can be used for self-instruction.

Source: J.B. Lippincott

Preparing a Child for Appendectomy (filmstrip and audiocassette)

Postoperative teaching techniques for a child who has undergone emergency appendectomy. The use of teaching tools to describe anatomy and physiology, procedures, wound appearance, and postoperative care is described.

Source: Campus Films

Discussion Questions

1. Gastrointestinal anomalies in newborns often require surgery early in life. What are ways you can help parent—child bonding despite this early surgery?

2. The frequency of both ulcerative colitis and Crohn's disease is rising in children. Many of these children have a colostomy or ileostomy performed. How would you help an adolescent accept this?

3. Many children are admitted to a hospital for an emergency appendectomy. What emergency steps should you take to make this a safe admission?

Written Assignments

1. Parents may have a difficult time understanding why it is dangerous to use tap water as an enema solution with infants. Write a paragraph explaining why water intoxication occurs. How would parents make a normal saline solution at home?

2. Trying to avoid the use of wheat, oats, and rye grains in cooking can be difficult. Make out a day's menu including your favorite foods. Inspect it for grains. List how many foods would be contraindicated in a celiac child's diet. How would you modify your meal plan to eliminate these grains?

3. Children who cannot digest fat cannot digest fat-soluble vitamins. What are these vitamins and what is the effect of deficiencies in a diet?

Laboratory Experiences

1. Assign students to a client care service where children with gastrointestinal disorders are admitted for care. Ask students to focus their assessment on discovering the effect a nutritional disorder in one member of a family has on the entire family.

2. Ask a parent whose child was diagnosed as having Hirschsprung's disease and who had a colostomy performed to come to a postconference and discuss how difficult or easy the parent found caring for an infant with a colostomy. How could health care providers have been more helpful?

3. Many parents are unsure how serious diarrhea is in an infant. Assign students to create a teaching display at a parent's class on the importance of parents notifying a health care provider at the first sign of diarrhea in an infant.

Care Study: An Infant With Pyloric Stenosis

Jack Weintraub is a 6-week-old infant brought to the hospital emergency room by his father.

Health History

- Chief Concern: "He throws up after every feeding."

- History of Chief Concern: Child was breast fed until 1 week ago when he was changed to formula (Carnation with iron, 4 oz, 6 times per day) when his mother was hospitalized. Almost immediately, child began vomiting at least half of each feeding. Vomitus is sour but no mucus or blood is present. Vomiting was projectile this pm. Father thinks child has lost weight; stools are yellow and formed.

- Family Profile: Parents are married. Family lives in a 2-bedroom apartment. Mother was admitted to hospital 1 week ago for multiple trauma from automobile accident. Father is having difficulty caring for infant and working and visiting wife in hospital. Admits to "feeding in a hurry" to "get it over with" so he can take child to babysitters. Finances are "about to be ruined" because of hospital bills.

- History of Past Illnesses: No major illnesses. No hospitalizations. Child had skin tag in front of left ear removed by ligation at 1 week of age; no sequelae. An IVP done at birth was normal. Child was seated in infant seat a week ago when mother's car was struck by a taxi cab. Infant was seen in the emergency room and discharged as uninjured. Weight at visit: 4.5 kg.

- Pregnancy History: Pregnancy was planned. Mother was diagnosed as having placenta previa at 20 weeks by sonogram; this persisted throughout pregnancy so infant was delivered by cesarean birth. Apgars 7 and 9; breathed spontaneously.

- Growth and Development: Social smile: 6 weeks; lifts up head when on abdomen.

- Family Medical History: Paternal grandmother: Raynaud's disease. Maternal aunt: diabetes mellitus.

- Review of Systems: Negative except for chief concern.

Physical Examination

- General Appearance: Rangy-appearing, crying, 6-week-old male. Weight: 4.0 kg. Height: 57 cm.

- Head: Normocephalic. Anterior fontanelle palpated at 33 cm, slightly sunken. Posterior: barely palpable.

- Eyes: Red reflex present; child follows right and left; not past midline.

- Ears: Normal alignment. TMs pink; landmarks identified; no cerumen. Attunes to examiner's voice.

- Nose: Midline septum; no discharge; mucous membrane pink; nares patent.

- Mouth and Throat: No teeth; mucous membrane dry; hard and soft palate intact; gag reflex present.

- Neck: Full range of motion; no palpable lymph nodes.

- Chest: Lungs: Respiratory rate: 22/min. Clear to percussion and auscultation.

- Heart: Rate 132/min; no murmurs.

- Abdomen: Skin turgor poor; rapid bowel sounds all quadrants. Liver and spleen both palpable 1 cm below costal margins. Palpable olive-sized mass in right epigastric region; when fed a bottle of glucose water, visible peristaltic waves left to right were visible on abdomen. Child vomited feeding with force.

- Genitalia: Circumcised male; testes descended; midline meatus.

- Extremities: Full range of motion; skin turgor on thighs poor.
- Back: Midline vertebrae; no tufts or dimples on spinal column.
- Neurologic: Moro, sucking, parachute, step-in-place tested and intact; Babinski flaring.

Care Study Questions

1. This infant had an intravenous pylogram done at birth. What was the associated finding which was the basis for this?

2. Jack was seen in the emergency room a week ago and weighed 4.5 kg. Today he weighs 4.0 kg. What is the percent of his weight loss?

3. Jack was diagnosed as having pyloric stenosis. Complete a nursing care plan that would identify and meet his needs.

Nursing Care of the Child With a Disorder of the Kidneys or Urinary Tract

Chapter 46 discusses care of the child with a urinary or renal disease. The chapter begins with a nursing process overview to help students improve their assessment and select nursing diagnoses specific to children with these disorders. Discussion is focused on care of the child with congenital disorders such as hypospadias and ureteral reflux as well as acquired disorders such as urinary tract infection, glomerulonephritis, and the nephrotic syndrome. The nurse's role in caring for the child on hemodialysis, peritoneal dialysis, and post—kidney transplant is included.

Many of the concepts gained from care of the adult client with a renal or urinary tract illness apply to care of the child with these disorders. Students need to review basic anatomy and physiology in order to help them adapt care when their client has a smaller urinary system than an adult's that is more prone to infection.

Chapter Objectives

After mastering the contents of this chapter, students should be able to:

1. Describe common renal and urinary disorders that occur in children, such as urinary tract infection (UTI), nephrosis, and glomerulonephritis.
2. Assess a child for a renal or urinary tract disorder.
3. Formulate nursing diagnoses related to a renal or urinary disorder.
4. Plan nursing care related to urinary or renal disorders, such as teaching about the importance of perineal hygiene to prevent infection.

5. Implement nursing care for the child with a renal or urinary disorder, such as assisting a child with glucose or protein urine analysis.
6. Evaluate outcome criteria to ensure that nursing goals have been achieved.
7. Identify national health goals related to renal or urinary tract disorders and children that nurses can be instrumental in in helping the nation achieve.
8. Identify areas related to care of the child with a renal or urinary disorder that would benefit from additional nursing research.
9. Use critical thinking to analyze methods for making nursing care of the child with a renal or urinary disorder more family centered.
10. Synthesize knowledge of renal and urinary disorders with nursing process to achieve quality maternal and child health nursing care.

Key Points

- Many urinary tract disorders such as cystic kidneys, urethral obstruction, and bladder exstrophy are evident on fetal sonogram. Early identification in this way allows therapy to begin immediately at birth.
- Many urinary tract disorders such as infection or chronic renal insufficiency are long-term conditions requiring years of therapy. Be certain that parents are well informed about the child's condition so they can continue to participate in planning the child's care.
- Diminished kidney function leads to both fluid and electrolyte imbalances. Creative techniques are necessary to encourage children to continue to ingest a high protein diet to counteract protein losses in urine.
- Congenital structural abnormalities of the urinary tract are patent urachus, exstrophy of the bladder, hypospadias, and epispadias. Surgical correction is required for all of these.
- Urinary tract infections tend to occur more often in girls than boys. ''Honeymoon cystitis'' refers to a UTI occurring with first sexual relations.
- Vesicoureteral reflex is the backflow of urine into ureters with voiding. It occurs because the valve that guards the entrance to the ureters is defective. Surgical correction may be necessary to prevent repeated urinary tract infection.
- Renal dysfunction can occur from structural reasons such as kidney agenesis, polycystic kidney, and renal

hypoplasia. Acute poststreptococcal glomerulonephritis is inflammation of the glomeruli following a streptococcus infection. It is characterized by an acute episode of hematuria and proteinuria.

- Nephrotic syndrome is a immunologic process that results in altered glomeruli permeability. Nursing diagnoses associated with this are "Altered nutrition," "High risk for altered skin integrity," and "Knowledge deficit."

- Renal insufficiency can occur in an acute or chronic form. Peritoneal dialysis or hemodialysis may be used to remove body waste until kidney function can be restored.

- Kidney transplantation may be a therapy option for some children with kidney disorders. This is extensive surgery and requires the child to remain on immunosuppressive therapy to counteract transplant rejection.

Definitions of Key Terms

acute transplant rejection: an immediate reaction that occurs after organ transplantation indicating rejection

Alport's syndrome: a progressive chronic nephritis inherited as an autosomal dominant disorder

azotemia: excessive accumulation of nitrogen wastes in the bloodstream

dialysis: the removal of body waste products through the use of a semipermeable membrane

enuresis: involuntary discharge of urine

exstrophy of the bladder: a congenital disorder in which the bladder is exposed on the anterior surface of the abdomen

glomerular filtration rate: the rate at which body wastes are excreted by the kidney

glomerulonephritis: inflammation of the glomeruli of the kidney

hydronephrosis: distention of the pelvis of the kidney with urine as a result of obstruction of the ureter

hypospadias: opening of the urethra on the ventral surface of the penis

patent urachus: an open connection between the bladder and umbilical cord

polycystic kidney: a condition in which normal kidney tissue is displaced by fluid-filled cysts

postural proteinuria: protein in urine present on standing in an upright posture

prune belly syndrome: a congenital disorder marked by kidney involvement and a flaccid abdominal wall

vesicoureteral reflux: back flow of urine from the bladder into the ureters on voiding{/GL}

Nursing Process Overview

The Nursing Process Overview in this chapter concentrates on suggestions for helping the student assess urinary tract and renal disease and to select nursing diagnoses that reflect a family focus, since many urinary system disorders become long term and so involve the entire family.

Study Aids

Boxes

Focus on Nursing Care: Medications frequently prescribed with urinary or renal disorders

Tables

Table 46-1: Kidney functions

Table 46-2: Average urine output in a 24-hour period in children

Table 46-3: Normal urine analysis findings

Table 46-4: Comparison of features of acute glomerulonephritis and the nephrotic syndrome

Table 46-5: Foods high in potassium

Table 46-6: Possible complications of CAPD

Displays

Focus on National Health Goals

Focus on Family Teaching

Focus on Nursing Research

Focus on Cultural Awareness

Critical Thinking Exercises:

1. Mary is a 12-year-old who is admitted to your hospital unit because of her third urinary tract infection this year. Her mother asks you if there is anything she should be doing to help prevent these. How would you answer her?

2. Charlie is a child with end stage renal disease awaiting a kidney transplant. He tells you he hopes he has been good enough to deserve being chosen for the next kidney available. What would you want to teach Charlie about the transplant selection process?

3. Beth is 6-year-old who has continuous ambulatory peritoneal dialysis. She wants to go to her church camp this summer. Her parents ask you if this would be a good experience for Beth. What factors would you want to know about the camp? About Beth? About her procedure?

Media Resources

Obtaining a Clean-Catch Urine Specimen (9-minute videocassette)

The appropriate methods for collecting urine specimens from male and female clients are shown. The various types of equipment necessary and a step-by-step demonstration of the procedure are included.

Source: Health Sciences Consortium

A Life Without Kidneys, A Second Chance at Living (15-minute film)

A nephrologist and a 12-year-old dialysis patient share their experiences.

Source: NAPHT, Inc.

Dialysis: an Overview (14-minute slide/audiocassette)

The principles and techniques of hemodialysis and peritoneal dialysis are illustrated. Discussion includes the nurse's role in the care of the client on dialysis.

Source: Trainex Corporation

New Concepts in Urinary Tract Infections (15-minute film)

The diagnosis and treatment of urinary tract infections.

Source: Vacumate Corporation

Preparing a Child for Renal Transplant (filmstrip with audiocassette)

A child's reactions to preoperative teaching for a renal transplant. A discussion of kidney anatomy and physiology is given along with dramatic play techniques and psychologic reactions associated with hemodialysis, transplant, and post-operative body image changes.

Source: Campus Films

End Stage Renal Disease (15-minute slides/audiocassette)

Living with kidney disease, renal failure, peritoneal dialysis, hemodialysis, and kidney transplant is discussed. The disease processes and treatment procedures for renal disease are described. Patient interviews describe feelings and coping responses.

Source: Health Sciences Consortium

Teaching a Child About Nephrosis (Filmstrip with audiocassette)

The use of body outlines and hospital equipment can help to teach children about nephrosis, diagnostic tests, and management of the disease. A scenario of a child who has not been prepared for hospitalization and refuses to cooperate with procedures is dramatized to emphasize the importance of preparation.

Source: Campus Films

Patients Who Need Help with Urinary Elimination (CAI)

Patient situations that require nursing strategies for assistance with urinary function are presented. These include adults with chronic glomerulonephritis, cystitis, and renal colic, as well as a care study of a 6-year-old girl with nephrosis.

Source: J.B. Lippincott Company

Discussion Questions

1. Dana is a child in chronic renal failure. How does such a disease affect a family? Or a child's feelings about herself?

2. Caring for a child with nephrotic syndrome is complicated because the child has extensive edema. What special measures should you teach the parents concerning this?

3. Hypospadias can interfere with body image in early life and fertility in later life. How would you prepare a 3-year-old for surgery?

Written Assignments

1. Parents may not be familiar with the process of osmosis and so be unable to quickly understand the process of peritoneal dialysis. Write a paragraph detailing how you would explain this to a parent.

2. Parents may have difficulty keeping a child on limited protein diets with end-stage renal disease. Write out a typical day's diet that would fit a low protein criteria you think a child might enjoy.

3. Nocturnal enuresis can become a family problem. List methods parents can use to help a child achieve night-time bladder control.

Laboratory Experiences

1. Assign students to a clinical area where children with renal or urinary tract disorders are cared for so they can learn appreciation for the concern these disorders cause the entire family, not just the individual child.

2. Allow students to perfect urine testing by making sets of "urines" that test positive for various substances. Tea serves as the base; add Karo syrup for glucose; gelatin powder for protein; vinegar to produce ketones.

3. Assign students to observe for a day at a hemodialysis center or with a home care nurse who cares for clients on ambulatory peritoneal dialysis so they can better understand these therapies.

Care Study: A School-Age Child With Nephrotic Syndrome

Lynda Maggio is a six-year-old admitted to the hospital with a diagnosis of nephrotic syndrome.

Health History

- Chief Concern: "Her kidneys aren't working right."

- History of Present Concern: Child began "gaining weight" a week ago and becoming irritable. Yesterday, her face appeared "very puffy." Urine was tested at pediatrician's office and found to be 4 **for protein.**

- Family Profile: Child has four older siblings (all brothers) ages 16, 15, 11, and 8. Family intact and lives in a private home. Father is a brick layer for a construction company; mother is homemaker. Finances are rated as "tight but okay."

- Pregnancy: Planned pregnancy; mother fell at fifth month during pregnancy and fractured wrist; x-rays were taken of wrist and mother was concerned during pregnancy that she had hurt the baby. Vertex, vaginal delivery under epidural anesthesia. Breathed spontaneously; discharged with mother at 2 days postbirth.

- Growth and Development: Child met infant and pre-school developmental milestones. Currently attending first grade (age appropriate). Enjoys school; doing well although tends to be "shy" in large crowds. Plays softball (T-ball) in city league.

- Past Medical History: No childhood infectious diseases. Bitten on hand by neighborhood dog 1 year ago; no rabies vaccine given as dog was observed and found not rabid. Circular scar still present on child's hand.

- Family Medical History: Both parents overweight; both paternal and maternal grandmothers overweight. Paternal grandfather died of cerebral vascular accident 2 years ago.
- Review of Systems: Neuropsychiatric: Tends to be "shy" in crowds. No seizures.

  Eyes and Ears: Hearing and vision tested in school during last year; both normal.

  Gastrointestinal: Has always had a tendency to be overweight.

  Extremities: Scar present on hand from dog bite.

Physical Examination

- General Appearance: Obese-appearing 6-year-old in no apparent distress. Weight: 30 kg. Height: 115 cm. Blood pressure: 115/60.
- Head: Normocephalic. Hair: good quality; facial edema marked.
- Ears: Red reflexes present; follows to all fields of vision; conjunctivae not inflamed.
- Ears: TMs pink; good movement on pneumoscopy; brown cerumen in left canal. Child identified sound of watch ticking bilaterally.
- Nose: Midline septum; nares patent; no discharge; mucous membrane pink.
- Mouth and Throat: Both central upper incisors missing; no cavities. First year molars erupted. Midline uvula; no erythema of throat or tonsils.

- Neck: Midline trachea; no palpable lymph nodes.
- Lungs: respiratory rate: 22/min. No adventitious sounds.
- Heart: 100/min. Grade II systolic murmur heard in left recumbent position.
- Abdomen: protuberant; no masses; bowel sounds present in all four quadrants. Fluid level percussed.
- Genitalia: Normal female; Tanner 1. Vulva edematous and reddened.
- Extremities: Full range of motion present. Regular gait. Marked dependent edema (4 over tibia) present.
- Neurologic: Patellar and brachial reflexes 2. **Sensory and motor function grossly intact.**

Laboratory Findings

- Urinalysis: 4 protein, many casts.

Care Study Questions

1. Lynda appears to have severe involvement and yet her parents have just brought her in for care. Why do you think this happened?

2. Nephrotic syndrome causes severe edma; the therapy (prednisone) can cause a "cushingoid" syndrome or an overweight appearance. Lynda is already reported to be shy. How will these disease symptoms affect her? Are there measures that could be taken to help her?

3. Complete a nursing care plan that would identify and meet Lynda's needs.

Nursing Care of the Child With a Reproductive Disorder

Chapter 47 discusses the care of the child with both a congenital reproductive disorder such as ambiguous genitalia, cryptorchidism, or hypospadias and acquired disorders such as delayed or precocious puberty, testicular cancer, menstrual and breast disorders, and sexually transmitted diseases. Educating children about reproductive illnesses so they can play a part in prevention is stressed.

Students may not be aware of the number of reproductive disorders that can occur in children. They need to review reproducitve system anatomy and the potential of children to develop with either male or female body organs to understand such disorders as ambiguous genitalia.

Chapter Objectives

After mastering the contents of this chapter, students should be able to:

1. Describe common reproductive disorders in children.
2. Assess the child with a reproductive disorder.
3. Formulate nursing diagnoses related to a child's reproductive illness.
4. Plan nursing care related to preventing reproductive disorders in children, such as teaching about ways to avoid vaginal infections.
5. Implement nursing care for the child with a reproductive disorder, such as caring for the child with undescended testes.
6. Evaluate outcome criteria to be certain that nursing goals have been accomplished.
7. Identify national health goals related to reproductive disorders and children that nurses can be instrumental in in helping the nation to achieve.
8. Identify areas related to care of children with reproductive disorders that could benefit from additional nursing research.
9. Use critical thinking to analyze ways that nursing care for the child with a reproductive disorder can be more family centered.
10. Synthesize knowledge of reproductive disorders in children with the nursing process to achieve quality maternal and child health nursing care.

Key Points

- The cause of ambiguous genitalia is unknown but may be related to the level of testosterone produced in utero. The true sex of children is established by a sex chromatin test (Barr body determination) or a karyotype of chromosomes.

- Precocious puberty is the development of breast or pubic hair before age 8 years. Girls may be treated with a synthetic analogue to luteinizing hormone-releasing hormone to reduce development. Such children are at high risk for body image disturbance without effective support.

- Delayed puberty is the failure to develop secondary sex characteristics by age 17. Girls may be administered estrogen to promote development.

- Balanoposthitis (inflammation of the glans and prepuce) and phimosis (constricted foreskin) are conditions seen in boys. Phimosis can be treated with circumcision.

- Cryptorchidism is failure of one or both testes to descend during intrauterine life. The condition is surgically corrected to prevent malignancy development later in life.

- Testicular cancer is a rare malignancy but tends to occur in young adults. Boys need to be taught self-testicular examination for early detection.

- Dysmenorrhea is a menstrual disorder which occurs frequently in adolescent girls. Therapy for this is a prostaglandin inhibitor such as ibuprofen.

- Endometriosis (the abnormal growth of extrauterine endometrial tissue) can lead to infertility later in life if not treated. Therapy is administration of danazol or a synthetic androgen, or surgery to reduce the size of the abnormal tissue.

- Children whose mothers took diethylstilbestrol (DES) while the child was in utero may be susceptible to adenitis or vaginal cancer if girls; cystic testes if boys.

They need follow-up by health care personnel to detect these disorders.

- Vulvovaginitis (inflammation of the vulva) or pelvic inflammatory disease are infections that can occur in adolescents. These need therapy to prevent scarring of fallopian tubes and infertility later in life.

- Breast disorders such as fibrocystic breast disease can occur as early as adolescence. Adolescent girls need to learn self-breast examination to detect abnormalities that could mean breast cancer.

- Sexually transmitted diseases such as candidiasis, trichomoniasis, Chlamydia trachomatis, genital warts, herpes genitalis, gonorrhea, and syphilis are increasing in incidence in the adolescent population. An important health teaching area with children is the need to follow safe sex practices. Girls need to be taught, in addition, ways to avoid toxic shock syndrome (TSS).

- STDs do not confer immunity and so can be contracted more than once. Also, protection against pregnancy such as an oral contraceptive does not offer protection against STDs.

- Children who are born with a reproductive tract disorder frequently adjust well when young. They may need counseling at puberty or when they become aware of the impact of their disorder on their ability to reproduce.

Definitions of Key Terms

adenocarcinoma: a malignant epithelial cell tumor of a gland

adenosis: a disease of a gland

amenorrhea: absence of menstrual flow

anovulatory: without ovulation

colposcopy: an examination utilizing a colposcope

cryptorchidism: undescended testes

dysmenorrhea: painful menstruation

endometriosis: abnormal implantation sites of endometrial cells outside the uterus

fibrocystic breast disease: benign fluid-filled cysts of the breast

gynecomastia: excess development of male breast tissue; a transient occurrence in normal adolescence

hermaphrodite: an individual with both testes and ovaries

hydrocele: a collection of fluid in the sac surrounding a testis

menorrhagia: an excessively profuse menstrual flow

metrorrhagia: vaginal bleeding between normal menstrual cycles

mittelschmerz: pain in the middle of a menstrual cycle

orchiectomy: excision of one or both testes

orchiopexy: surgical fixation of an undescended testis into the scrotum

pelvic inflammatory disease: the inflammation of the internal female reproductive organs

premenstrual syndrome: a cluster of symptoms such as irritability and headache experienced prior to menstrual flow

pseudohermaphrodite: an individual with the external features of both sexes

sexually transmitted disease: an illness spread by sexual relations

toxic shock syndrome: infection occurring during the menstrual flow from organisms entering through the vagina

varicocele: dilation of a blood vessel of the spermatic cord

vulvovaginitis: inflammation of the external female reproductive organs

Nursing Process Overview

The Nursing Process Overview in this chapter concentrates on assessing adolescents for sexually transmitted diseases and assisting with a first pelvic examination in girls. Related nursing diagnoses stress the importance of maintaining self-esteem. The importance of educating children about reproductive disorders is stressed.

Study Aids

Boxes

Box 47-1:   Gynecologic history questions

Box 47-2:   Symptoms of TSS

Box 47-2:   Methods to reduce the risk of TSS

Tables

Table 47-1:   Common vulvovaginitis infections

Table 47-2:   Comfort measures for vulvitis

Displays

Focus on National Health Goals

Focus on Family Teaching

Focus on Nursing Research

Focus on Cultural Awareness

Critical Care Questions:

1. Ralph is a 16-year-old who tells you he is sexually active but is not practicing safe sex practices because he does not believe with only sporadic sexual relations, he will contact a disease. Is Ralph being realistic? Are the measures you would want to discuss with Ralph?

2. Chris is a 15-year-old who has no breast development and also has not menstruated as yet. She asks you if it is time to worry. how would you counsel her?

3. Timothy is a 12-year-old who was born with undescended testes. He had surgery for this at 2 years. He is concerned now that he is high risk for testicular cancer. How would you counsel him regarding this?

Media Resources

Venereal Disease: The Hidden Epidemic (27-minute film)

The epidemic of sexually transmitted diseases from a variety of perspectives is presented. The history of syphilis and gonorrhea, changing attitudes toward these diseases, and evolution of treatment are reviewed. Prevention is stressed.

Source: Encyclopedia Britannica Education

Half a Million Teenagers (20-minute film)

Syphilis and gonorrhea are discussed, including the symptoms, methods of transmission, problems resulting from nontreatment, methods of diagnosis, importance of follow-up, and the need for informing sexual contacts. A situation of an adolescent who contracts an STD is portrayed.

Source: Churchill Films

Then One Year (14-minute videocassette)

The physiologic changes in the reproductive systems of both boys and girls are explained. Social and emotional adjustments to puberty are discussed.

Source: Churchill Films

Discussion Questions

1. Educating adolescents helps to prevent the spread of sexually transmitted diseases. What signs and symptoms of these diseases would you teach adolescents to observe for?

2. Surgery for cryptoorchidism has the potential to be a traumatic procedure for children. What special precautions would you take to make it less so?

3. Fibrocystic breast disease causes concern for women because it causes palpable lumps in breasts. What steps should a girl with fibrocystic breast disease take on discovering a new lump in her breast?

Written Assignments

1. Many high school girls have some degree of dysmenorrhea. What are practical steps a girl should take to relieve this discomfort?

2. Ask students to explore what sex education program is offered by the local school system. Have them write a paragraph describing whether they think this is adequate preparation or not.

3. Testicular cancer in males and breast cancer in females are cancers that can be discovered early by self-examination. Describe the steps for self-breast examination; self-testicular examination.

Laboratory Assignments

1. Assign students to an ambulatory setting which cares for adolescents. Ask them to survey adolescents as to their knowledge of sexually transmitted diseases and how many of them are practicing safe sex.

2. Assign students to observe circumcisions in a newborn setting. Ask them to evaluate whether parents were fully informed as to the risks and benefits of this procedure.

3. Assign students to experience in a college health service. Ask them to initiate a program on prevention of sexually transmitted diseases.

Care Study: A Preschooler With Hypospadias

Peter Kalulopidus is a 3½-year-old admitted to the hospital for 1-day surgery for hypospadias.

Health History

- Chief Concern: "He's having his penis fixed."

- History of Present Concern: Peter was born with midshaft hypospadias with chordee. Has had no urinary tract infections. Has had IVP showing normal kidneys and ureters. Is not circumcised. Has been prepared for surgery by mother.

- Family Profile: Family intact. Father, 19 years old, is an Army motor pool technician stationed in Saudi Arabia. Has been absent from family for 8 months. Mother works as a clerk in a downtown department store. Mother describes finances as "okay" because both sets of grandparents help out. Family lives in 2-bedroom base housing unit. Child attends day-care center on base.

- Pregnancy History: Pregnancy was not planned but not undesired. Parents were married as soon as pregnancy was confirmed. No complications during pregnancy; no rashes or falls. Mother drank a few beers early in pregnancy before she realized she was pregnant; no recreational or prescription drugs during pregnancy. Vaginal vertex birth; weight 8 lb, 6 oz. Apgars: "High." Hypospadias was diagnosed in birthing room.

- Growth and Development: Child met infant and preschool milestones. Sat at 8 months; walked at 11 months. Spoke in sentences at 2 years; toilet trained at 3 years. Currently attends day care 5 days a week 8 to 5 pm. Adjusted to experience readily. Feeds self and puts on most of own clothing.

- Past Medical History: No major illnesses. Seen regularly by Army base clinic. Received immunizations there.

- Family Medical History: No other children with congenital anomalies in family. Paternal grandfather has COPD (was a heavy cigarette smoker). Father has persistent acne. Mother had Crohn's disease from 13 to 18 years.

- Review of Systems: Ears: Otitis media at 12 months; treated with antibiotic with no recurrence.
  Eyes: Never formally tested but mother feels sight is good.
  Genitourinary: No UTIs, no circumcision. IVP at birth normal; no difficulty with toilet training.

Physical Examination

- General Appearance: Relaxed-appearing, well-proportioned 3½-year-old white male. Weight: 14 kg. Height: 95 cm. Blood pressure: 100/60.

- Head: Normocephalic; fontanelles closed.

- Eyes: Red reflexes present; PERLA. Extraocular muscles intact.

- Ears: Normal alignment. TMs pink. Landmarks evident. Hearing is equal to examiners.

- Nose: Midline septum; no discharge.
- Mouth and Throat: 20 deciduous teeth; no cavities. Midline uvula; mucous membrane moist; no erythema.
- Neck: Midline trachea; full range of motion.
- Lungs: Clear to auscultation and percussion; rate: 24/min.
- Heart: Rate 88/min; no accessory sounds. PMI: third left intercostal space.
- Abdomen: Soft; not tender to touch; no masses. Liver palpable 1 cm under right costal margin.
- Genitalia: Testes descended bilaterally; urinary meatus present at mid shaft on ventral surface of penis; no erythema at meatus. Chordee producing marked curve in penis shaft noted.

- Extremities: Full range of motion; normal gait.
- Neurologic: Patellar reflexes 2 bilaterally. Oriented to place and name.

Care Study Questions

1. Peter is at an age when fear of mutilation is at a peak. What are the implications of this when preparing him for surgery?

2. Mrs. Kalulopidus asks you why this could have happened to her son? Did she have unusual risk factors? Is there any reason to think this birth defect occurred other than by chance?

3. Complete a nursing care plan that would identify and meet the needs of the Kalulopidus family.

Nursing Care of the Child With an Endocrine Disorder

Chapter 48 discusses the care of children with a common endocrine disorder. The chapter begins with a review of nursing process and the modifications necessary, because these are long-term disorders. Hypo- and hyper-dysfunctions of thyroid, pituitary, and adrenal glands, and hypodysfunction of the pancreas and parathyroid glands are discussed. The potential for prenatal diagnosis for many of these disorders is included. The need for long-term supervision and the effect this can have on families are stressed.

In order to understand endocrine disorders, students must call on knowledge gained from anatomy and physiology courses so they can appreciate the effects of negative feedback. Reviewing this information can be tedious and delays the ability of students to plan care until it is reviewed.

Chapter Objectives

After mastering the contents of this chapter, students should be able to:

1. Describe the different endocrine glands and their functions.
2. Assess a child with a disorder of endocrine function.
3. Formulate nursing diagnoses for the child with altered endocrine function.
4. Plan nursing care for the child with altered endocrine function, such as planning health teaching for the child with hypopituitary dysfunction.
5. Implement nursing care for the child with endocrine dysfunction, such as teaching insulin administration to the child with diabetes mellitus.
6. Evaluate outcome criteria established to be certain that goals of nursing care were achieved.

7. Identify national health goals related to endocrine disorders and children that nurses could be instrumental in in helping the nation achieve.
8. Identify areas related to care of children with endocrine disorders that could benefit from additional nursing research.
9. Use critical thinking to analyze ways that care of the child with altered endocrine function can be family centered.
10. Synthesize knowledge of endocrine dysfunction and nursing process to ensure quality maternal and child health nursing care.

Key Points

- Hypopituitary dwarfism results in children who are short in stature. Therapy for children is the injection of human growth hormone. Children can experience altered self-esteem if they don't receive adequate emotional support from significant others.

- Other pituitary disorders are pituitary gigantism and diabetes insipidus. With gigantism there is overproduction of growth hormone. With diabetes insipidus there is decreased release of adrenal hormone. Urine becomes dilute and large amounts are excreted. Therapy is administration of desmopressin (DDAVP), which is an arginine vasopressin. Children with this are at high risk for fluid volume deficit.

- Congenital hypothyroidism occurs as a result of an absent or nonfunctioning thyroid gland. The condition is discovered by a blood test at birth. The therapy is oral administration of synthetic thyroid hormone.

- Thyroiditis (Hashimoto's disease) is an autoimmune phenomenon that interferes with thyroid gland production. Therapy is administration of synthetic thyroid hormone.

- Acute adrenal cortical insufficiency can occur in children from causes such as overwhelming infection in which there is hemorrhage destruction of the adrenal gland. A more common disease in children is congenital adrenal hyperplasia. This is inherited as a autosomal recessive trait. Girls are born masculinized; either sex may be unable to retain sodium, resulting in rapid fluid loss. Therapy is administration of corticosteroids. Without therapy, children are prone to altered self-esteem and high risk for fluid volume deficit.

- Cushing's syndrome is overproduction of cortisol by the adrenal gland. This usually results from a tumor in the gland. Children appear abnormally obese. Therapy is surgical removal of the tumor.

- The most frequently seen pancreatic disorder is type I diabetes mellitus. This may be an autoimmune process in which there has been destruction of insulin producing islet cells. Therapy is administration of insulin. Nursing diagnoses associated with this are ''Health-seeking behaviors,''''High risk for parental anxiety,'' and ''Altered nutrition.''

- Hypocalcemia, a parathyroid gland disorder, results in lowered blood calcium. Children develop tetany. Therapy is the administration of calcium.

- Endocrine disorders are almost all long-term disorders. Helping parents and children remember to take medicine on a long-term basis is an important nursing responsibility.

- Children with endocrine disorders often develop height or weight discrepancies. Help children continue to feel high self-esteem by concentrating on those things they are able to do despite growth lag, not those they cannot do.

- Children with endocrine disorders are often identified first through routine height and weight measurements. Weighing babies at birth may detect the salt-losing form of adrenal genital syndrome. That makes this measurement one of the most important ones that nurses make. Weight loss is often an early sign of diabetes mellitus in children and may be identified first by a nurse at a pediatric clinic or office. School nurses may be the first to discover hypopituitary growth problems through yearly school assessments.

Definitions of Key Terms

carpal spasm: a convulsion or twitching of the wrist

exophthalmos: a marked protrusion of the eyeballs

glycosuria: the presence of glucose in the urine

hormones: a chemical substance possessing a regulatory effect

hyperfunction: excessive function

hypofunction: lessened function

hypoglycemia: less than normal level of glucose in blood

hypothalamus: the tissue of the floor of the third ventricle which exerts control over visceral activities, water balance, temperature, and sleep

ketoacidosis: acidosis accompanied by ketones in the body

latent tetany: neuromuscular irritability as a result of a lowered calcium level

manifest tetany: twitching of the muscles as a result of a lowered calcium level

pedal spasm: convulsion or twitching of the foot

polydipsia: excessive thirst

polyuria: excessive urine production

sella turcica: the depression of the sphenoid bone which contains the pituitary gland

Somogyi phenomenon: the situation in which a child with diabetes mellitus needs less insulin but has symptoms suggesting insulin lack

Nursing Process Overview

The Nursing Process Overview in this chapter concentrates on helping students plan care for children with long-term illnesses. Formulating nursing diagnoses and planning nursing interventions that include the entire family are stressed.

Study Aids

Boxes

Box 48-1:   Teaching points for long-term medicine administration{/UL}

Tables

Table 48-1:   Comparison of type I and type II diabetes

Table 48-2:   Acceptable target blood glucose levels for young children

Table 48-3:   Common types of insulin

Table 48-4:   Comparison of hypoglycemia and hyperglycemia symptoms

Table 48-5:   Assessment for hypocalcemia

Displays

Focus on National Health Goals

Focus on Family Teaching

Focus on Nursing Research

Focus on Cultural Awareness

Critical Thinking Exercises:

1. Lea is a 12-year-old girl with hypopituitary dwarfism. She is only three foot high at present and probably will achieve a final growth of not over 4 foot 6 inches. Her parents tell you they find her ''''cute'' so do not want her to receive growth hormone. How would you approach this family? How much should Lea be able to contribute to this decision?

2. Caroline is a newborn diagnosed as having salt-dumping adrenogenital syndrome. What would be the most important measure to teach her parents before Caroline is discharged from the hospital?

3. Shawn is a 16-year-old who has been diagnosed as having diabetes mellitus since he was seven. You have been following him in an ambulatory clinic. You notice that although he was in good control for years, over the last 6 months, he has ''forgotten'' to take his insulin at least once a week. Since he obtained his driver's license, he has been eating many meals away from home and indulges in rich desserts. What health teaching does Shawn need? Why is this happening at this time of life?

Media Resources

Pituitary Disorders (21-minute filmstrip)

The anatomy and physiology of the pituitary gland and alterations in function are discussed. Dwarfism, gigantism, Cushing's disease, Graves' disease, and diabetes insipidus are discussed.

>   Source: Medical Electronic Educational Services

Evaluation of the Child with Small Stature (27-minute videocassette)

The use of growth charts, history, physical examination, and diagnostic tests for evaluation of small stature in children is discussed. Common syndromes of growth disorders are reviewed.

>   Source: University of Michigan

Juvenile Diabetes: One Family's Story (23-minute videocassette)

Issues of concern to families of children with diabetes including the relationship with health care providers are discussed. The psychologic stages a family and child pass through following diagnosis is presented. The mother of a 7-year-old with diabetes elaborates on these topics by relating her family's reactions. A discussion of the symptoms and possible causes of diabetes is included.

>   Source: Health Sciences Consortium

Amy—An Adolescent with Diabetes (15-minute slides/tape)

Problems frequently seen in the adolescent who has diabetes include noncompliance, lack of knowledge, rebellion, family conflicts, and lack of independence. An interdisciplinary approach to care is demonstrated.

>   Source: University of Michigan

Living with Chronic Illness (29-minute videocassette)

Three 12-year-olds are interviewed, one with diabetes, one with hemophilia, and one with rheumatoid arthritis. Children are asked questions about the effects of the diseases on their personal lives, the effects of the illnesses on their families, their feelings about their doctors, and advice they would offer to others.

>   Source: Public Television Library

Listen to the Kid: Adolescents Talk about Diabetes (15-minute videocassette)

The special psychosocial problems faced by the adolescent with insulin-dependent diabetes are presented. The tape could be used as a client educational program to help adolescents better adapt to their illness.

>   Source: University of Michigan Medical Center

Discussion Questions

1. The therapy for many endocrine disorders involves long-term administration of medicine. What special things do you want to review with parents about long-term administration of medicine?

2. Endocrine disorders are often difficult to explain because parents are not aware of endocrine gland function. What teaching aids could you use to make teaching more effective?

3. Diabetes mellitus is an endocrine disorder that is growing in frequency. Set up a teaching plan for an adolescent child in contrast to a 6-year-old. Explain how your teaching would differ for these two children.

Written Assignments

1. Parents have difficulty distinguishing between hypoglycemia and hyperglycemia in a child with diabetes mellitus. List the ways that these two conditions differ.

2. Children with hyperthyroidism may first come to the attention of nurses because they begin to exhibit behavior problems in school. List the behaviors that occur with hyperthyroidism that you would want classroom teachers to report to you that might suggest the problem is occurring.

3. Children with hypopituitarism may not be able to reach a usual height if their condition is not discovered early. What are measures a family could take to increase self-esteem in a child who is abnormally short?

Laboratory Experiences

1. Assign students to observe for a day with a diabetes teaching nurse so they can better appreciate the type and number of questions parents ask about this illness.

2. Assign students to interview children who have attended a specialized diabetic summer camp as to why they did or not enjoy it. Did it make them feel ''special'' or ''different''?

3. Invite the parent of a child with an endocrine disorder to come to a postconference and discuss his/her reaction at the diagnosis of the illness and the problems the family is encountering with the child's therapy, explaining the illness to neighbors, or helping the child learn to think of himself/herself as a well person.

Care Study: A Toddler With Hypothyroidism

Ashley McGray is a 2-month-old seen at a well child conference.

Health History

*   Chief Concern: ''She seems constipated; otherwise is good.''

*   History of Present Concern: Child is a foster child brought to clinic by foster mother. Foster mother states infant is ''easy to care for; rarely cries.'' Child has a bowel movement only every other day and that is only because mother uses ½ glycerin suppository to initiate this. Stool is hard; yellow in color; no blood in stool.

*   Family Profile: Baby was placed in foster care at birth because mother has been incarcerated for a 6-month jail term. Baby has lived with foster mother for 1 month. Foster mother has taken care of six other foster infants; has four children of her own who are high school and

college age. Foster mother is a homemaker; father works as a Navy recruiter. Finances are "comfortable." Home is equipped for infant care. Infant has crib in section of room of a daughter away at college.

- Past Medical Illnesses: None known.

- Growth and Development: Child "sticks out tongue" in place of a social smile. Lifts head when prone and looks at objects although it is "difficult to get child interested in toys."

- Nutrition: Child takes 3—4 ounces SMA with iron every 4 hours. Rarely cries to be fed, although sucks well when formula is presented.

- Family Medical History: Unknown. Natural mother apparently in good health.

- Review of Systems: Integumentary: Child had severe diaper area rash when first placed in foster care; now resolved; skin is dry; foster mother adds Nivea baby oil to bath water and does not use soap to improve this. No immunizations at present.

  Weight: 13 lbs. Height: 22½ inches.

Physical Examination

- General Appearance: Sleepy, well proportioned, slightly obese 2-month-old.

- Head: Normocephalic; hair is blonde, feels thin to touch and without luster. Anterior fontanelle palpated at 23 cms; posterior fontanelle palpated at ½ cm. Head circumference: 40 cms.

- Eyes: Red reflex; follows right and left.

- Ears: TMs pink; landmarks present; good movement on pneumoscopy. Normal alignment of pinna.

- Nose: Midline septum; no nasal flaring; nares patent.

- Mouth and Throat: No teeth; midline uvula. Gag reflex intact. Tongue appears large in relation to oral cavity. Child extrudes it over lower teeth while sleeping.

- Neck: Midline trachea; thyroid not palpable; full range of motion present.

- Lungs: Clear to auscultation; respiratory rate: 18/min.

- Heart: Heart rate: 100/min. No murmurs.

- Abdomen: Scaphoid; bowel sounds in all quadrants. Hard mass palpable in left lower quadrant; cord site well healed.

- Genitorectal: Normal female; no discharge. Rectal exam reveals hard yellow stool in rectum.

- Neurologic: Moro, tonic neck, step-in-place tested and intact. Unable to elicit a social smile. Head lag obvious on pull to sit; steadies poorly in sitting position.

Care Study Questions

1. Ashley is diagnosed as having hypothyroidism. What signs or symptoms does she have that suggest this?

2. Ashley has been born into a family with economic and disorganizational problems. What can be the consequences of this on managing a long-term illness?

3. Complete a nursing care plan that would identify and help meet Ashley's needs.

Nursing Care of the Child With a Neurological Disorder

Chapter 49 discusses the nursing care of children with common neurologic disorders. The chapter begins with a Nursing Process Overview that discusses the nursing diagnoses pertinent to neurologic disorders and the importance of encouraging families to continue the long-term care necessary with these disorders. Care of the child with recurrent convulsions, cerebral palsy, spinal cord injury, and neurofibromatosis is discussed.

Students need to review their knowledge of the nervous system, particularly in relation to upper and lower neuron function, before they can appreciate what type of motor dysfunction (spasticity or laxicity) will result following a spinal cord disorder. Learning the effect of increased intracranial pressure enlarges the student's ability to care for clients in coma as well as those who have suffered a head injury.

Chapter Objectives

After mastering the contents of this chapter, students should be able to:

1. Describe common neurologic disorders in children.
2. Assess a child with a neurologic disorder.
3. Formulate nursing diagnoses for the child with a neurologic disorder.
4. Plan nursing care for the child with a neurologic disorder, such as teaching a child about the importance of taking anticonvulsant medication consistently.
5. Implement nursing care (eg, perform a neurologic assessment) for the child with a neurologic disorder.
6. Evaluate outcome criteria to be certain that nursing goals were achieved.
7. Identify national health goals related to neurologic disorders and children that nurses could be instrumental in in helping the nation achieve.

8. Identify areas related to care of children with neurologic disorders that could benefit from additional nursing research.
9. Use critical thinking to analyze ways that care of the child with a neurologic disorder could be optimally family centered.
10. Synthesize knowledge of neurologic disorders and nursing process to achieve quality maternal child health nursing care.

Key Points

- Increased intracranial pressure arises from an increase in the CSF volume, from blood accumulation, cerebral edema, or space-occupying lesions. Neurologic changes such as increased temperature and blood pressure and decreased pulse and respiration rates that occur with this are subtle. Always compare assessments to previous levels to detect that a consistent, although minor, change is occurring.

- Cerebral palsy is a nonprogressive disorder of upper motor neurons. The exact cause is generally unknown, but the condition is associated with anoxia before, during, or shortly after birth. Four major types are identified: spastic (there is excessive tone in the voluntary muscles), athetoid (abnormal involuntary movement), atonic (decreased muscle tone), and mixed (symptoms of both spasticity and athetoid movements are present). Nursing diagnoses identified for this are ''Knowledge deficit,'' ''High risk for disuse syndrome,'' ''Self-care deficit,'' ''Altered growth and development,'' ''Altered nutrition,'' and ''Impaired verbal communication.''

- Meningitis is infection of the cerebral meninges. It is caused most frequently by bacterial invasion. Nursing diagnoses identified for this are ''Pain'' and ''High risk for altered tissue perfusion.'' Children need follow-up afterward to monitor for hearing acuity and undersecretion of antidiuretic hormone.

- Encephalitis is inflammation of brain tissue. This is always a serious diagnosis because the child may be left with residual neurologic damage such as seizures or mental retardation.

- Reye's syndrome is acute encephalitis with accompanying fatty infiltration of the liver, heart, and lungs. Once common, the disease is now rarely seen, as it tends to follow the administration of acetylsalicylic acid (aspirin) to a child who has a viral infection. Cautioning parents not to administer aspirin has caused the illness to decline in incidence.

- Guillain-Barré syndrome is inflammation of motor and sensory nerves. The reaction may be immune mediated following an upper respiratory illness. Temporary demyelinization of the nerve sheaths occurs with loss of function.

- Botulism occurs when spores of Clostridium botulinum produce toxins in the intestine. Honey and corn syrup may be sources of the organism and they should not be given to infants.

- Recurrent convulsions are involuntary contractions of muscle caused by abnormal electrical brain discharges. Common types seen in children are infantile spasms, X, focal absence, and tonic-clonic. Seizures may occur from fever in children under 7 years. Therapy is administration of anticonvulsant drugs. Nursing diagnoses associated with recurrent convulsions are "High risk for injury" and "Altered family processes." Anticonvulsant medications need to maintain a serum level to be effective. Help children plan ways to remember to take them consistently and to plan ahead so they have them available for vacations, camp, holidays, etc.

- Spinal cord injury is occurring at increased rates in children from sports and motor vehicle injuries. Children pass through a first, second, and third recovery phase following the injury. Nursing diagnoses associated with this are "High risk for altered mobility," "Self-care deficit," "Altered respiratory function," "Altered skin integrity," "Altered urinary and bowel elimination," and "Grieving."

- Many neurologic disorders cause problems with balance. Be certain that children are capable of ambulating safely before allowing them out of bed without assistance. Some children need to wear a helmet to protect their head from trauma if they should fall.

- Nerve cells are unique in that they do not regenerate if damaged. This makes neurologic disease a long-term type of illness. Parents and children alike need support from health care providers to cope with problems that continue to occur over a long period of time.

Definitions of Key Terms

asterognosis: the inability to identify objects by touch

autonomic nervous system: the division of the nervous system that regulates involuntary body organs

central nervous system: the brain and spinal cord

cerebrospinal fluid: the fluid surrounding the spinal cord

decerebrate posturing: a position with the arms extended, internal rotation of the wrists, and feet in plantar flexion

decorticate posturing: a position with the upper and lower extremities rigidly flexed

diplegia: bilateral paralysis of any part of the body

graphesthesia: inability to identify a pattern drawn on the skin

hemiplegia: paralysis of one side of the body

kinesthesia: the perception of one's own body parts, weight, and movement

neuron: a nerve cell

paraplegia: motor or sensory loss of the lower extremities

peripheral nervous system: the division of the nervous system outside the central nervous system

quadriplegia: paralysis of the arms, legs, and trunk

stereognosis: the ability to recognize an object by touch

Nursing Process Overview

The Nursing Process Overview in this chapter concentrates on suggestions for nursing diagnoses pertinent to disorders of the nervous system. Planning and implementations focus on ways that care can be modified to accommodate the needs of the child with a long-term illness.

Study Aids

Boxes

Box 49-1:   Classifications of seizures

Box 49-2:   Safe administration of anticonvulsants

Tables

Table 49-1:   Normal findings of cerebrospinal fluid

Table 49-2:   Cranial nerve function

Table 49-3:   Signs and symptoms of increased intracranial pressure

Table 49-4:   Physical findings that suggest cerebral palsy

Table 49-5:   Anticonvulsants

Table 49-6:   Functional ability after spinal cord injury

Table 49-7:   Characteristics of upper and lower motor nerve lesions after spinal shock phase

Displays

Focus on National Health Goals

Focus on Family Teaching

Focus on Nursing Research

Focus on Cultural Awareness

Critical Thinking Questions:

1. Beverly is a 2-year-old diagnosed with bacterial meningitis. She has severe neck pain when she is moved. Her mother asks you not to worry so much about intake and output so her daughter can rest. How would you answer her mother? Suppose you call Beverly and she doesn't answer you? Why is this a particular cause of concern with a child with meningitis?

2. Bill is a highschool senior and your neighbor. He tells you that he thinks he has the flu and that he took some aspirin for it. When you tell him it isn't wise for children to take aspirin for flu-like symptoms, he tells you that advice is "just for babies." Would you pursue the matter with Bill?

3. A spinal cord injury can cause severe disability in adolescents. If you were designing a program to teach measures to prevent spinal cord injury, what topics would you include in your presentation?

measures to prevent spinal cord injury, what topics would you include in your presentation?

Media Resources

Neurological Assessment of the Pediatric Patient (28-minute videocassette)

The basic neurologic examination for infants and children including level of consciousness. Glasgow Coma Scale scoring is demonstrated. Age and developmentally appropriate examination and responses as well as signs of acute neurologic deterioration are shown. Techniques to adapt the examination for developmentally delayed and handicapped children are included.

Source: AJN Educational Services

Assessing Levels of Consciousness: The Glasgow Coma Scale (7-minute videocassette)

A nurse demonstrates the Glasgow Coma Scale to assess the level of consciousness in an adolescent experiencing drug overdose. The scoring system is explained, including descriptions of abnormal decorticate and decerebrate posturing.

Source: Health Sciences Consortium

Complications of Spinal Cord Impairment (28-minute videocassette)

Immobilization of the spine after an accident is demonstrated. The differences between spinal and hypovolemic shock are illustrated. Respiratory, urologic, gastrointestinal, cardiovascular, and autonomic system alterations associated with different levels of spinal cord impairment are described. Nursing management of the patient with a spinal cord injury is included.

Source: AJN Educational Services

Neonatal Problem Series: Seizures (25-minute slide/audiotape)

The causes of seizures in the neonate including metabolic, infection, and drug withdrawal are presented. Diagnoses and treatment modalities are described.

Source: Health Sciences Consortium

Seizure and Movement Disorders in Children (26-minute videotape)

Actual episodes of a variety of seizures and movement disorders in neonates and children are shown. Types of seizures are identified including discussion of evaluation and diagnosis. Illustrations of seizure activity are included.

Source: Ross Laboratories

Nursing Management of Increased Intracranial Pressure (10-minute videocassette)

A neurologic nursing assessment of an adult is used to explain increased intracranial pressure. Interventions of monitoring, prevention of infection, and nursing care are included. The discussion of the effects of nursing care procedures on a patient's intracranial pressure level is dramatic.

Source: AJN Educational Services Inc.

Cerebral Palsy (12-minute videocassette)

The usual causes and criteria for classifying cerebral palsy disorders are presented. Various types and degrees of muscular dysfunction are described and illustrated through examination of children with cerebral palsy. A multidisciplinary approach to treatment is discussed.

Source: Health Sciences Consortium

Introduction to Coma (25-minute slide/audiocassette)

The basic anatomy and physiology of the central nervous system are presented, along with the oxygen and energy requirements of neural cells during coma and possible causes of coma.

Source: Crisis Communications Corporation

Like You Like Me Series: Let's Talk It Over (6-minute film)

Sandy, an animated character, has epilepsy. Her condition is explained and the way a child copes with epilepsy is illustrated.

Source: Encyclopaedia Britannica Educa Corporation{/

Cerebral Palsy (12-minute videocassette)

A basic introduction to cerebral palsy. The classification of the various types of cerebral palsy and the etiologic and therapeutic management of the disorder are shown. The use of a multidisciplinary team approach is stressed.

Source: Health Sciences Consortium

Intermittent Catheterization: Self-Care (12-minute slide/audiocassette)

Basic functions of the urinary system are described followed by the steps of self-catheterization. Problems associated with overdistention and delayed bladder emptying are identified.

Source: AJN Educational Services

Discussion Questions

1. Bob is a 4-year-old with severe cerebral palsy. He has two younger unaffected siblings. In what ways would his disorder affect family life? What suggestions could you make to his family to maintain family integrity?

2. Recurrent convulsions are a disorder that is still ''strange'' to many people. How would you explain to first graders that a new classmate has this disorder?

3. Meningitis is a frightening condition for both children and their parents. What are important aspects of nursing care for children with meningitis?

Written Assignments

1. Children with head injuries leading to increased intracranial pressure must be assessed quickly in an emergency room. List the signs and symptoms that identify increased intracranial pressure.

2. A complete neurologic examination includes assessment of cranial nerves. List these and describe how you would test each one.

3. Spinal cord injuries are serious injuries in childhood. List safety precautions the school-age child and adolescent should take to prevent these from happening.

Laboratory Experiences

1. Assign students to a clinical area where children with neurologic disorders are cared for so they can gain an appreciation for the subtle signs and symptoms that occur with these disorders.

2. Ask a parent of a child with a disorder such as recurrent convulsions to come to a postconference and discuss how difficult it has been for the child to adjust to school. How could health care providers have been more helpful?

3. Assign students to perform a neurologic examination on a laboratory partner to grow better acquainted with the technique of such an examination.

Care Study: A School-Age Child With Cerebral Palsy

Joey Century is an 8-year-old admitted to the hospital to have a heel cord lengthening because of cerebral palsy.

Health History

- Chief Concern: "Surgery to lengthen heel cord."

- History of Present Concern: Joey has left-sided unilateral spasticity of muscles. He presently walks only on his tiptoes on left side because of a shortened Achilles tendon on that side.

- History of Past Illnesses: Chalasia severe enough to result in weight loss for the first 6 months of life. Surgery for strabismus at 3 years. Subluxated hip that occurred as a result of muscle spasticity treated with hip spica cast for 2 years. Health maintenance by private pediatrician.

- Family Medical History: Maternal grandmother has rheumatoid arthritis. Paternal grandfather died of colon cancer. Father has "allergies to almost everything."

- Pregnancy History: Infant was born of a G1P0 mother at 7 months of pregnancy following premature rupture of the membranes and premature labor. Child was maintained on a ventilator for 1 month in hospital ICU before discharge.

- Growth and Development: Child showed unilateral spasticity of lower extremities as early as 1 month of age. Weight below average even with "set-back age." Turned over at 6 months. Sat steadily at 10 months. Walked at 20 months. Language: first word (da-da) at 6 months; sentences at 2 years. Articulation of words is still poor; difficult for strangers to understand him.

- Review of Systems; Neuropsychiatric: Child "agitates easily." Vomits if too upset.

  Head: Has had frequent falls from unsteady gait in which he has hit head. One grade behind in school because of learning disability.

  Eyes: Strabismus of right eye repaired at 3 years and now straight.

Ears: Otitis media 1 at 5 years.

Extremities: Child "clumsy with hands;" various black and blue marks on legs always present from bumps and falls.

Physical Examination

- General Appearance: Alert-appearing 8-year-old male who walks with an uncoordinated gait and on ball of left foot.

- Head: Prominent occipital prominence; hair well nourished. One keloid scar present on left forehead.

- Eyes: Red reflexes present; eye alignment straight by Hirschberg's sign; right eye doesn't follow well into superior lateral position.

- Ears: TMs pink; landmarks and cone of light well defined. Child's hearing comparable with examiner's.

- Nose: Midline septum; patent nares.

- Mouth and Throat: Teeth in good repair; 1 filled cavity. Right upper central incisor is a prosthesis. Mucous membrane moist. Uvula midline.

- Lungs: Lungs clear to auscultation and percussion; respiratory rate: 20/min.

- Heart: Heart rate 90/min; no murmurs.

- Abdomen: No masses; no tenderness; bowel sounds present in all four quadrants; abdominal reflexes present.

- Genitalia: Testes descended; circumcised male; midline meatus.

- Back: Slight lateral curvature (10 degrees) of spine, deviated to right noted; curve more pronounced on bending forward.

- Extremities: Arms: Full range of motion in right arm; left arm has extension of elbow reduced by 20 degrees.

- Hips: Full range of motion on right side; left hip has external rotation limited to 120 degrees.

- Knees: Full flexion of right knee; left knee is 10% limited in flexion.

- Ankles: Full range of motion on right side; child holds left foot plantar flexed. Dorsiflexion severely restricted; no clonus elicited.

- Neurologic: DTRs: 4 **on left side; 2 on right. Babinski: flares on left; plantar flexes on right.**

Cranial nerves:

I Olfactory: Able to identify the odor of oranges bilaterally.

II Optic: Has color perception both eyes; vision 20/30 bilaterally.

III, IV, VI Oculomotor, trochlear, and abducens: Child follows light into all fields on left side; unable to follow to superior lateral position on right.

V Trigeminal: Mastication lessened on right; sensory innervation intact bilaterally.

VII Facial: Facial movement equal on both sides.

VIII Vestibulocochlear: Child hears a watch ticking. bilaterally.

IX and X Glossopharyngeal and Vagus: Uvula elevates bilaterally; gag reflex intact.

XI Accessory: Poor trapeze resistance on left side.

XII Hypoglossal: Tongue protrudes at midline; no tremors.

Romberg: Negative.

Finger to Nose: Accurate on right side; great deal of difficulty on left side.

Care Study Questions

1. Joey was born at 7-month gestation and was cared for in an intensive care nursery for 1 month. Is there an association between low birth weight and cerebral palsy?

2. Joey's spasticity mainly affects his left side. What modifications in self-care would you want to explore with his mother in light of this?

3. Complete a nursing care plan that would identify and meet Joey's needs.

Nursing Care of the Child With a Disorder of the Eyes or Ears

Chapter 50 discusses care of the child who is experiencing a disorder of vision or hearing. The chapter begins with a nursing process overview that concentrates on assessment of these disorders and nursing diagnoses specific for this area. Vision concerns include astigmatism, strabismus, amblyopia, eye trauma, cataract, congenital glaucoma, and infection. Auditory concerns resulting from external and internal otitis media and colesteatoma are also included. Care of vision- and hearing-impaired children in the hospital is presented.

Students may need to review the techniques of vision and hearing screening discussed in Chapter 26 in order to understand the level of hearing or vision possible in these children.

Chapter Objectives

After mastering the contents of this chapter, students should be able to:

1. Describe the structure and function of the eyes and ears and disorders of these organs that affect children.
2. Assess the child who has a disorder of vision or hearing.
3. Formulate nursing diagnoses related to the child with a disorder of vision or hearing.
4. Plan nursing interventions for the child with a disorder of vision or hearing, such as teaching parents about eye patching.
5. Implement nursing care to meet the specific needs of the child who has a disorder of the eyes or ears, such as preparing the child for eye surgery.
6. Evaluate outcome criteria to be certain that goals for nursing care have been achieved.

7. Identify national health goals related to vision and hearing disorders of children that nurses could be instrumental in in helping the nation achieve.
8. Identify areas related to care of children with vision or hearing disorders that could benefit from additional nursing research.
9. Use critical thinking to analyze ways that nursing care of children with dysfunctional vision or hearing could be more family centered.
10. Synthesize knowledge of disorders of the eyes or ears in children with the nursing process to achieve quality maternal and child health nursing care.

Key Points

- Refractive errors of vision such as myopia and hyperopia are the most common eye disorders in children. Amblyopia (lazy eye) is subnormal vision in one eye. Children with these disorders need correction at the time the disorder is recognized to prevent further vision distortion.

- Coloboma is congenital incomplete closure of the pupil or lower eyelid. Ptosis is the inability to open the upper eyelid normally. Ptosis needs correction to avoid development of amblyopia.

- Strabismus is unequally aligned eyes. Like ptosis, it may lead to amblyopia if not corrected.

- Infections of the lids such as styes or chalazions can occur in children. Conjunctivitis (inflammation of the conjunctiva) often presents with acute symptoms. An antibiotic is necessary for therapy.

- Children need to be taught to avoid eye injuries by using proper eye protection during sports or work. Eye injures such penetration by a foreign body need follow-up to be certain that vision remains adequate.

- Children with either vision or hearing impairment need special preparation and orientation for a hospital or ambulatory health visit so they can fully understand what is going to happen at the visit.

- Help children with vision impairment work through new experiences by letting them feel equipment as much as possible. Guide their hands through the steps of a new procedure you are teaching them.

- Otitis media (middle ear infection) is a common childhood illness. Children need therapy with antibiotics to correct this. With serous otitis media, some children have myringotomy tubes placed to relieve pressure and supply air access to the middle ear.

- Photos, drawings, or demonstration should be used more often than normally with hearing-impaired children to help them learn new skills. Contact a signing interpreter as appropriate to be certain the child understands instructions.

- Teaching preventive measures to avoid eye and hearing injury (wearing goggles or ear protection as appropriate) and screening children for sensory impairments are important nursing roles.

Definitions of Key Terms

accommodation: adjustment of the eye for various distances

amblyopia: reduced vision in one eye

astigmatism: an uneven cornea

chalazion: inflammation of a meibomian gland of the eyelid

cones: the structures of the retina that allow for visualization of color

convergence: the coordinated movement of the two eyes toward fixation of the same point

diplopia: double vision

fovea centralis: the location on the retina where cones are concentrated

globe: the shape of the eye

goniotomy: an operation to increase the flow of aqueous humor from the anterior chamber of the eye

hyperopia: farsightedness

light refraction: the deviation that occurs when a ray of light strikes a fluid; allows light rays to fall on the retina for sight

myopia: nearsightedness

myringotomy: an incision into the tympanic membrane

nystagmus: rapid irregular eye movements

orthoptics: eye exercises designed to correct visual control of binocular vision

photophobia: sensitivity to light

ptosis: an abnormal condition in which an upper eyelid does not fully open

rods: the retinal structures that perceive light

stereopsis: vision fusion

strabismus: deviation of an eye

stye: an infection of a sebaceous gland of the eyelid

tympanocentesis: an incision into the ear drum{/GL}

Nursing Process Overview

The Nursing Process Overview in this chapter focuses on identifying signs and symptoms of vision and hearing impairment and nursing diagnoses that reflect not only the actual problem (perhaps sensory deficit) but also the impact of the defect on the child and family (perhaps ineffective coping). The importance of planning teaching strategies to prevent vision and hearing disorders is stressed.

Study Aids

Tables

Table 50-1:   Levels of hearing impairment

Displays

Focus on National Health Goals

Focus on Family Teaching

Focus on Nursing Research

Focus on Cultural Awareness

Critical Thinking Questions:

1. Jody is a 4-year-old who is going to have eye surgery. What special steps in preparation for surgery would you want to make for her? Is Jody old enough to appreciate the importance of seeing?

2. Fred is a 14-year-old who is deaf from developing meningitis as a preschooler. He uses sign language to communicate. How could you communicate effectively with Fred while hospitalized? What are Fred's rights as a patient in regard to having an interpreter provided for him?

3. You are going to teach a class to a first-grade class on ways to prevent eye and hearing injuries. What would you include in your class? Would this be different if the class was for 16-year-olds?

Media Resources

Acute Middle Ear Disease in Infants and Children. (slide/audiocassette)

The anatomic characteristics of children that predispose to middle ear disease are described, along with the development, pathogenesis, and symptoms of the disease. Acute middle ear disease is presented and must be regarded as a serious condition.

Source: National Audio Visual Center

Can Your Patient Hear? (32-minute videocassette)

Screening techniques for potential hearing impairments in children up to 6 years of age. Questions, anatomic and physical indicators, and conversational techniques are helpful tools during a routine history and physical examination to assess a child's hearing.

Source: Health Sciences Consortium

Children and Deafness (30-minute videocassette)

The needs of families with children who have profound hearing loss are discussed. Family reactions are explored, at the time of diagnosis and through acceptance of the condition. Options for treatment including the use of hearing aids, education, and systems of communication are described.

Source: Pyramid Films

Language and Hearing Impaired Children (15-minute videocassette)

The difference between normal language development and language development in the child who is hearing impaired is described. Vignettes of children in learning situations are used to describe a total communication approach to promote language, social, and motor development in children with alterations in hearing ability.

Source: Health Sciences Consortium

Sound of Sunshine, Sound of Rain (14-minute videocassette)

The world of sound and touch is shown as experienced by a 7-year-old who is blind. The sightless world of the child is contrasted to the world of reality as experienced by the child's sighted sister. The narrative is based on a children's book by Florence Parry Heide.

Source: Film Fair Communications

Discussion Questions

1. Many parents do not give a prescribed antibiotic for otitis media for the full, prescribed 10 days. What measures would you use to help parents do this more reliably?

2. A severely vision-impaired child can be very frightened by a hospital experience. What would you want to explain about a nursing unit to reduce this fright?

3. Many grade school children have myringotomy tubes inserted to aerate their inner ears. As a school nurse, what precautions would you want them to take to be certain they do not injure their middle ear?

Written Assignments

1. School nurses have an important role to play in preventing eye injury. What safety rules would you teach grade school children to follow to protect their eyes? What would you teach adolescents?

2. Joey is a 7-year-old with color blindness for blue and green. What are situations in which he will need to take extra precautions in order to be safe?

3. Heather is a 4-year-old with a hearing loss of 50 dBs. What are situations in which she would need to take extra precautions in order to be safe?

Laboratory Experiences

1. Assign students to observe a school nurse performing hearing and vision screening to give experience in learning these techniques.

2. Ask a parent of a child with a hearing deficit to come to a postconference and describe the problems of raising a nonhearing child in a hearing world. How could health care personnel be more helpful to her?

3. Assign students to experiences in an ambulatory clinic where children with vision disorders such as glaucoma or cataract are cared for in order that they can gain a better understanding of the importance of sight to normal development.

Care Study: A School-Age Child With Conjunctivitis

Loreen Coach is an 8-year-old seen in the emergency room.

Health History

- Chief Concern: "Her eye is bright red."

- History of Present Concern: Child complained yesterday that her right eye "itched;" mother was called by school headmaster today because sclera of Loreen's right eye was bright red and tearing.

- Family Profile: Child is one of identical twins; has a 12-year-old sibling. Family intact; father is a radiologist; mother is commercial artist. Finances are rated as "not a problem." Family lives in a private 4-bedroom home with a generous yard and play space.

- Pregnancy History: Planned pregnancy; twin pregnancy was diagnosed at 16 weeks into pregnancy; mother hospitalized for last 2 months of pregnancy to prevent premature birth. Infants born by cesarean birth because of transverse lie of second twin. Both infants breathed spontaneously; both discharged with mother at 5 days postbirth.

- Past Medical History: Chickenpox at 6 years; scarlet fever at 7 years. Fall from horse 2 months ago; no loss of consciousness. Seen in emergency room of local hospital. No x-rays or therapy given.

- Growth and Development: Met developmental milestones of infant and preschool period. Currently is in second grade in private school for girls; very interested in horses; attends a riding academy three afternoons a week after school.

- Family Medical History: Maternal grandmother: ovarian cancer (died 3 years ago).

  Father: Sinus headaches in March and April each year.

- Review of Systems: Head: fall as listed in past history.

  Eyes and Ears: No eye or ear infections; vision and hearing both tested in school last year and found to be normal.

  Hair: Head lice last fall; treated with Kwell with no return.

  Gastrointestinal: "Nervous" stomach when facing new experiences.

  Extremities: Strawberry hemangioma on right wrist that has not changed in size since she was 1 year old.

Physical Examination

- General Appearance: Well-proportioned school-age white female with reddened, watery right eye; blinking as if eye is sensitive to light. Weight: 28.5 kg. Height: 130 cms. Blood pressure: 104/58.

- Head: Normocephalic; fontanelles closed. Hair good texture.

- Eyes: Red reflex present bilaterally; PERLA; conjunctiva on right sclera is firey red; thick yellow discharge on lower conjunctival rim.

- Ears: TMs pink; landmarks evident. Hearing equal to examiner's.

- Nose: Midline septum; no discharge.

- Mouth and Throat: Front upper central incisors missing; permanant teeth can be palpated under gum. No caries; midline uvula. No erythema.

- Neck: Full range of motion. No palpable lymph nodes. Midline trachea.

- Lungs and Chest: Lungs clear to auscultation and percussion. Rate: 20/min. Breast development: Tanner 1.

- Abdomen: Soft; bowel sounds heard in all 4 quadrants. No masses.

- Genitalia: Deferred.

- Extremities: Bright red vascular nodule 2 cm 1 cm present on dorsal surface of right wrist; not tender to touch. Full range of motion in joints. Normal gait.

- Neurologic: Patellar and brachial reflexes 2. Oriented to person, place, and time.

Care Study Questions

1. Loreen has a reddened, inflamed eye. What is the usual reason for this in school-age children? Many children with eye infections are reluctant to let anyone examine their eye because they are afraid it will hurt. What would be an effective way to support such children?

2. Loreen has a strawberry hemangioma on her wrist that has not changed in size since she was a year old. Is this usual? Should it have faded by now?

3. Loreen was diagnosed as having a conjunctivitis of her right eye. Complete a nursing care plan that would identify and meet her needs.

Nursing Care of the Child With A Musculoskeletal Disorder

Chapter 51 discusses care of the child with a disorder of the muscular or skeletal system. The chapter begins with a nursing process overview detailing assessment of these disorders and suggesting nursing diagnoses that speak to the long-term problems often inherent in these disorders. Care of the child in a cast or in traction is discussed. Bone development disorders such as genu varum, Legg-Calve-Perthes disease, osteogenesis imperfecta, and scoliosis as well as muscular illnesses such as myasthenia gravis and muscular dystrophy are included.

Chapter Objectives

After mastering the contents of this chapter, students should be able to:

1. Describe common musculoskeletal disorders in children.
2. Assess the child with a musculoskeletal disorder.
3. Formulate nursing diagnoses related to the child with a musculoskeletal disorder.
4. Plan nursing care such as age-appropriate diversional activities for the child with a musculoskeletal disorder.
5. Implement nursing care for the child with a musculoskeletal disorder (eg, explain cast care to a school-age child and parents).
6. Evaluate outcome criteria to be certain that goals established for care were achieved.
7. Identify national health goals related to musculoskeletal disorders and children that nurses can be instrumental in helping the nation to achieve.
8. Identify areas related to care of the child with musculoskeletal disorders that could benefit from additional nursing research.
9. Use critical thinking to analyze ways that care of the child immobilized by a cast or traction can be more family centered.
10. Synthesize knowledge of musculoskeletal disorders with the nursing process to achieve quality maternal and child health nursing care.

Key Points

- Many children have casts applied to allow broken bones to heal. Nursing diagnoses identified in connection to cast care are "High risk for altered peripheral tissue perfusion," "Impaired tissue integrity," and "Parental health-seeking behaviors."

- Volkmann's ischemic contracture is a complication that occurs when an arm is casted in a bent position and the radial artery and nerve are compressed at the elbow. Frequent assessments that finger color and warmth remain adequate are safeguards that compression is not occurring.

- If broken bones are not easily aligned, children are placed in traction. Nursing diagnoses commonly associated with this are "High risk for altered nutrition," "Impaired physical mobility," "Altered skin integrity," "Infection," and "Altered growth and development."

- Developmental disorders that occur in children are flat feet (pronation), genu varum (bowlegs), and genu valgum (knock knees). The majority of these disorders are corrected naturally by normal growth.

- Slipped epiphysis is slipping of the femur head in relation to the neck of the femur at the epiphyseal line. It occurs most frequently in obese or rapidly growing boys.

- Osteomyelitis is infection of the bone. It can result in extensive destruction of the bone. Antibiotic therapy is necessary to combat the infection.

- Scoliosis is a lateral curvature of the spine. It is treated by bracing or surgery. Nursing diagnoses commonly identified for this are "Knowledge deficit" and "High risk for altered skin integrity and altered self-concept."

- Juvenile rheumatoid arthritis (JRA) occurs in a number of different forms: polyarthritic, pauciarticular, and systemic. Therapy is exercise, heat application, splinting, and administration of nonsteroidal antiinflammatory drugs or aspirin.

- Myasthenia gravis can occur in a transient form at birth from transfer of antibodies from a mother with the illness or as a primary form later in childhood. Therapy is administration of anticholinesterase drugs such as neostigmine (Prostigmin) which prolong acetylcholine action.

- Muscular dystrophy is the inherited progressive degeneration of skeletal muscles. Different types that can occur are congenital, facioscapulohumeral, and pseudohypertrophic. Children and parents alike need long-term support through the course of this long-term illness. Fortunately, due to new progress in gene replacement therapy, research is close to revealing a cure for this disease.

- A fracture or bruise of soft tissue could have resulted from child abuse. Be certain to secure a detailed history of an injury to be certain that the history is consistent with the degree of injury.

- Bone and muscle disorders tend to be long-term disorders. Children and their families need help to think through how the disorder will affect tasks of daily living to better help the child adjust to a cast or brace. Help children plan self-diversional activities as necessary so they continue to grow developmentally while confined to a cast or traction.

- As a rule, if a bone is broken, children need additional calcium in their diet to aid bone healing. If they are on strict bed rest, however, this should only be a moderate addition to their diet to prevent renal calculi from forming.

Definitions of Key Terms

cartilage: connective tissue

diaphysis: the shaft of a long bone

epiphyseal plate: the growth center of a long bone between the epiphysis and metaphysis

epiphysis: the head of a long bone

fracture: a break in a bone

long bone: a bone of the arm or leg

metaphysis: the point in bone at which diaphysis and epiphysis meet

myopathy: abnormality of skeletal muscles other than that caused by nerve degeneration

periosteum: the fibrous, highly vascular, covering of bone

petaling: application of adhesive tape to the edge of a cast to smooth the edges

sequestrum: a portion of dead bone detached from healthy bone

smooth muscle: muscle not under voluntary control, such as that in intestine

striated muscle: skeletal muscle; muscle under voluntary control

traction: aligning bone fragments by pulling on a body part in one direction against a counterpull exerted in the opposite direction

Nursing Process Overview

The Nursing Process Overview in this chapter focuses on helping the student assess children for orthopedic disorders and suggests nursing diagnoses that include the entire family, since caring for a child who is immobilized affects the entire family. Establishing both short- and long-term goals is stressed.

Study Aids

Boxes

Box 51-1:   Screening procedure for scoliosis

Tables

Table 51-1:   Neurocirculatory assessment for the child in a cast

Table 51-2:   Characteristics of different types of juvenile rheumatoid arthritis

Table 51-3:   Types of fractures

Displays

Focus on National Health Goals

Focus on Family Teaching

Focus on Nursing Research

Focus on Cultural Awareness

Critical Thinking Exercises:

1.   Judy is a 14-year-old who wears a Milwaukee brace 23 hours a day for scoliosis. During the last month, she turned down an invitation to the highschool prom and has dropped out of the highschool band and the one afterschool club she belonged to. She tells you is dropping activities to have more "time to study". Would you be concerned about Judy?

2.   Dominic is a 3-year-old with juvenile rheumatoid arthritis. You notice when he returns for a follow-up visit to arthritis clinic that the inflammation in his joints is worse than at his last visit. He has a great deal of pain. His mother tells you she has been giving him acetaminophen instead of aspirin for therapy because her primary doctor said not to give aspirin to children under 18. How would you explain these contradictory instructions? Why do children with JRA receive aspirin?

3.   Mrs. Howard has three athletically inclined boys in gradeschool. She is concerned with guiding them into sports that will be safe for them during their growing years. What advice would you give her?

Media Resources

Scoliosis (30-minute videocassette)

The screening, diagnosis, and treatment of scoliosis from a medical perspective are presented. Complications resulting from inadequate or lack of treatment are described. Case studies are included.

Source: Health Sciences Consortium

Spinal Fusion: What You Need to Know (18-minute videocassette)

A patient education program presents an adolescent recalling her experiences with spinal fusion surgery: preoperatively, immediately postoperatively, and during the period of immobilization while in a body cast after surgery.

> Source: University of Michigan

Children in Traction (27-minute videocassette)

The physical care needs of children in traction is presented. The film includes a thorough discussion of the psychologic problems imposed by immobilization and nursing care strategies to meet the psychologic needs of children in traction.

> Source: Health Sciences Consortium

Nursing Care of Patients with Casts (28-minute videocassette)

The purpose, types, application, and removal of casts with emphasis on nursing responsibilities. The priorities of care include preventing complications, reducing pain, increasing mobility, and providing information. Presentation is within a nursing process format.

> Source: AJN Educational Services

Orthopedic Assessment (28-minute videocassette)

The physical assessment of the musculoskeletal system of an adult. Special aspects of assessing children, emergency room patients, and persons with orthopedic deviations from the norm are included.

> Source: AJN Educational Services

Caring for the Child in a Hip Spica Cast (19-minute slide/audiocassette)

A parent education program describing the application of a hip spica cast and related care. Included are techniques for keeping the cast clean and dry, checking circulation, protecting the skin, planning play activities, and ensuring safety.

> Source: University of Michigan

Muscular Dystrophy and Related Diseases: a Differential Diagnosis (32-minute film)

The various types of muscular dystrophy are presented along with a discussion of diagnostic evaluation, clinical manifestations, methods of genetic transmission, age of onset, and progression of muscle involvement. The role of the genetic counselor is discussed.

> Source: National Audiovisual Center

Discussion Questions

1. Instructions for cast care are often given in ambulatory settings. What points would you review with the parents of a 7-year-old who has just had a cast applied to the forearm? With an adolescent?

2. Children with orthopedic disorders may be admitted to the hospital for long-term bed rest with traction. What activities would you plan to keep a 4-year-old interested for long periods? A 10-year-old? An adolescent?

3. Helping to maintain self-esteem for children in Milwaukee braces is a challenging task. What are specific ways to do this?

Written Assignments

1. Screening for scoliosis is an important role of school health nurses. List the steps of scoliosis screening.

2. When a cast is applied over the elbow, there is a danger that the nerve will be pinched causing permanent paralysis of the fingers. List the steps of assessment you would make to be certain this does not happen.

3. Siblings of a child with muscular dystrophy may worry that they too will contract this disorder. Describe the inheritance pattern of this disorder.

Laboratory Experiences

1. Assign students to a hospital unit where adolescents with scoliosis are admitted for spinal instrumentation and fusion so they can appreciate not only the care required but also the effect this disorder has on a child's self-esteem.

2. Assign students to an ambulatory clinic where children are seen for congenital orthopedic problems such as talipes defects in order to help them appreciate how having a child in a cast affects the entire family.

3. Assign students to an emergency room where they will see the care of clients with fractured bones from trauma. This allows them to appreciate the stress that this level of trauma places on families.

Care Study: A Girl With a Traumatic Injury

Mindy Goodhaven is a 12-year-old seen in the emergency room after a fall from the roof of the porch of her house.

Health History

- Chief Concern: "Can't bend my arm."

- History of Present Concern: Child fell from roof of a one-story house about 20 minutes ago. Had crawled up onto roof to fly a kite. Fall was stopped by thick hedge by side of house. Child is unable to bend right elbow; has pain and swelling in upper arm.

- Family Profile: Child lives with mother. Parents were divorced 2 months ago. Mother states Mindy has been difficult to live with for past 2 months; "acts out" by being disruptive in school and at home.

  Has two younger siblings, ages 8 years and 6 years. Mother works full time as a paralegal assistant. Mindy is expected to stay by self after school for 2 hours daily until mother returns home. Younger siblings are watched by a neighbor.

- Past Medical History: No childhood communicable diseases; no hospitalizations or surgery. Immunizations and health maintenance care up to date by private M.D.

- Growth and Development: Child attends parochial school in 7th grade (grade appropriate for age). Initially had difficulty reading in first grade and had to take an extra summer course; no further difficulty. Marks were As and Bs until divorce 2 months ago; marks now are Cs.

- Family Medical History:

    Maternal grandmother: adult onset diabetes

    Father: duodenal ulcer (under treatment)

    8 year old sibling: ureteral reflux repaired 1 year ago.

- Review of Systems:

    Eyes: Examined in school yearly; vision is 20/50, 20/70. Child wears contact lenses she cleans and cares for by herself. No eye infections.

    Ears: Hearing assessed in school and found to be adequate. No ear infections.

Physical Examination

- General Appearance: Distressed-appearing 12-year-old white female, holding right arm supported by left. Numerous dirt-smeared, linear abrasions with slight bleeding noticeable on forehead and right thigh. Weight: 40 kg. Height: 150 cms. Blood pressure: 112/60.

- Head: Normocephalic; linear abrasions as above.

- Eyes: PERLA; extraocular muscles intact. Red reflex present bilaterally.

- Ears: Normal alignment; TMs pink; no discharge present.

- Nose: Septum midline; no discharge.

- Mouth and Throat: 32 teeth; no caries; midline uvula; no erythema of mucous membrane.

- Neck: Full range of motion; one shotty lymph node present on left anterior cervical chain.

- Lungs: Clear to auscultation and percussion. Rate: 20/min.

- Heart: Rate: 90/min; no murmurs.

- Abdomen: No masses; bowel sounds present in all 4 quadrants; tender to touch in left lower quadrant.

- Genitalia: Deferred.

- Extremities: Normal gait; swollen, purple-blue ecchymotic area surrounding right elbow; elbow tender to palpation. Child unable to extend arm from bent 90-degree position.

- Neurologic: Patellar reflexes 2 bilaterally; oriented to name, place, and date.

Care Study Questions

1. Mindy's accident happened during the time she was unsupervised after school. Is 12 years old old enough to stay alone after school? How could you help Mindy better decide which activities are safe for time-alone play?

2. Mindy has been showing disruptive behavior for 2 months since her parents' divorce. Could trying unsafe activities be a part of this? How long is it ''normal'' for children to act this way following a disruptive life event?

3. Mindy is diagnosed as having a fractured radius. Complete a nursing care plan that will identify and meet her needs.

Nursing Care of the Child With a Traumatic Injury

Chapter 52 discusses care of the child following a traumatic injury. The Nursing Process Overview in this chapter reviews the importance of assessing vital organ function first in an emergency and the importance of including the entire family in nursing care, since the traumatic event that injured a child may have included other family members.

Conditions such as burns, head, dental, and abdominal trauma, drowning, poisoning, foreign body obstruction, and bites are discussed. The importance of teaching safety measures to parents and children in order to prevent accidents is stressed.

Chapter Objectives

After mastering the contents of this chapter, students should be able to:

1. Describe the causes and consequences of common accident and injuries in childhood as well as measures to prevent them.

2. Assess a child injured from an accident such as poisoning or burning.

3. Formulate nursing diagnoses related to the injured child.

4. Plan nursing care related to the injured child, such as teaching poisoning prevention.

5. Implement nursing care for the child with an injury, such as assessing circulation after casting.

6. Evaluate goal outcomes to be certain that nursing goals were achieved.

7. Identify national health goals related to children and trauma that nurses can be instrumental in in helping the nation to achieve.

8. Identify areas related to care of children with traumatic injuries that could benefit from additional nursing research.

9. Use critical thinking to analyze ways that accidents and injuries can be prevented in childhood.

10. Synthesize knowledge of injuries in childhood with nursing process to achieve quality maternal and child health care.

Key Points

• Children need total body assessment following a traumatic injury, since they may be unable to describe other injuries besides the primary one they may have suffered. Be certain that aseptic technique is maintained when caring for trauma victims so the child doesn't develop an additional unnecessary infection.

• Head injuries are always potentially serious in children. Skull fractures, subdural hematoma, epidural hematomas, concussion, and contusions can occur. Nursing diagnoses identified in association with this are ''High risk for fluid volume excess'' and ''Altered growth and development.''

• Coma (unconsciousness from which children cannot be roused) may be present in children following severe head trauma. Nursing diagnoses related to this are ''High risk for ineffective airway clearance,'' ''Altered skin integrity,'' and ''Altered nutrition.''

• Abdominal trauma resulting in splenic or liver rupture may occur in connection with multiple trauma.

• Near drowning can occur from salt or fresh water. Nursing diagnoses identified with this are ''High risk for infection'' and ''Fear.'' The physiologic basis for complications following drowning differs as to whether the water was fresh or salt water.

• Common substances children swallow that result in poisoning are acetaminophen (Tylenol) and salicylic acid (aspirin). Teach parents to keep the number of the local poison control center next to their telephone and to always call first before administering an antidote for poisoning.

• Lead poisoning most frequently occurs from the ingestion of lead chips from older housing. Preventing this is a major nursing responsibility.

• Burns are divided into three types: first, second, and third, depending on the depth of the burn. Burns produce systemic body reactions. Nursing diagnoses identified with this are ''High risk for altered tissue perfusion,'' ''Ineffective airway clearance,'' ''Altered patterns in urinary elimination,'' ''Altered nutrition,'' ''Infection,'' ''Social isolation,'' ''Altered family processes,'' ''Diversional activity deficit,'' and ''Self-esteem disturbance.''

- Be aware that some trauma in children occurs from child abuse. Screen for this by history and physical examination.

Definitions of Key Terms

allografting: tissue grafting between two genetically dissimilar individuals

autografting: surgical transplantation of tissue from one part of the body to another part

bougie: a cylindrical flexible instrument for insertion into a body cavity to dilate it

contrecoup injury: an injury to the opposite side of the brain from the side where a blow was struck

débridement: the removal of dirt, foreign bodies, or injured tissue from a wound or burn

drowning: asphyxiation because of submersion in water

escharotomy: surgical incision into the necrotic tissue formed after a burn

heterografting: tissue from another species used to temporarily cover a burned area

homografting: allografting

near drowning: the state of having inhaled water, but a condition short of asphyxiation

stupor: lethargy or unresponsiveness

Nursing Process Overview

The Nursing Process Overview in this chapter focuses on formulating nursing diagnoses that relate specifically to the injured child yet meet the needs of the family as well. Important points include asking other family members if they were also injured and the meaning of the accident to the family.

Study Aids

Boxes

Box 52-1:   Scoring for Glasgow coma scale

Focus on Nursing Care: Drugs used to counteract poisoning

Tables

Table 52-1:   Most frequent accidents in children by age group

Table 52-2:   Important assessments on initial examination of an injured child

Table 52-3:   Levels of salicylate poisoning

Table 52-4:   Classification of lead poisoning risk

Table 52-5:   Degrees of frostbite

Table 52-6:   Classification of burns

Table 52-7:   Characteristics of burns

Table 52-8:   Fluid shifts after thermal injury

Table 52-9:   Comparison of open and closed burn therapy

Procedures

Procedure 52-1:   Gastric lavage

Displays

Focus on National Health Goals

Focus on Family Teaching

Focus on Nursing Research

Focus on Cultural Awareness

Critical Thinking Questions:

1. Jeremy is a 6-year-old who is admitted to the hospital in coma. What special precautions would you want to take to insure he maintains a patent airway? That he maintains skin integrity?

2. Susan is a 3-year-old seen in the emergency room for acetaminophen poisoning. Her father tells you they normally lock all medicine away carefully. His wife left acetaminophen on the counter because she was hurrying to take some and lie down because she had a migraine headache. Would you want to discuss the necessity of poisoning prevention with these parents or should they have learned from this experience that their actions were not safe?

3. Chris is a 10-year-old who has third-degree burns on her legs from lighting a fire to burn leaves. She will probably have a lengthy hospitalization and may need skin grafts to improve healing. What precautions does Chris need to prevent infection until healing is complete?

Media Resources

The ABCs of Pediatric Trauma Nursing (28-minute videocassette)

A systematic approach to assessment and stabilization of the child with multiple injuries. The ways in which the pediatric trauma patient's needs differ from the adult's needs are shown. The need for special pharmacologic considerations and psychosocial care is stressed.

Source: AJN Educational Services

Nursing Management of Acute Head Injuries (28-minute videocassette)

The differences between minor and major head injuries are shown using illustrations and nursing diagnosis statements. Neurologic assessment, Glasgow Coma Scale scoring, and ICP monitoring procedures are detailed.

Source: AJN Educational Services

Emergency Assessment of the Traumatized Child (46-minute videocassette)

Assessment of the injured child is presented. The importance of developing a systematic, disciplined approach to the examination of a child who presents with trauma is stressed.

Source: Medical Electronic Education Services, Inc.

First Aid: Newest Techniques (filmstrip or videotransfer)

First aid emergencies are shown in the form of vignettes that are interrupted at critical points with a series of alternative interventions; the viewer is allowed to choose the most appropriate action. Artificial respiration, bleeding, poisoning, shock, burns, fractures, frostbite, heat and cold exposure, choking, sudden illness, bites, and head and multiple injuries are included.

Source: Career Aids

Eye Trauma (28-minute videocassette)

An adolescent who develops a retinal detachment is presented. Emergency room care as well as follow-up is included. Basic structures of the eye, common injuries, and assessment are illustrated. Nursing diagnoses and interventions for physical and psychologic problems associated with eye trauma are discussed.

Source: American Journal of Nursing Educa Services

The Other Child: Burns in Children (50 minute videocassette)

The physical and psychologic impact of severe burn injury on children and families is illustrated through interviews with burned children and health professionals. Burn treatment and reconstuctive surgery are both discussed. The importance of helping parents to face the final outcome of their child's injury is stressed.

Source: American Journal of Nursing Educa Services

Nursing Care of Burn Patients (45-minute videocassette)

An overview of nursing care in the first 72 hours following a major burn injury is presented. Oxygenation, fluid and electrolyte balance, wound care, complications, and pain management for the immediate burn period are discussed. Débridement, topical medications, skin grafting, and nutrition are illustrated and discussed. Psychologic reactions to burns are included.

Source: American Journal of Nursing Educa Services

Discussion Questions

1. Injuries are always frightening times for parents and children. What are some methods you can use to quickly calm children or parents in emergencies?

2. Dental trauma is a common injury in children. What steps should parents take after a tooth is dislodged?

3. Lead poisoning is a major problem with inner city children. What steps should parents who are refurbishing an older home take to keep children from being affected by lead?

Written Assignments

1. The fluid shifts that occur after severe burns change the type of nursing care required. What are these shifts and how does nursing care differ depending on whether fluid is shifting toward or away from the burned area?

2. Abdominal injury after an accident often presents silently. What observations would you make of a child seen in an emergency room to detect if an abdominal injury is present?

3. Drowning differs in nature if it occurs in salt rather than fresh water. How does this influence nursing care?

Laboratory Experiences

1. Assign students to clinical experiences in emergency rooms where they can see children who have been injured being given immediate treatment.

2. Assign students to observe at a school or park playground and document the number of accidents about to happen in order to appreciate the importance of preventive guidance in this area.

3. Construct a display in the practice laboratory area with a doll mannequin to show unsafe practices such as a crib rail down, pillow in crib, etc. Hold a contest and give a prize donated by a local fast food restaurant to the student who names the most potential accidents in the display.

Care Study: A Girl With a Head Injury

Missy Long is a 12-year-old seen in the emergency room following a head injury.

Health History

*   Chief Concern: "She was hit by a hockey puck."

*   History of Present Concern: Child was hit in the head by a hockey puck while playing indoor ice hockey after school. The puck struck her forehead; she was unconscious about 3 minutes following accident; has been sleepy since then; states "everything looks double;" has vomited 3 times since accident. Child was not wearing a helmet at time of accident.

*   Family Profile: Intact family; 2 younger siblings, 6-year-old twins. Mother works as a computer analyst; father is an editor for evening newspaper. Family lives in a home in north suburbs; finances are described as "adequate."

*   History of Past Illnesses: Frequent otitis media as an infant; serous otitis media beginning at age 5. Had myringotomy tubes placed at 9 years; removed 6 months ago.

Chickenpox at age 7 years.

Four stitches in chin at 8 years for fall at playground.

*   Pregnancy History: Pregnancy was planned; birth was induced at 42 weeks for post-term pregnancy. Baby's presentation was vertex. Breathed immediately. Mother unfamiliar with term "Apgar." No alcohol, smoking, or recreational drug use during pregnancy. Mother took ASA for frequent headaches throughout pregnancy.

*   Growth and Development: Child met infant and preschool milestones. Currently in 7th grade (age appropriate). Participates in indoor ice hockey and soccer. Parents state child is doing well in school. Is happy and friendly with peers. Menarche 3 months ago. Menses irregular; flow scant.

*   Family Medical History: Paternal grandfather and father both have had bipass surgery; a cousin was born with an atrial septal defect.

A paternal aunt has breast cancer.

Mother has a positive tuberculin reaction following exposure from a fellow worker; had a negative x-ray 1 month ago.

- Review of Systems: Negative but for chief concern and past illnesses.

Physical Examination

- General Appearance: Slim, well-proportioned, difficult to rouse 12-year-old. Two-inch bleeding laceration in center of forehead surrounded by edematous area. Height: 150 cms. Weight: 40.6 kg. Blood pressure: 135/70.

- Head: Normocephalic; laceration as above.

- Eyes: Left pupil dilated in comparison to right and reacts slowly to light. Inability to follow light into superior oblique field; red reflex bilaterally. No ptosis. Funduscopic examination: no papilledema; disc edges distinctive. AV ratio 2/3.

- Ears: TMs pink with landmarks and cone of light present. Difficult to document hearing because of difficulty in rousing child; tear evident in right tympanic membrane with clear fluid drainage in external ear canal.

- Nose: Midline septum; nares patent. No discharge.

- Mouth and Throat: Midline uvula; no malalignment of or broken teeth. Mucous membrane moist.

- Neck: Full ROM; no palpable lymph nodes; midline trachea.

- Lungs: Respiratory rate: 16/min; no adventitious sounds.

- Heart: Heart rate: 68/min; no murmurs; marked sinus arrhythmia.

- Abdomen: Soft; no masses; bowel sounds in all quadrants. Liver palpated 1 cm under right costal margin.

- Genitalia: Normal preadolescent female; Tanner 4.

- Extremities: Full range of motion. One old ecchymotic bruise on calf of left leg (yellow-brown); one on anterior surface of right lower leg (purple-red). Not asked to walk because of mental confusion.

- Neurologic: DTRs: 1 patellar and brachial on left; 2 on right. Sensory: responds to painful stimuli. Motor: equal bilaterally. Babinski: flares on left foot. Kernig's sign: negative.

Finger to Nose: Abnormal; Romberg: not attempted because of inability to stand steadily.

Care Study Questions

1. Missy required stitches to her chin because of a previous sports injury. Does she sound like a child who takes unnecessary risks or are these expected injuries?

2. Missy was diagnosed as having a concussion. A skull x-ray revealed a linear fracture of the frontal bone. Complete a nursing care plan that would identify and meet Missy's needs.

Nursing Care of the Child With Cancer

Chapter 53 discusses care of the child with a malignancy. The chapter begins with a Nursing Process Overview that details the subtle ways that symptoms of cancer in childhood present and also suggests nursing diagnoses that speak to the total body involvement that occurs with cancer. Care of children receiving common cancer therapy such as radiation and chemotherapy are discussed. Leukemia, the lymphomas, neoplasms of the brain and bone and muscle, eye and kidney are included. Helping parents to view cancer as a long-term but not necessarily fatal illness is stressed.

Students may need to discuss their preconceived ideas and personal feelings about cancer in children before they are prepared to shift their focus to one of optimism before beginning care.

Chapter Objectives

After mastering the contents of this chapter, students should be able to:

1. Define terms related to tumor growth such as neoplasm, benign, malignant, sarcoma, and carcinoma and describe normal cell growth and theories that explain how cells are altered to become neoplastic in children.

2. Assess the child with a neoplastic process, such as a rhabdomyosarcoma, neuroblastoma, Wilms' tumor, and leukemia.

3. Formulate nursing diagnoses related to the child with a malignancy.

4. Plan nursing care specific to the child with a neoplasm such as measures to prevent nausea and vomiting from chemotherapy.

5. Implement nursing care for the child undergoing cancer therapy, such as providing mouth care for the child with stomatitis.

6. Evaluate outcome criteria to be certain that nursing care goals were achieved.

7. Identify national health goals related to the care of the child with cancer that nurses can be instrumental in in helping the nation to achieve.

8. Identify areas related to care of children with cancer that could benefit from additional nursing research.

9. Use critical thinking to analyze ways that nursing care for the child with a neoplasm can be more family centered.

10. Synthesize knowledge of abnormal cell growth in children with the nursing process to achieve quality maternal and child health nursing care.

Key Points

- Radiation is an important treatment modality in cancer therapy. Immediate side-effects that occur are anorexia, nausea, vomiting, and hair loss if radiation is to the head. Long-term effects may be growth retardation or learning disabilities.

- A chemotherapeutic agent is one capable of destroying malignant cells. Nursing diagnoses that may apply to children receiving Chemotherapy are High risk for altered nutrition, Fluid-volume deficit, Self esteem disturbance, Altered oral mucous membrane status, Altered patterns of bowel elimination, Diversional activity deficit, and Infection.

- Help children to use time during chemotherapy in constructive ways, such as completing a project or writing a short story, in order to keep them mentally stimulated and advance emotional development.

- Be aware of the need to use gloves when preparing chemotherapy drugs to protect yourself from adverse effects of the medication.

- Leukemia is the distorted and uncontrolled proliferation of white blood cells and is the most frequently occurring type of cancer in children. About 90% of children with an initial good prognosis will now have long-term survival. Common nursing diagnoses identified for this are "High risk for infection," "Fluid-volume deficit," "Pain," and "Altered health maintenance."

- Hodgkin's disease is a malignancy of the lymphatic system. It occurs most often in adolescents. The initial symptom is often one painless, enlarged lymph node. Therapy is with radiation and chemotherapy.

- Non-Hodgkin's lymphoma is a malignant disorder of the lymphocytes. Therapy is chemotherapy.

- Brain tumors are the most common solid tumors to occur in childhood. Beginning symptoms are usually those of increased intracranial pressure. Therapy is surgery, followed by radiation and chemotherapy.

- Bone tumors occur in two main forms: osteogenic sarcoma and Ewing's sarcoma. These tumors tend to be fast growing because of the ready blood supply to bone. Nursing diagnoses identified for these are "Anticipatory grief related to possible amputation," "High risk for fluid-volume deficit," "Pain," and "Health-seeking behaviors related to life adjustments." Therapy is surgery, followed by radiation and chemotherapy. Amputation is much less frequent today than formerly.

- Neuroblastomas are tumors that arise from the cells of the sympathetic nervous system. They are the most common abdominal tumor in childhood. Therapy is surgery and radiation and chemotherapy.

- Rhabdomyosarcomas are tumors of striated muscle. The peak age of incidence is 2 to 6 years. Therapy is surgery and chemotherapy.

- Wilms' tumor (nephroblastoma) is a malignancy that arises from the metanephric mesoderm cells of the kidney. It is usually discovered early in life. Therapy is surgery, followed by radiation and chemotherapy.

- Retinoblastoma is a malignant tumor of the retina of the eye. It may be inherited as an autosomal dominant pattern. Therapy is radiation, chemotherapy, and possibly enucleation.

- After the diagnosis of cancer, help parents and children to change their thinking about cancer, from an older concept of it as an always painful, fatal disease to a newer concept of it as a condition where there is therapy and hope.

- Because the therapy for cancer involves so many return hospitalizations and so much parental concern, the siblings of children with cancer may begin to feel left out of family activities. Remind parents to incorporate the entire family in activities, when possible, to help them grow as a family during the course of therapy.

- Skin cancer is a type of malignancy that begins in childhood. Cautioning children about sensible sun exposure can be an important health promotion role for nurses.

Definitions of Key Terms

benign neoplasm: an innocent, noncancerous tumor

biopsy: the surgical removal of tissue cells for laboratory analysis

chemotherapeutic agent: a chemical used to treat disease that affects the causative organism of the illness but does not harm the host

Ewing's sarcoma: a malignant tumor of the midshaft of long bones

leukemia: a malignant process of blood-forming organs characterized by an overproduction of white blood cells

lymphoma: a neoplasm of lymphoid tissue, usually malignant

malignant neoplasm: a cancerous tumor

metastasis: the process by which tumor cells are spread to distant body parts

neoplasm: an abnormal growth of new tissue

neuroblastoma: a malignant tumor of nervous tissue

oncogenic virus: an organism capable of causing tumors

osteogenic sarcoma: a malignant tumor of the epiphysis of long bones

rhabdomyosarcoma: a malignant tumor of striated muscle

sarcoma: a malignant neoplasm of the soft tissue

tumor staging: a method to determine the extent of malignant involvement in order to determine and guide therapy

Nursing Process Overview

The Nursing Process Overview in this chapter focuses on ways to help parents adjust to the diagnosis of cancer in their child and maintain an optimistic viewpoint. The importance of establishing both short-term and long-term goals is stressed as well as the importance of continuous evaluation so care can be kept current.

Study Aids

Boxes

Box 53-1:   The seven danger signs of cancer

Focus on Nursing Care: Guidelines for care of the child receiving radiation

Focus on Nursing Care: Guidelines for care of the child with neutropenia

Tables

Table 53-1:   Phases of the cell cycle

Table 53-2:   Commonly used chemotherapeutic agents

Table 51-3:   Sample protocol for the treatment of acute lymphocytic leukemia

Table 51-4:   Common sites and symptoms of rhabdomyosarcoma

Table 51-5:   Staging of Wilm's tumor

Table 51-6:   Staging of retinoblastoma (Reese-Ellsworth system)

Displays

Focus on National Health Goals

Focus on Family Teaching

Focus on Nursing Research

Focus on Cultural Awareness

Critical Thinking Exercises:

1. Jose is a 6-year-old you see in a well-child setting. His mother tells you he wakes up every morning with a headache. He also vomits almost every morning just after he wakes up. She says this began just after he started school so she is certain it is related to this. The school nurse suggested Jose have his eyes examined. What additional questions would you want to ask to see if you should pursue this problem further?

2. Nancy is a 2-year-old who is going to be receiving chemotherapy following surgery for a neuroblastoma. How would you prepare her for this? What activities would you propose to keep Nancy occupied while an intravenous solution is infusing?

3. Salvatore is an adolescent who has been diagnosed as having Hodgkin's disease. How would you explain this disease to him? He is active in a school sports program and works part-time as a grocery store clerk. Will he need to halt these activities?

Media Resources

A Sense of Hope (13-minute film)

The daily activities of a boy with leukemia during a period of remission are presented. Research findings and cure rates are discussed as well as the role of bone marrow transplants. The boy's ability to participate in home, school, and organized recreational activities is stressed.

Source: Leukemia Society of America

Nursing Management of Children with Cancer (20-minute videocassette)

}The definition, incidence, treatment, and prognosis of Wilms' tumor, acute lymphocytic leukemia, and rhabdomyosarcoma are presented. The side-effects of chemotherapy and the psychologic care of the child and family are discussed.

Source: American Cancer Society

Bone Marrows and Spinal Taps: A Child's View (12-minute videocassette)

The experience of an 11-year-old boy brought to the hospital for blood work, a bone marrow aspiration, and spinal tap are presented. Techniques that are stressed are those which can be used with pediatric oncology patients to reduce fear of procedures.

Source: Carle Medical Communications

Title: Only One Road: Three Families Coping with Childhood Cancer (53-minute videocassette)

Interviews were made of three children, ages 5 to 9, who are undergoing therapy for cancer. Vignettes of daily interactions in home, school, and hospital settings are shown. Their families were able to adapt to a serious diagnosis with the help of special resources for coping.

Source: University of Michigan

The Show Must Go On (17-minute videocassette)

A clown puppet interviews pediatric oncology patients in an attempt to encourage them to discuss their feelings. Leukemia is the major illness discussed although there is some discussion of solid tumors. Side-effects of cancer therapy and the difficulties children have dealing with these are shown.

Source: Miller Children's Hospital Child Life Department

People You'd like to Know Series: Diana (10-minute film)

Diana, an adolescent, had her leg amputated because of a cancerous tumor. Diana discusses her adjustment to her handicap and the adjustment of others around her. She is shown participating in vigorous activities such as skiing.

Source: Encyclopedia Britannica Educational Corporation

Caring for the Myelosuppressed Child (28-minute videocassette)

The cellular alterations and signs of myelosuppression in children receiving chemotherapy are presented. Transfusion therapies and nursing interventions for different managements, support, and evaluation of a child are key topics.

Source: AJN Educational Services

Coping with Cancer (20-minute videocassette)

The developmental coping responses of children with cancer and their families are presented. Strategies for nurses to use to promote understanding, reduce fear, and facilitate coping are included.

Source: AJN Educational Services

Julie and John (20-minute videocassette)

Two terminally ill adolescents with cancer discuss their thoughts and feelings from two different perspectives. Julie is shown in a music video which she developed; John is shown in a series of edited tapes discussing his thoughts on his illness.

Source: Health Sciences Consortium

Discussion Questions

1. Children receiving chemotherapy often lose their hair. How would you prepare a 3-year-old for this? A 16-year-old?

2. Children with brain tumors may develop high fevers as their temperature control mechanism is affected. What are measures to help reduce fever in such a child?

3. Children with cancer therapy have a need for therapeutic play. What particular play materials would you encourage to help them express how they feel about their therapy?

Written Assignments

1. Children receiving chemotherapy may become dehydrated and malnourished because of nausea and vomiting with therapy. List techniques you would use to decrease nausea and vomiting with chemotherapy administration.

2. The parents of a child with a compromised immune system from chemotherapy need to be careful that the child is not exposed needlessly to infectious diseases. What precautions would you urge parents to take to accomplish this?

3. Children with a diagnosis of cancer may become depressed as they contemplate the possible outcome of

their illness. What are signs and symptoms of depression in children important to observe?

Laboratory Experiences

1. Assign students to inpatient units where children with cancer are cared for so students can have experience in assisting with chemotherapy administration.

2. Assign students to ambulatory settings where children with cancer return for care so they can better appreciate the long-term prognosis for children.

3. Ask a parent with a child diagnosed with cancer to come to a postconference and describe how taxing it has become and how family resources have become stretched thin when a child has a long-term illness such as cancer.

Care Study: A Child With Lymphoblastic Leukemia

Mark Ralston is a 5-year-old seen in an ambulatory clinic for loss of weight.

Health History

- Chief Concern: "He hasn't been himself since Christmas."

- History of Chief Concern: Child has had a series of upper respiratory infections with accompanying herpes simplex infections and otitis media since mid-winter. Has lost 5 pounds during spring months. Mother has noticed "easy bleeding for last two weeks." Child has 5 ecchymotic areas on arms and 7 on legs. Gums bleed easily as well.

- Family Profile: Family intact. Child is youngest of 4 children (others are 19, 16, and 14 years). Father works as self-employed landscaper. Mother works part-time as a substitute language teacher. Finances "vary depending on season of year" but are generally "good." Family tries to plan to do at least one activity together on weekends.

- Pregnancy History: Pregnancy unplanned but not undesired. Delivered by cesarean birth for failure to progress; Apgars 7 and 9; spontaneous respirations. Mother took no recreational nor prescription drugs, only prenatal vitamins during pregnancy. Some concern with elevation of blood pressure late in pregnancy (130/80) but no treatment was given for this.

- Growth and Development: Child met developmental milestones: sat at 6 months, walked at 11 months. Spoke in sentences as early as 15 months; parents feel coordination for such games as baseball is well ahead of sibling's. Nutrition: Likes all foods; appetite loss noticed during spring months. Child takes 1 multivitamin tablet daily.

  Attends kindergarten at local consolidated school; is bused to full-day program; has missed 32 days since start of second semester from illness or "tiredness."

- Past Medical History: Child wore Denis Browne splints for 11 months for "toeing in" of left foot while an infant. No childhood communicable diseases.

  Was hit by car while crossing street 1 year ago; had spleen removed to halt bleeding. Received hemophilus and pneumococcal vaccines to protect against respiratory illness since surgery. No hospitalizations except for surgery after accident.

- Family Medical History:

  Paternal grandfather: glaucoma and arthritis.

  Father: had pyloric stenosis surgery as an infant.

  A 19-year-old sibling has asthma.

- Review of Systems:

  General Health: Child complains constantly of "growing pains" or "being tired." Mother asking whether loss of spleen could be causing this.

  Eyes: Tested in pre-K program last fall and vision found to be 20/20; 20/50. Child wears patch over right eye for amblyopia.

  Ears: Hearing tested in pre-K program: normal.

  Heart: Has innocent heart murmur heard since infancy.

- Allergies: None known.

- Immunizations: Preschool series given by private M.D.

Physical Examination

- General Appearance: Listless-appearing, pale 5-year-old white male; eyepatch in place over right eye. Four ecchymotic areas approximately 3 cm 2 cm obvious on arms. Child appears tired; had been sleeping in waiting room. Nose draining clear fluid; holding hand over left ear. Height: 110 cms. Weight: 32 lbs. Blood pressure: 102/60.

- Head: Normocephalic; fontanelles closed.

- Eyes: PERLA. Extraocular muscles intact; red reflex present bilaterally; mucous membrane pale.

- Ears: Left TM reddened and bulging forward; landmarks unclear. Hearing: Weber test lateralizes to left ear.

- Nose: Clear rhinitis present; mucous membrane reddened and swollen.

- Mouth and Throat: Mucous membrane pale; 20 deciduous teeth present; no caries. Mucous membrane at gumline bled when touched with tongue blade. Gag reflex intact; slight erythema of throat; tonsils not enlarged; midline uvula.

- Neck: Full range of motion; midline trachea. Several enlarged lymph nodes on both sides.

- Lungs: Moist rhonchi present in right and left upper lobes. Respiratory rate: 22/min.

- Heart: Grade I systolic murmur heard at second left intercostal space; no thrill or radiation. Heart rate: 104/min.

- Abdomen: Soft; no masses; surgery scar present in left upper quadrant. Liver palpable 2 cms below right costal margin.

- Extremities: Ecchymotic areas as noted in chief concern; area 22 cm of scattered petechia on left elbow. Full range of motion in joints but with pain experienced on movement of left knee. Right leg tender to touch over distal tibia.

- Genitalia: Normal male; midline meatus; testes descended bilaterally.
- Neurologic: Patellar reflexes 2 bilaterally; normal but listless gait. Overall mood quality: whining and irritable.

Care Study Questions

1. Mark has numerous symptoms (easy bleeding, frequent infections, leg pain) that should have alerted his parent earlier that he was ill. What are reasons that a parent delays this long before seeking care?

2. Mark was diagnosed as having acute lymphoblastic leukemia. Complete a nursing care plan that would identify and meet Mark's needs.

Nursing Care of the Child With a Cognitive or Mental Health Disorder

Chapter 54 discusses care of the child with a cognitive disorder such as mental retardation and mental health disorders such as autism. The chapter begins with a Nursing Process Overview to help the student apply nursing process to these disorders. Care is discussed for children with disruptive behavior disorders such as hyperactivity, anxiety disorders such as separation anxiety, and eating disorders such as bulimia. The importance of continued evaluation in order to keep therapy and interventions current is stressed.

Chapter Objectives

After mastering the contents of this chapter, students should be able to:

1. Describe common cognitive and mental health disorders in children.

2. Assess a child for a cognitive or mental health disorder.

3. Formulate a nursing diagnosis related to the cognitive or mental health disorders of childhood.

4. Plan nursing care for the child with a cognitive or mental health disorder, such as helping parents plan a behavior modification program.

5. Implement nursing care for the child with a cognitive or mental health disorder, such as teaching parents about the need for a safe environment.

6. Evaluate outcome criteria to be certain that nursing goals established for care were achieved.

7. Identify national health goals related to cognitive or mental health disorders that nurses can be instrumental in in helping the nation achieve.

8. Identify areas related to cognitive or mental health that could benefit from additional nursing research.

9. Analyze ways that care of the child with a cognitive or mental health disorder can be more family centered.

10. Synthesize knowledge of childhood cognitive and mental health disorders and nursing process to achieve quality maternal and child health nursing care.

Key Points

- Both mental retardation and mental illness pose long-term care concerns for children and their families.

- Mental retardation still carries a stigma in many communities; therefore, parents may have a more difficult time accepting this in their child than they would a physical illness. Help parents to gain the insight that mental retardation occurs in a proportion of infants in every population, and that having a child with this is not shameful but merely reflects a chance occurrence.

- Most children with mental retardation benefit from early schooling. Urge parents to enroll children in early education programs so the child has a ''head start'' on schooling.

- Mental illness often begins subtly in children and is first manifested as a behavior problem in school. Assess thoroughly any child referred for disruptive behavior in class for the possibility that he or she has a serious emotional problem.

- Infantile autism is a pervasive developmental disorder that has a syndrome of behaviors such as fascination with movement, nonverbal communication, and insensitivity to pain. Early identification is important to avoid placing unreal expectations on the child.

- A number of disruptive behavior disorders such as attention deficit with hyperactivity disorder (ADHD) may occur in childhood. Such children may be treated with methylphenidate hydro(Ritalin) to reduce the hyperactivity and allow them to achieve better in school and interact better at home.

- Eating disorders seen in childhood are pica, rumination, anorexia nervosa, and bulimia. All these disorders can lead to loss of weight and electrolyte imbalances if left unrecognized and untreated.

- Children who are depressed are at high risk for committing suicide. They need thorough assessment and close observation to be certain this does not happen.

- Tic disorders are abnormalities of semi-involuntary movement thought to result from dysfunction of the basal ganglia. Tourette's disorder is an example of this.

- Encopresis is the repeated passage of feces in places not culturally appropriate for that purpose. Therapy is both physiologic and psychologic.

Definitions of Key Terms

anhedonia: the inability to feel pleasure or happiness from events normally experienced as such

catatonia: a state manifested by immobility and inability to communicate

choreiform movements: rapid uneven movements of extremities

complex vocal tics: Rapid repetitive movements such as facial gestures or grooming behaviors

coprolalia: excess use of obscene language

echolalia: a meaningless repetition of words

expressed emotion: the outward showing of feelings

flat affect: no outward sign of emotion

graphesthesia: the inability to recognize a figure drawn on the skin

hyperactivity: excess driven behavior

labile mood: a rapidly changing mood

motor tics: rapid repetitive muscle movements such as rapid eye blinking

palilalia: rapid repetition of the same word

stereognosis: the ability to identify an object by touch

vocal tics: a spasmodic action manifested by a verbal response

Nursing Process Overview

The Nursing Process Overview in this chapter concentrates on the necessity to observe children with cognitive or mental health disorders over time, to obtain a full evaluation of a child. Nursing diagnoses speak to family as well as individual concerns, since these disorders become family problems.

Study Aids

Boxes

Box 54-1:   Common causes of mental retardation

Box 54-2:   Common symptoms in the child with autism

Box 54-3:   Nonproductive approaches to care of the child with anorexia nervosa

Tables

Table 54-1;   Guidelines for the mental health interview of the child

Table 54-2:   Disorders usually first evident in infancy, childhood, or adolescence

Displays

Focus on National Health Goals

Focus on Family Teaching

Focus on Nursing Research

Focus on Cultural Awareness

Critical Thinking Exercises:

1. Bethany is a 3-year-old with Down syndrome who is critically ill with pneumonia. It is difficult to believe that her mother didn't recognize sooner how ill the child was becoming and bring her sooner for care. What questions would you want to ask the mother to confirm if this is true or not? Why would a parent have reacted this way?

2. Todd is a second grade student with attention deficit disorder with hyperactivity. His family feels "at their wits end" because his attention span is so short and his behavior is so disruptive. What suggestions could you make to his mother to help him adjust better to the family routine?

3. Barry is an adolescent whose parents tell you seems increasingly depressed, so much so that he sleeps almost all day on weekends. Does Barry need a referral or is he just demonstrating usual adolescent behavior? What questions would you want to ask to be able to tell confidently?

Media Resources

Jennifer (19-minute film)

The life of a child with Down syndrome is presented. Her school experience and her prognosis in terms of future skills and employment are explored.

Source: Films, Inc.

Sara has Down's Syndrome (16-minute film)

The life of 6-year-old Sara, a child with Down syndrome is presented. Aspects of both Sara's home and school life and her family's reactions to her are shared, along with a general discussion of the behavior and development of a child with Down syndrome.

Source: Educational Development Center

People You'd Like to Know Series: Paige (10-minute film)

Paige, a child with Down syndrome, is portrayed during the course of her daily activities. She is seen attending a grade school mainstreamed class and competing in athletic activities in the Special Olympics.

Source: Encyclopedia Britannica Educational Corporation

Adolescent Depression (filmstrip/video)

The differences between normal adolescent mood swings and serious depression are discussed. Case studies are used to illustrate personality traits and social dynamics that can lead to depression.

Source: Guidance Associates

Psychiatry Learning System: Disorders of Infancy, Childhood, and Adolescence (42-minute videocassette)

The causes, manifestations, and therapy of several psychiatric disorders are presented, including autism, pica, anorexia, Tourette disorders, and bulimia. Examples are given to aid understanding.

Source: Health Sciences Consortium

Schizophrenia: Removing the Veil (filmstrip/audiocassette)

The causes, symptoms, and treatment of schizophrenia are discussed, with graphic examples of the major diagnostic categories. A discussion of childhood schizophrenia is included.

Source: Human Relations Media

Wasting Away: Understanding Anorexia Nervosa and Bulimia (videocassette)

A series of vignettes illustrating typical anorectic and bulimic behaviors. Adolescent stressors, personality types, and family/social situations that can lead to these disorders are shown. The physiologic effects of anorexia and bulimia are discussed in detail.

Source: Guidance Associates

The Enigma of Anorexia Nervosa: Delusion and Discord (18-minute videocassette)

}An overview of the history of anorexia nervosa and approaches to treatment. The video stresses the need to view the condition from a biopsychosocial approach.

Source: Carle Medical Communications

Understanding Autism (19-minute videocassette)

The nature and symptoms of autism and treatment based on behavior modification principals are discussed. Three families with autistic children are featured.

Source: Fanlight Productions

Discussion Questions

1. Anorexia nervosa is a major problem of adolescents. What is the effect of media advertising on adolescents with this syndrome?

2. A child with Tourette's syndrome can be disruptive in a classroom if peers don't understand his or her illness. How would you explain the cause of coprolalia to school-age children?

3. The overanxious child can be extremely threatened by a hospital experience. What are concrete steps you could take to make such an experience easier for him or her?

Written Assignments

1. Children with autism are fascinated with moving objects. What are special "childproofing" measures parents of these children must take to be certain they are safe?

2. It can be exhausting to be the parent of a child with an attention deficit disorder. What are suggestions you could make to parents to make parenting more enjoyable for them?

3. Depression occurs in children the same as in adults. What are the symptoms of depression you would observe for to detect this in children?

Laboratory Experiences

1. Assign students to a preschool setting where children with mental retardation are enrolled in order to help them appreciate the extra time parents of these children spend encouraging development.

2. Ask parents of children with mental retardation to come to a postconference and discuss their experiences with raising their child. Encourage them to speak about how health care personnel could have been more helpful to them at the time of diagnosis.

3. Assign students to an ambulatory psychiatric setting or a crisis intervention center that cares for children with emotional or mental disorders. Ask students to evaluate the impact of this disorder on family functioning.

Care Study: A Newborn With Down Syndrome

Natasha Berlinger is a newborn who is diagnosed as having Down syndrome.

Health History

- Chief Concern: "Baby was diagnosed as being retarded at 20 weeks of pregnancy."

- History of Present Concern: Mother is a 39-year-old single woman who learned at 16 weeks of pregnancy after a feto-alphaprotein serum analysis that "something was wrong with the baby." The diagnosis of Down syndrome was made by sonogram at 20 weeks of pregnancy. Mother was given the option to abort pregnancy at that time but chose not to do so.

- Family Profile: Mother lives with and is supported by a female friend. They live in restored Victorian home in center of city. Together they own a home decorator service; mother resigned position during pregnancy to be full-time mother. Finances are reported as "good."

- Pregnancy History: Mother was artificially inseminated (donor insemination) because she wanted to have a child and had no male companion. Was counseled on the risk of Down syndrome with pregnancy at her age. Mother had premature labor at 7 months of pregnancy; contractions were controlled with magnesium sulfate and she returned home. She self-administered oral turbutaline during remainder of pregnancy. Infant born at term after 10 hours of labor. Vertex position. Breathed spontaneously. Apgars 7 and 8.

- Family Medical History: Maternal grandmother has insulin-dependent diabetes; an aunt has uterine cancer. Paternal history: no known family illnesses.

- Review of Systems: Gastrointestinal: Infant has vomited three times since birth 2 hours ago. Vomitus: greenish-black in color.

  Neurologic: Infant "seems limp." Sucks poorly for breast feeding.

Physical Examination

- General Appearance: Hypotonic-appearing white female newborn with extra epicanthal fold present bilaterally, simian creases present on both palms; loose connective tissue on back of neck.

- Head: Normocephalic; anterior fontanelle, 44 cm; posterior fontanelle, 23 cm. Sagittal suture line overriding.

- Eyes: Epicanthal fold present at medial aspects of both eyes; red reflex present; small white specks in iris of both eyes; small conjunctival hemorrhage around cornea of left eye.

- Ears: Top of pinna ½ inch below usual position of line from inner to outer eye canthus. Child startles at loud noise as if hearing is intact.

- Nose: Midline septum; nares patent bilaterally.

- Mouth: No teeth; one small glistening fluid-filled cyst present on soft palate; tongue protrudes from mouth in resting position. Gag reflex intact; uvula midline.

- Neck: Full range of motion; loose fold of tissue at back of neck.

- Lungs: Rhonchi heard in all four lobes; Respiratory rate: 30/min.

- Heart: Diastolic murmur grade II heard at left sternal border. Rate: 162/min.

- Abdomen: Liver palpable 3 cms under right costal margin; spleen palpable 1 cm under left margin. Bowel sounds present in left upper quadrant; no bowel sounds heard in other quadrants. Facial ring at umbilicus 3 cms in diameter; cord drying; clamp in place.

- Genitalia: Normal female.

- Extremities: Joints are hyperflexic; clinodactyly present bilaterally. Wide space present between first and second toes and first and second fingers bilaterally. Simian creases present bilaterally on palms of hands.

- Neurologic: Deep tendon reflexes intact; Moro intact. Tonic neck and step-in-place: unable to demonstrate.

Care Study Questions

1. Natasha's mother knew from early in pregnancy that her child had a chromosomal disorder. Does knowing from early on about a disorder make acceptance of the disorder easier or more difficult?

2. Natasha is having emesis of greenish-black fluid. What are the possible implications of this? Why do newborns with Down syndrome need to be observed carefully for emesis?

3. Complete a nursing care plan that would identify and meet Natasha's family's needs.

The Family in Crisis: Child and Domestic Abuse

Chapter 55 discusses the nurse's role in relation to the many forms of human abuse. The chapter begins with a Nursing Process Overview stressing the nurse's responsibility for remaining aware of the possibility of abuse and the responsibility for reporting it. Physical and emotional abuse as well as physical and emotional neglect and sexual abuse are discussed. As it can lead to extreme emotional consequences, rape is included as well. Viewing abuse as a family problem and rape as a couple's problem are stressed.

Students have an awareness that abuse and rape exist but are usually amazed and sobered by the statistics on the extent of the two problems. This awareness increases their ability to continue to assess for abuse as they advance to other clinical areas and to grow in their ability to counsel clients under extreme stress.

Chapter Objectives

After mastering the contents of this chapter, students should be able to:

1. Discuss the types of abuse seen in families and the theories explaining their occurrence.
2. Assess a physically or emotionally abused family.
3. Formulate nursing diagnoses related to the abused family.
4. Plan nursing care for the abused family such as ways to role-model better parenting.
5. Implement nursing care for the family in which abuse occurred, for instance, assisting with immediate trauma care or counseling to prevent further abuse.
6. Evaluate outcome criteria to be certain that goals of nursing care were achieved.
7. Identify national health goals related to the abused family that nurses can be instrumental in in helping the nation achieve.
8. Identify areas related to care of the abused child that could benefit from additional nursing research.
9. Use critical thinking to analyze ways that nurses can be instrumental in preventing child abuse.
10. Synthesize knowledge of family abuse with nursing process to achieve quality maternal child health nursing care.

Key Points

- At least 10% of children seen for traumatic injury received their injury from child abuse. A high suspicion for abuse should be present when burns, head injury, or rib fractures are present or when the history of the accident seems out of context for the injury.

- Child abuse may exist in many forms. It may be physical, emotional, or sexual neglect or abuse.

- In infants, a ''shaken baby syndrome'' results in retinal or intracranial hemorrhage. Babies with this syndrome may appear groggy or unresponsive in an emergency department.

- A triad of a ''special parent, special child, special situation'' is characteristic of the family in which child abuse occurs.

- Failure to thrive is a syndrome in which an infant falls below the third percentile for weight and height on a standard growth chart. It is associated with a disturbance in the parent—child relationship.

- Children who comfort parents in emergency settings may just be sensitive children or they may be demonstrating ''role reversal,'' a behavior characteristic of abused children.

- In families in which a child is abused, the mother may also be a victim of abuse. Ask enough questions at health care visits to be certain that this problem doesn't exist as well.

- Child abuse is legally reportable. Nurses can initiate reporting as an independent action or through their health agency's referral network.

- Methods to prevent abuse that nurses can actively participate in include teaching about the expected growth and development of children, educating teenage parents for parenting roles, and teaching ''empowerment'' or a sense that children have control of their own lives.

- Sexual abuse of children can be prevented by teaching children to recognize abnormal advances and to know it is right to speak out about wrongs against them.

- Abuse is a family, not an individual, problem. Therapy must include all family members to be effective.

Definitions of Key Terms

abuse: to attack or injure

battered child syndrome: a child who has been physically, sexually, or emotionally abused

disorganization phase: a time period in which individuals are unable to organize thoughts clearly

failure to thrive: retarded growth and development of a child for nonorganic reasons

incest: sexual relations between members of the same family

learned helplessness: a behavioral state of a person who believes he or she is ineffectual and unable to achieve

mandatory reporters: individuals designated as ones who must report child abuse

molestation: unwelcome sexual involvement such as oral--genital contact, genital fondling, viewing, or masturbation

Munchausen syndrome by proxy: a situation in which a parent repeatedly brings a child to a health care facility for care when the child is actually well

pedophile: a person with an abnormal interest in children

permissive reporters: individuals who may report child abuse

rape trauma syndrome: a series of predictable behaviors resulting from having been raped

reorganization phase: a time period in which a person reestablishes his or her ability to think clearly

shaken baby syndrome: an infant who has been repetitively, violently shaken

silent rape syndrome: the predictable behaviors of an individual who was raped but allowed the rape to be unreported

Nursing Process Overview

The Nursing Process Overview for this chapter elaborates on the common findings of abuse, nursing diagnoses pertinent to this area, and strategies for caring for children and their parents after abuse. The nursing diagnosis "Rape trauma syndrome" for women and adolescents who have been raped is included.

Study Aids

Boxes

Box 55-1:   Women at high risk for potential child abuse or neglect that can be identified in the pregnant or postpartal period

Box 55-2:   Observations to be made at postpartum and pediatric check-ups to detect child abuse

Box 55-3:   Goals of crisis intervention for families of rape victims

Box 55-4:   Levels of wife abuse

Tables

Table 55-1:   Incidence of reported child abuse in the United States

Table 55-2:   Common specimen procedures following rape

Table 55-3:   Areas to explore in rape counseling

Displays

Focus on National Health Goals

Focus on Family Teaching

Focus on Nursing Research

Focus on Cultural Awareness

Critical Thinking Exercises:

1.   You weigh a baby at a well child conference and discover that the infant's weight is below the 2nd percentile on a standardized growth chart. What questions would you want to ask the mother to see if you can account for this? What particular areas would you want to assess on a physical exam?

2.   You are working in an emergency room and a father brings in a two-year-old because he can not move his arm. An x- ray shows the humerus to be broken. You notice in the chart that the child has been seen twice before; once for an ulnar fracture and once for a scald burn on his hand. The resident in charge of the emergency room dismisses the injuries as "typical of boys". What would be your action if you believe that there is suspicion of child abuse? What would be your legal responsibility?

3.   Tanya is a 4-year-old who is seen in an ambulatory clinic for a purulent vulvovaginitis. A culture reveals this is from gonorrhea. What questions would you want to ask Tanya to determine how she contracted this? Suppose her parents are influential people in your community. Would this influence what questions you ask?

Media Resources

Child Abuse (28-minute videocassette)

The nurse's role in prevention, detection, and management of child abuse is presented. Statistical information, high-risk parent profiles, and therapeutic programs are identified. The recognition, assessment, and emergency room presentation of various injuries are explained, and interviewing and observational strategies are offered for assessment of parents and children in suspected situations of child abuse. The legal responsibilities of the health care professional are stressed.

Source: American Journal of Nursing Educational Services

Violence in the Family (40-minute videotransfer)

The dynamics of family violence in American society are explored, including possible reasons for violence such as the relation between intimacy and violence, punishment of children, and society's fascination with violence. There are specific segments dealing with child abuse and neglect, battered wives, and adolescent abuse.

Source: Human Relations Media

Child Sexual Abuse: The Untold Story (30-minute videocassette)

Female victims of sexual abuse narrate their story. The film documents the effects of abuse on the girls' emotional and social development, their feelings and coping strategies, and their involvement in group therapy counseling programs.

Source: American Journal of Nursing Educational Services.

Sexually Misused Children: Identification, Documentation, Management (26-minute videocassette)

Physical and behavioral indicators of sexual misuse of children, guidelines for interviewing victims, physical assessment criteria, and appropriate documentation parameters are presented. A comprehensive program guide is included.

Source: University of Michigan

Child Abuse: Physical and Behavioral Indicators (28-minute videocassette)

Graphic examples of child abuse are shown. The role of the health professional in identification, initial management, and documentation of a child's injuries is discussed. Guidelines for family and child assessment are given and a study guide is included.

Source: University of Michigan

A Better Beginning (38-minute videocassette)

The social and emotional components of failure-to-thrive during the assessment and evaluation of two babies and their parents are presented. Included are guidelines for interventions to reverse negative parent—infant interactions. A study guide is also included.

Source: University of Michigan

Discussion Questions

1. Tom is a 4-year-old admitted to the hospital for child abuse. What approach would you use to establish an effective relationship with his parents?

2. Education for preventing child abuse begins during adolescence. What are specific areas to teach young people that would help prevent child abuse?

3. Spouse abuse has an effect on children as well as the adults in a family. What are common signs that spouse abuse is present?

Written Assignments

1. Nurses are designated abuse reporters. List the steps of the procedure for reporting and documenting abuse in your clinical agency.

2. Being able to offer support to rape victims is critical to emergency room nursing care. What special care would you give to a female adolescent who has been raped? To a male?

3. It may be possible to identify the potential for abuse in women during the postpartum period. List some mannerisms of women who may not be bonding well with their newborn.

Laboratory Experiences

1. Assign students for experiences in an emergency room where abuse and rape victims are cared for to increase their awareness of the role of the nurse in caring for these individuals.

2. Ask a member of a rape counseling team to come to a postconference and discuss various clients she or he has helped care for. Ask the counselor to discuss ways that health care personnel could be more helpful to counselors or clients.

3. Assign students to obtain the rape and abuse statistics for the local health department and analyze them as to differences that occur in local communities. Analysis of the statistics should strengthen the point that abuse occurs in all socioeconomic areas. Rape statistics, in contrast, should reveal that some communities have a higher incidence than others.

Care Study: A Child Who Has Been Abused

David Ludlow is a 2-year-old brought to the emergency room by his mother and her boyfriend.

Health History

- Chief Concern: "He fell and burnt his hand on the stove."

- History of Present Concern: Mother was watching child earlier in the day when child "tripped on a throw rug." As he reached out his hand to stop his fall, he put it into a gas flame on top of the stove. Posterior side of hand has a blackened, denuded, and extremely painful area 44 cm. Forehead is ecchymotic from hitting head on stove front.

- Family Profile: Mother is a 24-year-old single parent; works part-time as a city bus driver. Boyfriend and mother share an apartment over a neighborhood delicatessen. Boyfriend is not the father of David; he works as a hospital orderly; has lived with the family for 6 months. Father is the one who insisted that child be examined.

- Past Medical History: Child seen in emergency room at 1 year for febrile convulsion. Seen 3 months ago for fall down a flight of apartment stairs. Had "colic and crying" for almost all of first year. Health maintenance by well child conference has been sporadic. Mother unsure how many immunizations child has received.

- Pregnancy History: Pregnancy not planned. Mother had heartburn all through pregnancy. Gained 70 lbs and lost none of the weight afterwards. States "he ruined my figure for life." No falls or x-rays during pregnancy. Mother continued to smoke and continued drinking "beers on Saturday night." Smoked marijuana "occasionally." Unsure whether she used cocaine during pregnancy. "May have still used it once" after pregnancy confirmation. Birthweight was "seven-something." Length: Unknown. Apgars: Unknown. Child was a vaginal cephalic presentation. Labor 37 hours long.

- Growth and Development: Mother unable to remember milestones; child presently walks well; is not toilet trained. Mother not certain if he speaks in sentences; boyfriend is sure he does. Is able to feed self; boyfriend describes him as a "cute kid." Mother describes him as a "bratty kid."

- Nutrition: Eats table food; mother does not prepare anything specially for him.

- Review of Systems: Head: Had "lumpy scaly" scalp condition as infant. "Looked like he had lizard skin." Treated with mineral oil and crusts disappeared.

  Ears: Otitis media 3; mother states he doesn't come when she calls him; "If he's not deaf, he acts like it."

  Eyes: No infections; mother feels he sees all right.

  Nose: Had bleeding nose from a fall earlier in this day. Enough he "ruined mother's blouse with blood."

  Mouth: A lot of fussiness with teething as an infant. Mother gave him whiskey to keep him from crying and keeping her awake.

  Genitalia: Persistent diaper rashes.

Physical Examination

- General Appearance: Rangy-looking, crying, distressed 2-year-old. Blackened 44 cm area present on dorsum of right hand; ecchymotic area present around eyes and on forehead.

- Head: Normocephalic; fontanelles closed; one 33 space over right parietal area where hair is missing. Scalp erythematous at area; no scaling present. Large 35 cm dark ecchymotic area with underlying edema on center of forehead. Ecchymotic area extends to surround both eye globes. An older yellow-green fading ecchymotic area is on left temple.

- Eyes: Red reflex; follows to all fields of vision. Small subconjunctival hemorrhage in left sclera. Vision not formally tested but child reaches for object presented to him.

- Ears: TMs pink, landmarks present; dark brown cerumen in right external canal. Hearing not tested but child

follows instructions as if he has normal conversation level. Difficult to evaluate language since child is in pain and crying.

- Nose: Nares patent; midline septum.

- Mouth: 20 deciduous teeth; no cavities; midline uvula; gag reflex intact, membrane moist.

- Neck: Midline trachea; 1 palpable lymph node in anterior left cervical chain. Full range of motion.

- Lungs: Respiratory rate: 24/min (crying). Rhonchi in upper lobes.

- Heart: Rate: 120/min; no murmurs.

- Abdomen: Liver and spleen both palpable 1 cm below costal margins; ecchymotic area (purple-red) 43 cms present over left mid-abdomen; no masses palpable. Tenderness elicited at ecchymotic site.

- Genitorectal: Circumcised male; testes descended. Midline meatus. Reddened, irritated area in diaper area; skin covered with caked feces.

- Extremities: Full range of motion; pain elicited on movement of left elbow; joint slightly reddened and swollen. Four fading ecchymotic areas on legs (green-yellow). Blackened 44 cm area with white central area surrounded by erythema and blisters on dorsum of left hand. Painful to touch.

- Neurologic: patellar reflex 2. Sensory and motor nerves grossly intact.

Care Study Questions

1. Child abuse can occur because of poor bonding at birth. Does David's history suggest this may have occurred?

2. A mark of child abuse is that the history of an accident is inconsistent with the physical findings of the injury. Is this the case in David's history?

3. David was diagnosed as a victim of child abuse. Complete a nursing care plan that would identify and meet David's needs.

The Family Coping With Long-Term or Fatal Illness

Chapter 56 discusses care for the child who has a long-term or fatal illness. The chapter begins with a Nursing Process Overview stressing the necessity to make both long-term and short-term goals so that parent's energy can be sustained over time while they feel a sense of accomplishment in their care. Stages of grief as a reaction to both chronic illness and approaching death are reviewed. Care of the child coping with death and approaches to help the family move past this point are presented.

Content can be applied to care of children with many illnesses discussed in other chapters, including care of those children born with a congenital disorder. This chapter can also be used as an independent study when students are caring for a child with a chronic illness. Students may need discussion time to prepare themselves to think of children as having a long-term or fatal illness. They may need this preparation time before they can give more than superficial care to such children.

Chapter Objectives

After mastering the contents of this chapter, students should be able to:

1. Describe common concerns of parents of children with a fatal or long-term illness.

2. Assess adjustment of the child and family with a long-term or fatal illness.

3. Formulate nursing diagnoses for the child with a long-term or fatal illness.

4. Plan nursing care for the child with a long-term or fatal illness, such as planning for respite care.

5. Implement nursing care for the child with a long-term or fatal illness, such as supporting a family through a period of acute grief.

6. Evaluate outcome criteria to be certain that nursing goals established for care were achieved.

7. Identify national health goals related to children with long-term or fatal illnesses that nurses could be instrumental in in helping the nation to achieve.

8. Identify areas related to care of the child with a long-term or fatal illness that could benefit from additional nursing research.

9. Use critical thinking to analyze ways that nursing care of the child with a long-term or fatal illness can be more family centered.

10. Synthesize knowledge of long-term and fatal illness in children with the nursing process to achieve quality maternal child health nursing care.

Key Points

- Children with chronic illnesses need continual reassessment as their needs, like all children's, change as they grow older. Larger doses of medicine will become necessary; such things as additional muscle strengthening exercises may be necessary.

- Factors that make it easier for parents to accept chronic illness in a child are the presence of support people and being told about the disability at as young an age as possible.

- Chronic illness in a child is often most difficult for parents to accept at what would have been the child's "milestones" of development. Extra support for both the parents and child may be necessary at these times.

- Help children to do as much care for themselves as possible within the limits of a chronic illness. This empowers them to be as independent as possible.

- Children are about 9 years old before they are able to understand the meaning of death and that it is permanent.

- Children as well as parents are apt to need help to face a fatal diagnosis. Urge parents and the child to ask for help to see them through this very difficult time in their lives.

Definitions of Key Terms

anticipatory grief: mourning that precedes actual loss

death: the state of being without brain wave response on an electroencephalogram

grief process: the predictable mourning response to loss

vulnerable children: children whose parents were told that they would die who then subsequently lived

Nursing Process Overview

The Nursing Process Overview in this chapter focuses on assessment of the family as a whole in order to determine if the family will have adequate coping resources for this disastrous life event. Nursing diagnoses suggested are those that include the entire family. The importance of continued evaluation is stressed so that care can be kept current in light of changes in the child's condition.

Study Aids

Boxes

Box 56-1: Books about death for children

Box 56-2: Approaches to communicating with dying children

Tables

Table 56-1: Factors that make it easier for parents to adjust to a child's handicap

Table 56-2: Stages of grief

Displays

Focus on National Health Goals

Focus on Family Teaching

Focus on Nursing Research

Focus on Cultural Awareness

Critical Thinking Exercises:

1. Billy is a newborn who was born with a meningocele. His parents are both 40 years old; they live on a farm; finances are tight; they have no health insurance. Two grown children have expressed resentment at their parents being forced to spend so much time and money with a disabled child. How would you help this family? Do they have risk factors that might make adjusting to a disabled child more difficult than usual?

2. Tony is a 10-year-old who has an inoperable brain tumor. His parents have been told that he has only six more months to live. You notice Tony's parents in the waiting room of the hospital comforting a set of parents whose child was just hit by a car and killed instantly; you hear them say that losing a child suddenly is better than what they are experiencing. Why do you think Tony's parents feel this way? How could you help them with their feelings?

3. Adam is an adolescent with leukemia who wants to donate his corneas for transplant if he should die. His parents think this is totally wrong and say they will not allow it to happen. How would you counsel this family?

Media Resources

Seasons of Caring (40-minute videocassette)

The stressors and coping strategies of three families with preschool age children who have special health needs are presented. The families discuss the attitudes, approaches, and services they have found helpful. Issues encountered by school, social workers, physicians, and nurses are included.

Source: Association for the Care of Children's Health

Living with Chronic Illness...Reaching for Hope...Learning to cope (33-minute videocassette)

Vignettes of chronicallly ill children with rheumatoid arthritis, scleroderma, and systemic lupus erythematosus are presented. Methods of coping, common reactions to the diseases presented, and the needs of patients and their families are stressed.

Source: Health Sciences Consortium

Living with Chronic Illness: Reaching for Hope...Learning to Cope (28-minute videocassette)

Changes in daily living patterns experienced by the chronically ill child and family are presented. Vignettes help identify feelings and fears of children and families. Helping children cope effectively and guiding families toward acceptance of the child's condition are stressed.

Source: Health Sciences Consortium

The Dying Child: Focus on the Family (17-minute slide/audiocassette)

Professionals who have dealt with dying children discuss the reactions of families to the impending death of a child. Parental reactions and professional support by physicians and nurses are presented.

Source: Concept Media

The Dying Child: Focus on the Child (20-minute slide/audio-cassette)

A child's perception of death, sense of impending death, reactions to death, and home care during the terminal stages of an illness are all presented. Developmental changes in a child's ability to perceive death are shown. Ways that nurses can relate to dying children and responsibilities of nurses to dying children are illustrated and discussed.

Source: Concept Media

Where is Dead? (19-minute film)

The way in which children deal with and understand death is explored. When a 6-year-old's brother dies, her family's attempt to explain this event to her is described. The girl's reactions to the death and her questions about it are presented.

Source: Encyclopedia Britannica Corporation

Jeannie (6-minute videocassette)

The concerns of an 11-year-old girl who is admitted to the hospital for surgery to remove a cardiac tumor are presented. She expresses her fears about surgery and her inability to grasp the true meaning of death.

Source: Health Sciences Consortium

ABC Close-up: Can't It Be Anyone Else? (60-minute videocassette)

Three children with leukemia discuss their feelings about having a fatal disease. Vignettes show them in daily activities and how their illness affects members of their families.

Source: American Broadcasting Company

Discussion Questions

1. Mary is a 7-year-old dying of an inoperable brain tumor. You notice that her family visits very infrequently. What measures could you take to offer Mary the support she needs?

2. Charlie is a 6-year-old with cerebral palsy. His parents ask you to help them decide on a school placement for him. What principles would you use on which to base your advice?

3. A mother of a terminally ill child asks you whether she should admit him to hospice care or not. What are the advantages and disadvantages of hospice care you would explain to her?

Written Assignments

1. Being the sibling of a child with a chronic illness can be difficult. What are suggestions you could make to parents to help a sibling continue to feel equally loved?

2. Survey a group of grade school children as to their concept of death. At what age do they seem to have a grasp of the permanency of death?

3. Many parents experience chronic sorrow at the point their child would have reached a developmental milestone. What suggestions could you make to parents to ease their grief at these points?

Laboratory Experiences

1. Assign students to hospital units in which they will have experience caring for chronically ill or terminally ill children. Stress that caring for the family is a major part of their role.

2. Assign students to a hospice or for visits with a home care nurse to visit children with a terminal illness. Ask them to evaluate why this setting was best for this particular family.

3. Assign students to observe Saturday morning programming for children and analyze the message about illness or death the programs provide. How do these attitudes affect the thoughts of children who are terminally or fatally ill?

Care Study: A Child With Neuroblastoma

Scott Bergin is a 4-year-old diagnosed with neuroblastoma whom you visit at home.

Health History

- Chief Concern: "He's hardly ever awake any more."

- History of Present Concern: Scott was diagnosed as having a neuroblastoma 1 year ago. He was treated with chemotherapy following surgery until 3 months ago when his parents were told after "second look" surgery that his therapy had not been successful. His parents chose not to submit him to any more therapy and asked to care for Scott at home until his expected death.

- Family Profile: Scott is only child of a 26-year-old mother; father has 2 other children from a previous marriage who also live with them. Father is an ophthalmic resident at City Hospital; mother is homemaker and primary caregiver for child. A home care aide visits daily to assist with care; a home care nurse is case manager.

- Past Medical History: Child born with a skin tag anterior to right ear removed by ligation at 1 week. No childhood communicable diseases; no hospitalizations except for therapy for neuroblastoma.

- Family Medical History: Grandfather: cardiovascular heart disease; double bypass performed 2 months ago. Two maternal cousins were born with syndactyly.

- Review of Systems: Gastrointestinal: Child had constant nausea during chemotherapy; has had nagging abdominal pain since chemotherapy was halted.

  Urinary: Hemorrhagic cystic with chemotherapy; has catheter inserted now; no further problems.

  Neurologic: Gradually increased periods of deep sleep over last month.

Physical Examination

- General Appearance: Pale, thin-appearing 4-year-old male with nasogastric tube and urinary catheter in place; unresponsive except to painful stimuli. Height: 103 cms. Weight: 13.2 kg. Blood pressure: 70/50.

- Head: Normocephalic. Fontanelles closed.

- Eyes: Right pupil dilated; unresponsive to light. Child does not follow light due to unresponsiveness.

- Nose: Midline septum; nasogastric tube in place in right nostril. Crusting on nostrils present.

- Ears: TMs pink; landmarks visible; child does not respond to examiner's voice.

- Mouth: Geographic tongue; 20 deciduous teeth; no caries; uvula deviated to left.

- Neck: Full range of motion; trachea displaced to right; no palpable lymph nodes present.

- Lungs: Rhonchi present in all lobes; diminished breath sounds in left lobes. Respiratory rate: 14/min.

- Heart: Rate: 84/min. No murmurs.

- Abdomen: Distended; firm to palpation. Firm 45 cm mass palpable in left upper quadrant.

- Genitalia: Normal male; testes descended

- Extremities: Full range of motion; hips abduct to 180 degrees.

- Neurologic: Deep tendon reflexes 1; unresponsive to voice; Glasgow Coma Scale rating: 3.

Care Study Questions

1. Scott has two older siblings. What do you anticipate is the effect of Scott's home care on them?

2. Scott's parents made a decision to not allow him to have further surgery. What if you believe this was a wrong decision? How would it affect your care?

3. Complete a nursing care plan that would identify and meet the needs of Scott and his family.

Sources of Audiovisual Material

Abbott Scientific Products Division
820 Mission Street
S. Pasadena, CA 91030

ACOG Distribution Center
P.O. Box 91180
Washington, DC 20090-1180

Aims Media
6901 Woodley Avenue
Van Nuys, CA 91406

American Broadcasting Company
1313 Avenue of the Americas
New York, NY 10019

American Cancer Society
777 Third Avenue
New York, NY 10017

American Heart Association
8615 Director's Row
Dallas, TX 75247

American Journal of Nursing Company
555 West 57th Street
New York, NY 10019

American Lung Association
1740 Broadway
New York, NY 10019

Armstrong Medical Industries, Inc.
P.O. Box 700
Lincolnshire, IL 60069

Association for the Care of Children's
Health
3615 Wisconsin Avenue, N.W.
Washington, DC 20016

AVC Nursing Series
P.O. Box H
Novato, CA 94847

AWONN
P.O. Box 71437
Washington, DC 20024-1437

Birthways Childbirth Resource Center, Inc.
6313 159th Place, N.E.
Redmond, WA 98052

Cambridge Documentary Films
P.O. Box 385
Cambridge, MA 02139

Campus Film Distributors corporation
24 depot Square
Tuckahoe, NY 10707

Career Aids
20417 Nordhoff Street, Dept. HA
Chatsworth, CA 91311

Carle Medical Communications
510 W. Main Street
Urbana, IL 61801

Centre Films
1103 El Centro
Hollywood, CA 90038

Childbirth Graphics
P.O. Box 20540
Rochester, NY 14602-0540

Churchill Films
662 North Robertson Blvd.
Los Angeles, CA 90069

Communication in Learning, Inc.
2929 Main Street

Buffalo, NY 14214

Concept Media P.O.
Box 19542
Irvine, CA 90266

Crisis Communication Corporation
P.O. Box 904
Garden Grove, CA 92642

CRM/McGraw-Hill Films
110 Fifteenth Street
Del Mar, CA 92014

Cutter Biological
Cutter Laboratories, Inc.
Berkeley, CA 94710

Cystic Fibrosis Foundation
6000 Executive Boulevard, Suite 309
Rockville, MD 20852

Davidson Films, Inc.
165 Tunstead Avenue
San Anselmo, CA 94960

Educational Development Center
Distribution Center
39 Chapel Street
Newton, MA 02160

Educational Graphic Aids
2695 East Long Lane
Littleton, CO 80121

Encyclopedia Britannica Educational
Corporation
425 N. Michigan Avenue
Chicago, IL 60611

Fanlight Productions
47 Halifax Street
Boston, MA 02130

Feeling Fine
ASPO/Lamaze
P.O. Box 952
McLean, VA 22101

Film, Inc.
1144 Wilmette Avenue
Wilmette, IL 60091

Filmmakers Library
133 East 58th Street
New York, NY 10022

Film Fair Communications
10900 Ventura Blvd. Box 1728
Studio City, CA 91604

Films for the Humanities and Sciences
P.O. Box 2053
Princeton, NY 08543

Guidance Associates
Communications Park, Box 3000
Mount Kisco, NY 10549

Health Sciences Consortium
201 Silver Cedar Court
Chapel Hill, NC 27514

Human Relations Media
Room GC
175 Tompkins Avenue
Pleasantville, NY 10570

Indiana University
AudioVisual Center
Bloomington, IN 47401

J. B. Lippincott Company
227 East Washington Square
Philadelphia, PA 19106-3780

Kid's Corner
2027 N. Tejon
Colorado Springs, CO 80907

Leukemia Society of America, Inc.
800 Second Avenue
New York, NY 10017

Little Red Filmhouse
666 North Robertson Blvd.
Los Angeles, CA 90069

M.D.A. TV
M.D. Anderson Hospital
6723 Bertner Avenue
Mail Box 74
Houston, TX 77030

March of Dimes Birth Defects Foundation
1275 Mamaroneck Avenue
White Plains, NY 10605

Master Concepts
P.O. Box 5547
Huntington Beach, CA 92646

Mead Johnson Nutritionals
2404 W. Pennsylvania Street
Evansville IN 47721

MedCom Trainex
12601 Industry Street
P.O. Box 3225
Garden Grove, CA 92642

Medical Electronic Educational Services,
Inc.
Teaching Films, Inc.
930 South 4th Street
Edwardsville, KS 66113

Miller Children's Hospital
Child Life Department
2801 Atlantic Avenue
P.O. Box 1428
Long Beach, CA 90801

NAPHT, Inc. New York Chapter
220 E. 67th Street
New York, NY 10021

Nasco Health Care education Materials
901 Janesville Avenue
Fort Atkinson, WI 53538

National Audiovisual Center
8700 Edgeworth Drive
Capital Heights, MD 20743

National Foundation for Ileitis and Colitis,
Inc.
444 Park Avenue South
New York, NY 10016

National Hemophilia Foundation
35 West 39th Street
New York, NY 10018

Parents Magazine Films, Inc.
Communications Park
Box 3000
Mt. Kisco, NY 10549

Perennial Education, Inc.
930 Pitner Avenue
Evanston, IL 60202

Polymorph Films, Inc.
118 South Street
Boston, MA 02111

Prime Time School Television
108 West Grand Avenue
Chicago, IL 60610

Public Television Library
475 L'Enfant Plaza S. W.
Washington, DC 20024

Pyramid Film and Video
Box 1048
Santa Monica, CA 90406

Professional Research
930 Pitner Avenue
Evanston, IL 60202

Random House Media
Department 442
400 Hahn Road
Westminister, MA 21157

Rhode Island Office of Refugee
Resettlement
600 New London Avenue
Cranston, RI 02900

Ross Laboratories
Educational Services Department
625 Cleveland Avenue
Columbus, OH 43216

Time/Life Video Distribution Center
P.O. Box 644
Paramus, NY 07652

Trainex Corporation
P.O. Box 116
Garden Grove, CA 92642

Universal Education and Visual Arts
Division of Universal City Studios, Inc.
100 Universal City Plaza
Universal City, CA 90038

University of Arizona
Health Sciences Center
Tuscon, AZ 85724

University of California Extension Media
Center
2223 Fulton Street
Berkeley, CA 94720

University of Michigan Medical Center
Media Library
R4440 Kresge
Ann Arbor, MI 48109

University of Minnesota
Media Distribution
Box 734 Mayo Building
420 Delaware Street SE
Minneapolis, MI 55455

Vacumate Corporation
114 W. 26th Street
New York, NY 10001

Video Health Communications
6 Bigelow Street
Cambridge, MA 02139

Wayne State University
Systems Distribution and Utilization
5448 Cass Avenue
Detroit, MI 48202

Williams & Wilkins Electronic MEDIA
428 East Preston Street
Baltimore, MD 21202